Managing Care in Context

Edited by

Jeanette Henderson and Dorothy Atkinson
The Open University

Senior managers expect you to resolve problems without always having the opportunity to learn or get training – it's like finding your way through a maze at times.

(Team manager, manager consultations)

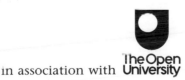

in association with **The Open University**

This book forms part of an Open University course K303 *Managing Care*. Details of this and other Open University courses can be obtained from the Course Information and Advice Centre, PO Box 724, The Open University, Milton Keynes MK7 6ZS, United Kingdom: tel. +44 (0)1908 653231, e-mail ces-gen@open.ac.uk

Alternatively, you may visit the Open University website at www.open.ac.uk where you can learn more about the wide range of courses and packs offered at all levels by The Open University.

To purchase this publication or other components of Open University courses, contact Open University Worldwide Ltd, The Open University, Walton Hall, Milton Keynes MK7 6AA, United Kingdom: tel. +44 (0)1908 858785; fax +44 (0)1908 858787; e-mail ouwenq@open.ac.uk; website www.ouw.co.uk

A

HV 100

First published 2003 by Routledge
11 New Fetter Lane, London EC4P 4EE

Simultaneously published in the USA and Canada by Routledge
129 West 35th Street, New York, NY 1001

Routledge is an imprint of the Taylor & Francis Group

Edited, designed and typeset by The Open University.

Printed and bound in the United Kingdom by the Cromwell Press Limited.

ISBN 0-415-29866-0 (hbk)

ISBN 0-415-29868-7 (pbk)

1.1

28185B/k303b1prelimsi1.1

Contents

Contributors

John Adams is a Senior Lecturer at Homerton College, Cambridge, School of Health Studies. His interests include gerontological nursing, health policy and health care ethics. He is currently completing a documentary study of the local administration of old-age pensions from 1908 to 1948, before embarking on an oral history-based account of the development of Fulbourn Psychiatric Hospital, Cambridgeshire.

Jane Aldgate is Professor of Social Care at The Open University. She has done a wide range of research about children and has worked closely with the Department of Health on several initiatives, including the development of the post-qualifying Award in Child Care and the Framework for the Assessment of Children in Need. She is co-author with June Statham of the Department of Health's overview of the Children Act 1989 research studies: *The Children Act Now – Messages from Research*.

Dorothy Atkinson is a Senior Lecturer in the School of Health and Social Welfare at The Open University. Her background is in social work and social care, including experience of working in mental health and learning disability services. Her work at the OU has involved writing for social care workers and social workers. Her research interests are in the history of learning disability, the use of narratives in social research and the development of advocacy in all its manifestations. Her publications include *An Autobiographical Approach to Learning Disability Research* (1997, Ashgate).

Ian Butler is a qualified social worker with considerable practice and managerial experience. He also worked as a parliamentary research assistant for members of the Labour Party before taking up a post as a lecturer in social work at Cardiff University. He is now Professor of Social Work at Keele University. His main research interests include children's accounts of their social worlds, the health care of looked-after children and the practice of substitute family care. He is also interested in the development of social policy as it affects children and young people.

Naomi Connelly did qualitative research during the 1980s, focusing on the development of social services' race equality policies and practices, and how social services departments and voluntary organisations took account of users' views. In 1989 she moved to social policy work, first in the Citizens Advice Bureau service and then at the National Institute for Social Work. Since 1994 she has been a freelance writer, researcher and editor and a tutor for Open University courses.

Celia Davies is Professor of Health Care in the School of Health and Social Welfare at The Open University. She is a sociologist by training, and her career in research and teaching has focused on the division of labour in health care, professionalism and the organisation of services. During the mid-1980s she worked at the UKCC on the Project 2000 reform of nurse education, and she has been involved recently in the early discussions about the NHS University. Her publications in this area include *Gender and the Professional Predicament in Nursing* (1995, Open University Press) and (with Abigail Beach) *Interpreting Professional Self-regulation: A History of the UKCC* (2000, Palgrave).

Angus Dawson is Director of Graduate Studies in the Department of Philosophy at Keele University. He is Course Director of the MA in the Ethics of Social Welfare, a course for working professionals in the broad area of social care. He has particular research interests in the theoretical and historical foundations of social work; ethical issues relating to children; and the concepts of 'competence' and 'capacity'.

Brian Dimmock is a Senior Lecturer in the School of Health and Social Welfare at The Open University. Until 1999 he was joint chair of the National Open Learning DipSW Programme. He has a background in social work practice and management, including periods working for Barnardos and the NSPCC. He was a trustee and chair of the National Stepfamily Association until 2000 and has worked extensively as a management consultant in a wide range of health and social care settings. His research interests cover family change and, more recently, how changes in the organisation of the health services will affect the provision of vocational and professional education.

Jeanette Henderson is a Lecturer in the School of Health and Social Welfare at The Open University and has experience of working in voluntary and statutory sector mental health services. Her research interests are in mental health, especially the meanings and constructions of 'care'. Recent publications include papers on the impact of policy on care within partnerships and implementing change in mental health services.

Ann McDonald is a Senior Lecturer in Social Work at the University of East Anglia in Norwich. She has a particular interest in community care, and in links between law and social work. She taught law at the University of Wales and Sheffield and was a tutor and consultant on the Open University course K269 *Social Care, Social Work and the Law (England and Wales)*.

Sara Meddings is a clinical psychologist with East Sussex County Healthcare (NHS Trust) Psycho-Social Rehabilitation Service. She is interested in how systems can be effected to promote the recovery of people disabled by serious, ongoing mental health problems. Her published papers include work on user perspectives, 'what getting better means', and hearing voices. She also manages her own recovery and disability caused by ME (chronic fatigue syndrome).

Barbara Murray obtained a degree in social work from the University of Melbourne in Australia. She has over 20 years of experience of social work in the UK as a practitioner, manager and guardian ad litem. She is currently Principal Social Work Manager for the London Borough of Richmond upon Thames.

Sheila Peace is a Senior Lecturer in the School of Health and Social Welfare at The Open University, where she has also been Sub-Dean (Research). She is both a geographer and a gerontologist with research interests in the environment and ageing, residential care services and the regulation of care services.

Mike Pinnock is a trained social worker and is currently Performance Manager for North Lincolnshire Social and Housing Services, where he manages policy, planning, performance review and staff training and development, covering child welfare services, social care and public housing. He is the Chief Executive's nominated champion for social inclusion and works part-time with the Child and Family Research Centre at Loughborough University, researching how outcome-based data can be used to inform the planning of services for children and families. He is an Honorary Fellow at the University of Hull.

Jill Reynolds is a Senior Lecturer in the School of Health and Social Welfare at The Open University. She has experience as a manager in the voluntary sector in the UK and Australia. Her research interests and publications include education, training and practice issues, feminist practice, and the meanings of care and support. Previous co-edited and co-published work includes *Health, Welfare and Practice* (1992, Sage), *Mental Health Matters* (1996, Macmillan) and *Speaking Our Minds* (1996, Macmillan).

Sheena Rolph is a Research Fellow in the School of Health and Social Welfare at The Open University, where she recently gained her doctorate with a thesis on the history of community care for people with learning difficulties in Norfolk from 1930 to 1980. She was previously a manager of an adult education centre for people with learning difficulties. She has published on the history of community care and learning disability, and is currently exploring through oral history the role of local Mencap societies in the development of community care in East Anglia.

Janet Seden worked as a probation officer and social worker and lectured at Leicester University before taking up her present post in 1999 as Lecturer in the School of Health and Social Welfare at The Open University. She is the author of *Counselling Skills in Social Work Practice* (1999, Open University Press), and has also published work on the assessment of children in need and their families; the provision of services for children and their families; social work processes; family assistance orders; parenting; children and spirituality; and practice teaching.

Emily Skye is a Gestalt psychotherapist with ten years of experience as a practitioner and a manager of volunteers in the field of health and social care. She works with adults and with children and families and is interested in addressing oppressive practice on a personal and an institutional level.

Barbara Waine is an Honorary Research Fellow in the Department of Health and Social Care at Royal Holloway, University of London. She was previously Reader in Public Sector Management at Middlesex University. Barbara has published extensively on public sector management in journals and is co-author (with Tony Cutler) of *Managing the Welfare State* (1997, Berg).

Steve Walker trained and qualified as a social worker in Glasgow. Since then he has worked as a practitioner, manager, trainer and researcher in the field of children and family social work. Stephen's publications include: (with J. Tunstill) *Developing the Partnership between Research and Practice* (1998, Socionomen); 'Children's perspectives on attending reviews', in Shemmings, D. (ed.) *Involving Children in Family Support and Child Protection* (1999, The Stationery Office); (with A. Cox) *The Family Pack of Questionnaires and Scales Training Pack* (2001, ACPP) and *The HOME Inventories: A Training Approach for the UK* (2002, Department of Health/ Pavilion); (with D. Shemmings and H. Cleaver) *Write Enough: A Training and Resource Pack on Recording in Child Care* (forthcoming, Department of Health); (with H. Cleaver and P. Meadows) *Research on the Implementation of the Framework for the Assessment of Children in Need and Their Families (working title)* (forthcoming, Department of Health).

Editors' acknowledgements

Writing an Open University book is a time-consuming process and usually involves the collaboration of many people in addition to those listed as editors and authors. We want to acknowledge the help we have had in the preparation of this book and, in particular, to thank the following people for their invaluable contributions.

First, the editors would like to thank the contributors who wrote or collaborated with the course team in writing the chapters: their details are given in full on pages vii–x. Our thanks also go to Stewart Black, Bob Sang and Dawn Wakeling, who offered ideas and suggestions during the early stages of the production process, and to Fran Orford for providing the cartoons in the text.

A huge debt of gratitude is owed to a very large number of people across the country who gave their time to work with us. They include the staff and service users who attended the numerous workshops and interviews that we set up in Belfast, Leeds, Leicester, Edinburgh, Newcastle, Durham, Stoke, Witney, York and Carlisle during 2000 and 2001. Their 'voices' are heard throughout the book. Thanks also to the workers and members at Redcar and Cleveland Mind. In Leicester thanks to City Social Services Family Centre and Children's Homes Managers (Child Care Resources), Family Service Unit, Homestart, the Rathbone Project, Compass Children's Services, the Centre for Deaf People, and The Carers Project. Also thanks to Milton Keynes Homestart, Surestart Mansfield and Coram Family for their help with interviews. Special thanks to the service users and managers at all these places whose stories appear throughout this book and to the managers who wrote or recorded their diaries for us, whose work we have quoted extensively.

We should take this opportunity to acknowledge the important role of critical readers and course testers in providing feedback not only on this book but also on all the K303 *Managing Care* course materials. They include Ganga Westwood and her equal opportunities group of Rohhss Chapman, Amerjeet Rebolo, Louise Townson, Judith Ward and Jude Wildwood, plus the critical readers group of Martin Armitage, John Burton, Kate Doyle, Robin Jackson, Ann Marsden, Lorraine Morgan and Christine Vigars, and the course testers group of Tim Clements, Sue Robson, Joan Green, Caroline Picking and Diane Savage. We have been greatly assisted by the comments of our external assessor, Richard Whipp of Cardiff Business School and Pro-Vice Chancellor of Cardiff University, whose encouragement has helped to shape the whole project.

The editors would also like to acknowledge the part played by their colleagues in the K303 *Managing Care* course team: Jane Aldgate, Brian Dimmock, Ingrid Jefferys, Jill Reynolds (the course chair),

Wendy Rose and Janet Seden; Anne Bullman (the course manager); Jenny Monk and Amanda Smith (the course editors); Siân Lewis (the graphic designer); Sara Hack (the graphic artist) and Kathy McPhee (the course team assistant). Also our thanks to other academic colleagues, in particular Mike Aiken, Ronny Flynn, Roger Gomm, Julia Johnson, Vivien Martin, Linda Miller, Anita Rogers, Fred Toates and Jenny Spouse for their academic input, comment and support.

Finally, we want to convey our thanks to the unsung heroes and heroines in The Open University who processed the text and to all the staff at Routledge who were involved in its printing and distribution.

Jeanette Henderson and Dorothy Atkinson, The Open University, September 2002

Acknowledgements

Grateful acknowledgement is made to the following sources for permission to reproduce material in this book.

Text

Chapter 4

Box 4.4: Home Office (2000) *Human Rights Act: An Introduction*, pp. 3–4. Crown copyright material is reproduced under Class Licence Number CO1W0000065 with the permission of the Controller of HMSO and the Queen's Printer for Scotland.

Table

Chapter 7

Table 7.1: James, A. (1994) 'Reflections on the politics of quality', *Performance Review in Social Care*, Jessica Kingsley Publishers.

Figure

Chapter 7

Figure 7.1: Joint Reviews of Local Authorities' Social Services: www.joint-reviews.gov.uk. © The Audit Commission of Local Authorities and the NHS in England and Wales 2000–2001.

Illustrations

Chapter 1

p. 5: Copyright © Harry Venning; *p. 17:* Copyright © Telegraph Group Limited 2001.

Chapter 6

p. 147: Copyright © Brendan Wilson.

Chapter 8

p. 196: Copyright © Ruth Jenkinson.

Chapter 12

Introduction

The pace of change in health and social care services is rapid and affects everyone, whether as a manager, service user, worker or citizen. Government policies demand accountability, quality and integration in health and social care services. The boundaries between health and social care are shifting and, some would say, merging. Nurses are employed as care managers and manage social workers. Social workers are employed by health trusts and voluntary agencies.

A central theme throughout this book is the importance of the context of management. That context is complex and challenging. We argue that managing people who deliver care services is fundamentally different from managing, for example, a factory or a retail organisation. The issues brought to managers by workers involved in safeguarding children from harm, or responding to the death of a resident in a nursing home, are rooted in practice. Practice – the way things are done – forms a strong link between everyone who works in care settings from workers (whether paid or unpaid, qualified or not) to managers and senior managers. We argue that it is essential to keep a firm focus on this practice context of managing in health and social care – the practice of managing the practice of others. We call this 'practice-led management', by which we mean that managers are continually aware of the demands and dilemmas, challenges and opportunities of practice situations.

Does having been a practitioner in one field give someone the mandate to manage people with different kinds of expertise? We suggest that understanding and awareness of practice situations are central to practice-led management. The main purpose of agencies concerned with health and social care is to ensure the best possible quality of life for the people who use their services. While strategic decisions by senior managers (preferably informed by consultations with members of their organisations, communities and service users) about the shape and kind of service will set the overall parameters, frontline managers are in touch with practice as it happens. Managers need an awareness of the impact on practitioners of working with people at times of great distress or need. Their own experiences as practitioners will be invaluable.

The detailed knowledge of particular contexts is, of course, distinctive. The steps that must be taken to apply for an emergency protection order to safeguard a young child are different from those for an application to detain someone under the Mental Health Act 1983. A manager must be knowledgeable about the legislative framework and the legal context governing practice. Equally important, however, is an awareness of the tensions faced by practitioners when implementing such legislation.

Frontline management in health and social care is challenging. Finding a route through a maze of changing service structures and professional groupings is a puzzle for managers to solve. It is also creative: forming new partnerships, and supporting and enabling workers to provide a better service for people who use care services. Frontline managers are often held responsible when good practice is lacking and when there are problems or complaints about services. Praise is scarce and managers rarely get the training or education they need to ensure they are best able to support staff and provide the managerial service that senior managers and service users expect.

There has been a lack of relevant material for managers in care settings and this book makes an important contribution to understanding the context of care provision and the orientation of managers. A multi-disciplinary Open University team compiled this volume, with additional contributions from academics, managers and practitioners. The text is informed by extensive consultations with managers, practitioners and service users (see the Appendix), and the examples are rooted in real experiences.

Structure of the book

This book is a core text for an Open University course. It is written in an accessible style, with helpful summaries of key points at the end of each section of a chapter. There is a logical progression that makes it worthwhile to read the chapters sequentially. However, the contributions are also written to make sense as independent chapters, so you may prefer to dip into different parts of the book. Each part has an introduction, which gives more detailed guidance on the themes of different chapters. The index can be used as a guide to key terms and discussions.

Part 1 Practice, Policy and the Law explores what managing to *care* means, in particular the requirements on managers to promote social inclusion. Influences on welfare practice and services range from global to local and they are many and varied. More people may require welfare services as they seek asylum from persecution, conflict and hardship in countries far from the UK. Residents within the UK may find their access to services affected by their location: whether they live in Scotland or England, an urban or a rural area, in Northern Ireland or South Wales. Social care may take place within large organisations, within an individual home and on the pavements with homeless people. Frontline managers may share offices with their team or project members or manage at a distance, having only occasional face-to-face contact with staff.

This part also charts the impacts on managers of a changing policy environment and 'managerialism': the application of management techniques borrowed from business and industry to enable the provision of effective services at lower cost. The message from government has shifted from competition to co-operation and partnership building. At the same time as developing an internal partnership between professionals within a team or project, frontline managers are required to develop partnerships with other agencies and organisations in their locality. External as well as internal partnerships are now a key feature of government policy in health and social care.

Part 2 The Contexts of Care examines organisations from three viewpoints. First, it explores how managers can work with different organisational structures and cultures. As in any relationship, new and developing agency partnerships bring with them particular challenges, often based around developing shared understandings of processes and practices, cultures and histories. Second, we look at organisations as environments. The interconnections between organisational structure and care services are shown in relation to the environment of a residential care home. Relationships between people who use the space – workers, residents and visitors – and how the manager can influence the caring environment lead into an assessment of recent moves towards the third focus: quality. We look at what 'quality' means to different people and how it might be achieved.

Part 3 People in Social Care draws on theories of understanding people, and theories of professional and managerial identity. A frontline manager in social care may have a professional background in, for example, nursing or social work (or neither), and may manage workers from several professional backgrounds alongside unqualified support workers. Is there any longer a place for professional identity? Service users want a service that best meets their needs. The profession of the person who delivers or co-ordinates that service is not the key issue for service users. More important for them is whether managers listen and respond to their views, the standard of service they receive, and whether they are treated with respect and dignity.

Just as the numbers of multidisciplinary teams grow, interdisciplinary training and education opportunities become more available. All this opportunity challenges traditional professional boundaries and allegiances. In some cases this results in an entrenched approach, a determination to reinforce a professional identity that took many years to achieve. In other cases the opportunity to draw on a variety of perspectives within a single team for an individual service user outweighs any challenges to professional identity. Managing a multi- or an interdisciplinary team may be a demanding task for a frontline manager, who needs to chart a way through an often turbulent course. It requires a high level of tact and diplomacy as well as skills in team building.

The state of knowledge about managing people and finding a balance between 'understanding' and 'getting the job done' is examined. Ethical managerial practice and dilemmas are explored, and the role of the manager in achieving good outcomes for individuals and families, services and the public is debated. The book ends by considering the relevance of trends in the management of care over the last century for today's manager and looking at prospects for the future.

Whatever the layers and length of lines of accountability and management in an organisation, the frontline manager is the closest person in the managerial hierarchy to the delivery of the service or the practice. The frontline manager forms a bridge or conduit between senior managers and practitioners. This operational role gives the frontline manager a unique perspective on the needs of practitioners and service users, the responses they give and receive and the extent to which responses meet needs.

A word about language

There are many terms used to describe people who receive care services. Generally, in this book the term 'service user' is our preferred term. However, this is a term that is contested and disputed by some critics. We use it here to identify people who by virtue of their needs might be eligible for some kinds of care service. Alternatives include 'client', 'user', 'customer' or 'survivor', each of which conveys a different kind of relationship with service providers. Some organisations refer to people who use their services as 'members' or 'residents'. Some people who have had contact with mental health services prefer the term 'survivor' or 'mental health system survivor'. Other approaches describe people's disabilities or impairments, such as people with learning disabilities or learning difficulties, mental health problems, and so on.

We acknowledge that 'service user' does present some problems as a term of general description. For example, are children who are looked after in care service users? Or are their parents? Are people detained against their will under the Mental Health Act service users? Managers need to be aware of the diversity of opinion and debates surrounding terminology and the power to define identity and experience.

Part 1 Practice, Policy and the Law

Introduction

Managing in care settings is qualitatively different from managing in other contexts. Health and social care services are not, as Aldgate and Dimmock argue in Chapter 1, a service industry. They do not provide the services offered by, for example, a bank, an insurance company or a hotel. Generally speaking, people cannot take their care needs elsewhere if they are dissatisfied with the service provided.

Managers of care services must deal with the ethical and practical implications of highly complex dilemmas and the decisions they make. A bank manager does not have to decide whether to enforce legislation in order to ensure that particular people use the services offered by that bank. If people are reluctant or refuse to accept care services, on the other hand, there can be compulsory interventions.

The importance of human relationships in the provision and management of care should not be underestimated or taken for granted. Relationships between managers and workers, service users and senior managers have an effect on the provision of care. Often care services are provided for people at times of distress, or as a result of transitions and changes in their lives and circumstances. People may welcome involvement but they may also reject it. The contexts in which care services are provided are constantly changing and, in the first part of this book, the relationship between contexts, people and management is explored.

A thread running throughout this part – and indeed throughout this book – is the tension caused by the dilemmas managers of care services face on an almost daily basis. Managers are asked to balance what appear to be incompatible needs. They need to work within the complexity of care services. Much is expected of care services – and much is achieved. However, whether managers of health and social care projects and teams have the power to tackle challenges such as promoting social inclusion within a wider context of unemployment, poverty and exclusion is open to debate.

One way to work towards an inclusive approach is through *partnerships*. These can be partnerships within and between organisations and sectors, and within local and national frameworks. Partnerships are developing between professions to create new forms of service provision. As service user involvement and consultation processes grow, partnerships between workers, managers and service users develop. For partnerships to flourish, however, there needs to be a commitment to sharing power and respect for the contributions all partners may make to the relationships. This commitment needs to be deep and embedded, not an optional part of the management task.

Dilemmas are posed by the need to manage performance and achieve outcomes and targets. For example, consider consultation and involvement with service users. It is possible to provide evidence of meeting the target and to tick the appropriate box on the audit trail. However, is this consultation to achieve the target merely in a nominal way or consultation to achieve real and meaningful change to services? One criticism levelled at managerialist approaches is that the measure of performance becomes more important than the impact of the performance itself.

The frontline manager forms a bridge between the complex and often competing needs of service users, workers – the people who directly use the services of frontline managers – central and local government, senior managers and the general public. The services accessed by this bridge have a legal foundation: managers and their organisations have powers and duties to provide care services.

In Chapter 1 'Managing to care', Aldgate and Dimmock set out to chart a route across the bridge that is frontline management in health and social care. They aim to provide an opportunity for reflection on the context in which managers in social care respond to the many challenges, demands and decisions they face every day. They explore the complexity of care and the connections between practice and management, introducing the concept of *practice-led management*, a theme running throughout this book. Another factor that has a continuing influence on the contexts of management in health and social care is *change*. The authors begin to explore the impacts of changes in care services and introduce topics – for instance quality and partnership – that are explored in more detail in other chapters.

Involvement of, and consultation with, service users has become part of quality assessment frameworks and standards. In Chapter 2 'What service users say about services: the implications for managers', Connelly and Seden locate this process within the context of user-defined needs and debates about the nature and role of care services. Services are structured around agency-designed specialist groupings, such as older people, disability or mental health, but service users do not see their own situations in such clear-cut categories. The authors suggest that managers must work to translate the often disparate views of people who use services and of their carers into acceptable and responsive service provision.

In Chapter 3 'Managers, managing and managerialism', Waine and Henderson argue that debates about managerialism have provided a powerful critique of the place of managers in social care and locate these debates within a wider policy context. They consider the impact and pace of changes to the operational, strategic and professional aspects of the management role, and highlight the complex framework within which managers must operate. They suggest there are positive outcomes as a result of the introduction of managerialist approaches to care services: the focus on improved quality of service for example. However, they go on to argue that the way such improvements are measured, through league tables, star ratings, and so on, is problematic. How do managers experience these techniques of managerialism and how does the practice-led manager respond?

In the final chapter of Part 1, 'Managers and the law', McDonald and Henderson give an overview of legislation as it impinges on the management task. Legislation affects and structures the way services are organised and assessed. Legislation may be overarching, such as the Children Act 1989, or specific, such as the Care Standards Act 2000, and their parallels in Scotland and Northern Ireland. The authors argue that managers need to be familiar with key legal concepts in order to work through the conflicts and dilemmas in the workplace and the duties that involve the proper interpretation of rights and responsibilities.

Chapter 1
Managing to care

Jane Aldgate and Brian Dimmock

1.1 Introduction

Many frontline managers will recognise the thoughts and feelings expressed in the following extract from a manager's diary.

SURRINDER'S DIARY

Wednesday 15th May

The rest of the morning was spent short-listing. I'm quite hopeful that out of fifteen candidates we shortlisted down to eleven. Set interview date and also sorted out the questions. In the afternoon sent all the original paperwork to Personnel about the senior nursery officer post and also faxed them the paperwork as well. I quickly had a bite to eat. At 1.30 p.m. did caseload supervision for lounge 3 ... (This) is specific supervision time allocated to look at and discuss with Keyworker(s) the children on their caseload ... After caseload supervision, did a review for a child's place (at the day centre). The place was continuing under the same objectives. Considering how the morning started with me feeling totally exhausted ... I feel like I have accomplished things today.

Thursday 16th May

I came out of the brief meeting with a parent at about 2.15 p.m. I looked at my desk and there were ten calls that I needed to return, so I started with a few of them. I quickly warmed up my pasta and came and sat down at the desk (to) follow up more calls. The rest of the afternoon was spent making calls, collating numbers of staff from other units, and writing up children's case records. I really feel for the two nursery officers - they have worked so hard this week, due to staffing levels. Fed back to the staff I appreciated all their hard work and said thank you ... It would be really nice, now and then, if someone acknowledged that for me.

Making time to plan and prioritise rather than just react is never easy. Care services in the UK are currently undergoing yet more change through the integration of health and social care under the banner of the government's reforms of the National Health Service (NHS) (Health Act 1999; NHS Plan 2000). In these circumstances it is difficult to escape the feeling that many services are permanently on the edge of chaos.

'Managing' may mean precisely what it says: that is, coping, surviving, rubbing along, and so on. 'I can manage – just about' is probably as close to a definition of the art of frontline management as most managers can get at present. Survival and doing your best for service users in difficult circumstances may be all that can be reasonably expected given resource limitations, increasing expectations and constant scrutiny, inspection and criticism.

In this chapter we take the position that there is something about people who devote their working lives to providing care services that enables them to transcend this permanent state of transition and change, or at least to survive it! Despite the difficulties, most managers and their staff still 'care' about the people who use their services. In this sense they are 'managing to care'. Although the world of care services may be increasingly complex, one aspect remains constant and simple: that is, the desire to help others, to recognise that everyone needs 'care' from time to time, and that the world is a better place if it is provided well and with generosity. It is this underlying ethic that makes care management distinctive and why it is not the same as managing a fast-food outlet.

We believe that care management is a human service, not a service industry. Weiner (1994) developed a definition of management in the domain of care ('human services', as he calls it) that involves caring *about* others and caring *for* others by attempting to improve the quality of their lives. It develops the idea of management being related to the values of care:

> Human services managers do not operate in a vacuum; they are the keepers and shapers of the modern welfare state. As such they need to have a clear vision of the ideological framework within which they operate. Regardless of personal political-economic philosophy, when accepting a position in human services management, one accepts a commitment to bring the highest quality of life to *all* inhabitants of our nation, particularly those with the greatest need.
>
> (Weiner, 1994, p. 21)

The aims of this chapter are to:

- examine what 'care' is and what this implies for those who 'manage' it
- outline the changes taking place through the integration of health and social care and to consider some of the implications of these changes for care managers
- explore 'practice-led' management as a model that is appropriate to this sector.

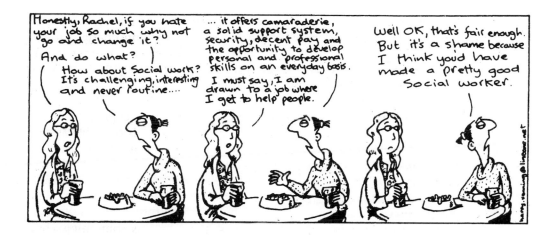

1.2 Setting the context for managing care

Dependence and independence

The starting point for anyone involved in managing care has to be their attitude (and that of the service for which they work) to dependence and independence. Do you see our dependence on each other as arising from the normal processes of human development and decline, coupled with particular events and circumstances through life that make us more or less dependent? Or is your thinking organised around the achievement and maintenance of 'independence' so that other states of being are considered at best unfortunate and at worst 'dehumanising'? Perhaps your focus is on how states of dependence come about. For example, some are part of a life stage, such as babyhood, or happen by chance or accident, such as illness or serious injury. What about those we 'bring on ourselves' through abuse of drugs and alcohol or reckless behaviour? Does some notion of 'deserving' and 'undeserving' creep into our thinking about dependence and how we should respond to it?

Jenny Morris, who has championed disability rights, argues for a rethinking of the terms 'dependence' and 'independence'. She asserts:

> Both terms need thinking about. The word dependence has both negative and positive connotations in that the state of dependence can be associated with helplessness and subordination *or* with reliability. In terms of the physical world, none of us – whether disabled or not – is completely independent in the sense we rely on nothing and nobody.
>
> (Morris, 1991, p. 137)

This would imply that our attitude to our dependence on other people should be informed by seeing it as a matter of degree – a measure of quantity rather than quality. In other words, when we are on the receiving end of care services, for whatever reason, it is an expression of our shared humanity, not an expression of our 'disability'. We should not become a separate 'class' of people ('the disabled', 'the elderly', and so on) when we receive care; we should experience it as something that helps to connect us with what we share with our fellow human beings, including those who are providing 'care' for us.

Morris (1995) advocates the approach exemplified by the Independent Living Movement. Their use of the word 'independent' does not imply that we should be able to do every task for ourselves. It is more concerned with maximising choice and control over how, when and who assists us. This is a major change from the tradition of 'the fortunate' giving help to 'the less fortunate' (for which, of course, they should be suitably grateful).

You may think that such a dichotomy no longer exists in these enlightened times but a close examination of many care services, their histories and traditions would suggest that old practices die hard. The fact that many services are provided by charities, however enlightened they may be, sits uncomfortably with the idea that care services are part of our rights as citizens (along with our responsibility to ensure that they are paid for and maintained to a high standard). Even the state services evolved out of charitable traditions. The values of the Charity Organisation Society (COS), formed in 1869, were echoed in some of the attitudes that prevailed since the formation of the modern welfare state after the Second World War. This is what Webb and Webb (1929) said about the COS:

> What was wrong about the COS, as may now be seen, was its deep-rooted censoriousness; its strange assumption that the rich were, as such, intellectually and morally the 'superiors' of the poor, entitled to couple pecuniary assistance with a virtual dictatorship over their lives.
>
> (Webb and Webb, quoted in Loney et al., 1991, p. 27)

People in the disability movement have fought hard to change attitudes and practices in service provision so that when we receive care services we are not 'dictated to'. Accepting the powerlessness that came with 'being looked after' might have been acceptable in 1944 when the welfare state was established but it is not good enough for us today. There is now active and successful lobbying by disability organisations, as well as by mental health groups. They reject the status of 'partial citizenship' in favour of a system that gives them full recognition as citizens with the right to enjoy assistance which they choose, defined on their terms.

From the perspectives of adults with learning disabilities, a clear message comes across about the unacceptability of care that assumes the dependence of those who are on the receiving end. Much has been written about this subject (for a helpful review see Reynolds and Walmsley, 1998 and Simons, 1998). The cumulative messages from both the research and the interest groups have now elicited a response from government and are highly relevant for managers both of residential and day care facilities and in the community. At the time of writing (May 2002), direct payment schemes with no age limit for either disabled or older people have been introduced (Department of Health, 1999a). In theory, they should address the concerns about choice and control of services by users. McDonald (2001) suggests that direct payments may offer 'freedom from local authority conventions on service delivery' but there are some caveats:

> The choice of personal assistants lies with the user as employer, although still subject to the local authority's assessment of need. In order that direct payments may be extended to all those potentially eligible, restrictive interpretations of who is 'willing' and 'able' to receive such payments need to be overcome; this is particularly important for people with learning difficulties.
>
> (McDonald, 2001, p. 149)

One of the major issues facing care services now is to adjust to a climate of fundamental human rights and citizenship exemplified by the challenges to established practice from service user organisations. Many people who are involved in service provision grew up with the welfare state being something for which they should be grateful (with due deference to be shown to important people such as doctors). The consumer movement and the growing power of service users are challenging the attitudes of service providers to those who use services as never before.

Care and humanity

Ann Brechin makes connections between the everyday and the professional view of care:

> Refusing to care what others think, what others want, what others need from you, is ultimately to turn your back on society and social engagement. 'To care', on the other hand, is to accept a host of moral responsibilities for your own and others' well-being. It is to accept that people matter. At the extreme, care can sustain or extinguish life itself. Even at its more routine, it can influence how people live their lives and the kind of people they become. Caring, therefore, really matters. It is fundamental to the pact involved in being human.
>
> (Brechin, 1998, p. 1)

Such strong words signal the importance of human relationships in the provision of care. What Brechin is saying is that 'care' should mean caring about people, and working in a way that values people: in other words, having caring values. This cannot be taken for granted, as she explains further:

> the way the concept of 'care' is used and understood reflects as well as influences actual experiences of care and caring and the consequences for quality of life.
>
> (Brechin, 1998, p. 3)

This may seem rather rarefied to people involved in hands-on management but it is evident in something as practical as providing a residential care home. This is what the Scottish Executive says about what people in Scotland want:

> people who use care homes seem united around a core of expectations and desires. They want a care home that respects them and treats them as individuals, enables them to retain as much control over their lives as possible, guarantees their privacy and enables them to have a choice about the location or type of home available to them. People in long stay care are concerned about the quality of their lives, of which the care they receive is only one, albeit important, part. Providers of homes need to refocus from a concentration on care alone and pay greater attention to the overall quality of life afforded to people who live in care homes.
>
> (Scottish Executive, 2001a, p. 3)

If managers are increasingly charged with listening to the users of their services, they must know more about the experience of being cared for and of receiving services. Of course, managers of care services, like anyone else, have their own experiences of care and what they would want for themselves and their loved ones. As well as the somewhat abstract issues of choice and self-determination, there are more down to earth issues of daily life, such as being listened to. The following questions help translate these value issues into reality. These are some of the questions that service users might want to ask themselves about the quality of their care. Although they were written in relation to older people, they could apply equally well to any adult receiving personal care services and, in most respects, to children and young people who are looked after by a local authority.

- How am I treated by staff when they are bathing me and helping me dress?
- How do they speak to me?
- Am I consulted in matters to do with my own care and matters that concern residents as a whole?
- Are my wishes respected?
- Are my views taken into account?
- Do staff regard me as a real person with desires, hopes and expectations just like them?

(Department of Health, 1999b, p. 16)

The words 'just like them' at the end of this quotation go to the heart of the changing culture in care service provision, from one that evolved from charity, through the early days of the welfare state, to a clearly articulated concept of citizenship and human rights. They imply an acceptance of equality between those providing and those receiving care because having our needs met (in most circumstances) is a right accorded by virtue of our status as citizens.

Power and vulnerability

During periods of our lives when our dependence on other people is high, usually we are more vulnerable to being abused or exploited. Being dependent on other people creates a potential imbalance of power. We may lack insight into our own circumstances (whether temporarily or permanently). We lose some of our ability to 'exchange' help or reciprocate. Indeed, reciprocity is probably central to everyday exchanges between people, and the loss of our ability to 'give back', or 'pay our way', can impact on our sense of dignity, self-respect and identity.

Those who are motivated to provide care are not usually saints but people who derive satisfaction from working with and for others. However, good intentions are not enough because power can be abused without this being the carer's intention. Managers have to go well beyond commonsense understandings of 'doing things for' or 'looking after' people to ensure that services enhance their human dignity, uphold their rights and improve the quality of people's lives. We have to remember that public concern about care services has been informed by many examples of such power being abused. Nowhere has this been more shocking than in the realms of sexual and physical abuse of children and adults in residential settings (Levy and Kahan, 1991).

Legislation relating to children stresses that *safeguarding* is an essential part of promoting welfare (Aldgate, 2001). One cannot be attended to without the other. Utting (1998) makes this point clearly with respect to providing residential and foster care (referred to here as 'accommodation for children'):

> Safeguards are an indispensable component to the child's security, and should be the first consideration for any body providing or arranging accommodation for children. Safeguards form the basis for ensuring physical and emotional health, good education and sound social development. These are the proper objectives of all institutions providing care and education for children.
>
> (Utting, 1998, p. 15, para. 1.23)

The same philosophy of safeguarding and promoting welfare applies to adults who are receiving care services. Protection from physical and sexual abuse is at one end but abuse through the neglect of dignity is another aspect that safeguarding must address. The implications of safeguarding therefore impose complex demands on frontline managers. Safeguarding has to be at the forefront of the daily routine of tasks.

Managers also face the responsibility of safeguarding staff. There are two elements here: protecting workers from violence and harm and ensuring that organisations do not abuse their staff. How safeguarding and promoting welfare are dealt with internally within an agency will affect the ability of managers and workers to care for and care about users of their services. Put more simply, the treatment by employers of their employees is part of what sets the tone for the treatment of service users.

Another perspective to be included in this debate about safeguarding is how managers reconcile the values of care with compulsory actions that are carried out on behalf of the state. Removing children who are at risk of significant harm from families and compulsory admissions under mental health legislation are two clear examples. Care services are frequently provided for people whose liberty has been restricted in their own or other people's interests. This can be through formal procedures of the court but there are also de facto restrictions exercised through everyday under-standings about the need to protect people considered to be 'at risk' of harm.

This imperative is at its clearest with respect to children. The belief is that their inexperience makes them vulnerable during their development, and that in day-to-day circumstances it is legitimate for adults in caring roles to protect them, if necessary by exerting power over them in some way. Giddens (1999) argues that in this case there is an implicit authority that legitimises the actions of adult carers but it still requires justification. He applies democratic principles to caring relationships (what he refers to as 'a democracy of the emotions'):

> A democracy of the emotions, it seems to me, is as important as public democracy in improving the quality of our lives. This holds as much in parent–child relations as in other areas. These can't, and shouldn't, be materially equal. Parents must have authority over children, in every-one's interests. Yet they should presume an in-principle equality. In a democratic family, the authority of parents should be based upon an implicit contract. The parent in effect says to the child: 'If you were an adult, and knew what I know, you would agree that what I ask you to do is legitimate'.
>
> (Giddens, 1999)

Giddens' position is that people caring for children (in this case, parents) have a responsibility to protect them that arises from democratic principles applied to caring exchanges. However, this responsibility has a clear ethical basis, and the authority is limited. If authority is exercised in a way that is not legitimate, it is an abuse of power. This is very different from a position based on a belief that children do not have rights and that 'adults know best' because there is increasing evidence that adults very often do not act in the best interests of children (Utting, 1998).

When we try to extend this idea of the carer 'knowing best' to adults (for example, people with a learning difficulty, degenerative illness or brain injury) we confront even more complexity. Monitoring the line between protecting people from their own lack of insight, restricting their liberties for the convenience of those who are providing care and committing straightforward abuse will be familiar to many readers. Most challenging of all is the issue of our attitude to adults who are vulnerable because of impairment of mind and a lack of insight that makes them a serious danger to themselves and/or other people if their liberty is not in some way restricted. For example, a person with dementia may become sexually disinhibited and touch staff, other service users or members of the public in ways that could easily cause considerable distress. They may lack insight into their behaviour to such an extent that on occasions their liberty has to be restricted to protect them and other people. With the exception of certain aspects of mental health practice, legislation is often very unclear in such circumstances.

Managers, care staff and other carers have to find a way of providing care to fellow adults who cannot, in any meaningful sense, participate in some, or even many, decisions about their lives. People in these circumstances are often left to struggle with the dilemmas this creates with little support and guidance and the fear that, if anything goes wrong, they will be blamed. This is an aspect of care practice and management that requires much more research and debate, and perhaps a greater degree of honesty. Should we take Giddens' approach to children and recognise that in most respects some adults' lack of 'ability' is such that it is foolish to pretend that carers and the people they care for are 'equal' in any meaningful sense? In this case authority would be exercised in a similar way to that suggested by Giddens for children, legitimated by acting on behalf of the adult to assert their rights and to protect them from harm. Tempting though this may be, it has enormous dangers. First, at what point is it decided someone has enough 'insight' to be assumed to be a full participant, and who decides? Second, this may represent the slippery slope to classes or degrees of citizenship. People with learning difficulties, acquired brain injury or degenerative brain conditions would be vulnerable if such an approach were adopted.

All we can do here is raise the issues, recognise how difficult it is for managers to work in such circumstances and repeat that the status differences between children and adults in terms of citizenship, rights and responsibilities do exist and must be recognised, however impaired and vulnerable an adult may be. In extreme cases the law can intervene, for example through the Court of Protection, but this usually does not happen. Carers, care staff and managers are left to cope with the ethical and practical implications of highly complex dilemmas. This is another reason why providing care services must be seen as more than just a service industry.

Exclusion and inclusion

Escaping from the Poor Law tradition whereby society was divided into 'the deserving' and 'the undeserving', presided over by 'the virtuous', has been less easy than the inventors of the welfare state may have believed. The intention behind the welfare state was to close the gap between what is good for people with choice and good enough for those without choice.

After 50 or more years, managers of care services still come face to face with inequalities and social disadvantage on a daily basis. Indeed, many of the early principles of the welfare state, notably universal provision, have been challenged to such an extent that they do not have much meaning (particularly in housing provision and financial provision for old age and education). One way of describing such inequalities is to use the term *social exclusion*. The Prime Minister Tony Blair is quoted as describing this as:

> A shorthand label for what can happen when individuals or areas suffer from a combination of linked problems such as unemployment, poor skills, low incomes, poor housing, high crime environments, bad health and family breakdown.
>
> (Department of Social Security, 1998, p. 23)

Policies of social inclusion imply that there is a desire to improve people's circumstances but there are dangers in this approach. Writers such as Levitas (1997) and Beresford and Wilson (1998) argue that the concept of social exclusion implies a need for excluded people to be subject to social control through coercive policies aimed at integrating them into the labour market to reduce their reliance on state benefits. As Levitas says:

> The 'real' society is not that constituted by the (unequal) 70 per cent, to which the poor are marginal or from which they are excluded. The real society is that made up of the whole 100 per cent, in which poverty is endemic.
>
> (Levitas, 1997, p. 19, quoted in Beresford and Wilson, 1998, p. 87)

Beresford and Wilson (1998) argue that to prevent policies aimed at social inclusion becoming a way of controlling people, it is very important that the voices of people labelled as excluded help to define social policy. This will promote what Lister (1998) calls 'sustained citizenship', where people not only have rights to vote but also feel that they are equal to others.

Bob Holman, a community worker in Easterhouse in Glasgow, speaks about social exclusion from direct experience as he describes how different elements join up to heighten the impact of social disadvantage on families living in poverty:

> The combination of escalating inequality and the deterioration of essential social services means that social exclusion is a characteristic of the lives of many residents of such neighbourhoods.
>
> They are excluded from the *physical safety* which is accorded to the affluent. Children in Social Class V are 16 times more likely than those in Social Class 1 to die from house fires. They are more liable to road accidents, illnesses and death. Overcrowded and damp homes, lack of gardens and inadequate nutrition all take their toll.
>
> They are excluded from the *family security* known to others. Children accommodated by public authorities are now overwhelmingly the children of the poor. As Bebbington and Miles (1989) concluded from

their large-scale study, a child whose family is not on income support, is in a two-parent family with three or fewer children, is white, and lives in a spacious, owner-occupied house, has only a 1 in 7,000 chance of entering care. A child from a large, one-parent family, living on income support, of mixed ethnic origin, and dwelling in a crowded, privately rented home, has a 1 in 10 chance.

This is not to say that the children of most poor parents go into care. It is to say that social deprivations make parenting much harder which, in time, can adversely affect the children. Just over the road from our flat is a family where both parents work 72 hours a week at £2 an hour: their long hours and low pay does not make it easy to look after their five children.

They are excluded from *amenities*. Youngsters from comfortable back-grounds have the money to travel to and can afford recreation and facilities. Those in deprived neighbourhoods have little money and few facilities. I have been encouraging a few people in Easterhouse to write. One mother with four children wrote: 'Easterhouse is not an easy place for teenagers. The Sports Centre is quite expensive and it is in the centre where a lot of kids will not go in case they get jumped.' After her teenage daughter was sexually assaulted, she is frightened to let her go out.

They are excluded from *jobs* ... They are excluded from the *good life* enjoyed by so many in our society ...

(Holman, 1998, p. 66)

If you were a manager providing services to the citizens of Easterhouse, what impact would Holman's analysis of exclusion have on your priorities? This begins to shift the focus away from the individual to social processes, which either create needs or at any rate exacerbate the problems of people living in deprived circumstances. Indeed, Holman argues that dealing with inequality and the deprivation this causes will release the energy and creativity of people who currently make heavy demands on public services. This will enable them to work together with local services to solve their own problems to a significant extent, reducing unnecessary dependence on services and enhancing their skills, dignity and self-respect in the process. At this point approaches to community development, community care, health provision and health promotion may overlap and change the relationship between the people who provide services and those who receive them.

For managers who play a key role in influencing the policy of their agencies, Holman's challenge is to consider their relationship with the communities they serve. Who decides on priorities? Where Morris (1991) advocates empowering people through direct payments for services, Holman argues for empowering whole communities through addressing fundamental inequalities in health, employment, education, community safety, leisure, and so on. What these approaches have in common is changing the relationship between service providers and service users to one of partnership and equality.

One particular process of social exclusion is very high on the government's agenda in 2002 and has been given added impetus by the Stephen Lawrence Inquiry Report (Home Office, 1999). The Race Relations (Amendment) Act 2000 (Home Office, 2000a), coupled with the Human Rights Act 1998 (Home Office, 1998a), changes the culture in which care services must operate. In particular, the UK government believes that public bodies must improve the way in which they develop and implement policies to ensure that racism and discrimination are not 'institutionalised' in how services are provided. Despite good intentions, many service users, or potential service users, are excluded from receiving care services through deeply rooted cultural ignorance as well as more overt forms of racial discrimination.

Managers have an important role in creating a positive staff culture through leadership and modelling good practice as well as encouraging openness, dialogue and constructive challenges to poor practice and behaviour. If they do not promote a positive culture this contributes to a climate where the abuse of service users and staff is possible (see Chapter 5 and Chapter 6 for more discussion of this). Cultures develop from shared experiences and traditions within teams and working groups. New staff often encounter a well-developed culture with established methods of welcoming staff into the team, allocating work and sharing jokes and humour. Are black and ethnic minority staff always expected to deal with black and ethnic minority service users? Is socialisation into the team inclusive of all staff, and are cultural and religious differences acknow-ledged and/or celebrated?

Individuals can be very influential in shaping the cultures of their organisations. Therefore, managers who have power as well as influence can shape the culture of the workplace either positively or negatively. Leadership means that managers need to 'walk the walk and talk the talk' when addressing diversity because it raises issues about:

- respecting dignity at work, and the rights and responsibilities of individuals
- identifying what is acceptable or not acceptable language and behaviour in the workplace
- creating an environment where debate and discussion are valued and where people refusing to learn is acknowledged as potential prejudice.

(Westwood, 2002)

The challenge to promote race equality takes us along the same path as that leading to the promotion of equity and social justice in general. It is an integral part of a manager's role in ensuring the quality of services.

Key points

- Attitudes to dependence and independence are the starting point for any person or organisation involved in managing care.

- Care means caring about and valuing people.

- Safeguarding and the promotion of welfare are needed to prevent the abuse of service users and staff.

- Social exclusion continues to be a problem and any social inclusion policy should take account of the views of the people affected.

- Managers need to promote a positive culture in which service users and staff cannot be abused.

1.3 Integrating health and social care

The permanence of change

In the 1980s and 1990s, policy was dominated by the attempt to separate the purchasing and providing of services and to apply the principles of market capitalism to the welfare state (Loney *et al.*, 1991). Since the election of the Labour government in 1997, and subsequently in 2001, the policy has shifted to one increasingly dominated by the integration of health and social care and breaking down the institutional and professional barriers to more efficient, 'user-friendly' services. Terms such as 'joined-up services' and 'modernising services' have become part of government rhetoric about its plans. What exactly is meant by 'joined-up' services? This is what the Social Services Inspectorate says:

> Being 'joined up' means recognising the wholeness of people's lives. Many people who use social services rely heavily on other public services: health, housing, employment services and benefit agencies. The problems that people experience are connected. Social services staff have to ensure that the people they work with receive all that they are eligible for or have a right to receive. Service delivery needs to be integrated such that our services move around the person, not the person around the service. People should experience their services as being well co-ordinated as well as making a difference to the quality of their lives.
>
> (Social Services Inspectorate, 2000, p. 64)

This idea is not new and was behind the reforms of the early 1970s that led to the creation of social services departments in England and Wales

(Seebohm, 1968). Thirty years later we are probably witnessing the end of social services departments, the focus now shifting to rigidities in the division between 'health' and 'social care' services. This is particularly stark in the current debate about the differences (or lack of them) between providing 'social' care and 'health' care for elderly people. Arguably, most of the distinctions are spurious and are largely administrative creations that prop up different ways of rationing resources. In 2001 the Scottish Parliament introduced measures to ensure that no older person needing residential nursing home care should pay for any social care within the home. Such an approach, it was argued, was justifiable in terms of need, in the same way in which health care needs have been met free at the point of entry. However, no such plans currently exist (in early 2002) for England, Wales or Northern Ireland. How does this fit with government plans for the integration of health and social care?

The government is trying to achieve two key changes through its policies for integration. First, it wants to devolve the planning and delivery of services to 'local' areas through the establishment of primary care trusts and hospital trusts (and some other local and regional arrangements). The government believes that this will improve participation and partnership between providers and users of services and release the creative energies of managers and professionals to get on with the job. Second, it wants to eliminate differences between areas in terms of standards of services, mainly through new inspection and standard-setting regimes.

One of the main challenges for managers is to ensure that criteria are fair and comparable with services in other parts of the country; but which 'country' are we talking about? So, the first point to be clear about is that comparability may sometimes apply across the UK but at other times it may need to be considered country by country. Whether the citizens of the UK or individual practitioners see it in that way is uncertain. The phenomenon of people moving house to benefit from better schools is well known, and we may yet see similar behaviour to take advantage of more or less generous care policies between the countries of the UK.

In the area of services for children, studies of family support services have shown tremendous variation in the interpretation of who is in need, to the point of stretching the boundaries of what is legal (Aldgate and Tunstill, 1995; Tunstill and Aldgate, 2000). In terms of services for adults, debates have been even more complex. The same issues of inconsistency of interpretation of eligibility criteria and lack of transparency of criteria are cited in government documents. The Joint Reviews Annual Report in 1998 notes:

> There appears to be no consistent link between referrals, assessments and services either between councils, or indeed between different services of the same council.
>
> (Quoted in Department of Health, 1998a, p. 23, para. 2.26)

Frontline managers find themselves addressing real tensions and issues, such as how to manage performance and achieve consistent outcomes at the same time as balancing day-to-day demands with an overall vision of care. One of the complexities of maintaining a particular vision is that there may be competing agendas between managers and their staff. This is particularly true for managers working with multidisciplinary teams. For example, Brechin (1998) notes that care in nursing has been influenced by nurses' desire to find a new professional identity that distinguishes them from 'the doctor's assistant'. The same might be said about care assistants and social workers, exemplified by the development of Scottish and National Vocational Qualifications (S/NVQs) and Occupational Standards, which attempt to define the professional elements of caring in terms of roles, tasks, values and skills.

The government is clearly impatient (on behalf of the public) with the excuses for professional resistance to change such as those noted above. It believes that a combination of more money and 'good management', allied to a clear strategy and a tight political timetable, ought to be sufficient to succeed where endless tinkering and a lack of consensus about public spending have failed in the past; but what does the government mean by 'good management'?

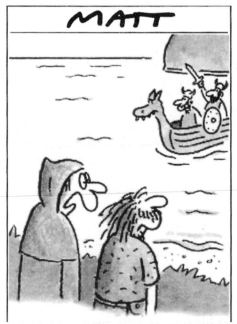

'I just hope they make an effort to fit in with our culture'

Changing cultures

Recent governments have had a great deal of faith in management and managers. What this means in the current context is that there is a need to look for the kind of leadership that can change values, attitudes, traditional ways of working and relationships; this is expressed in management theory as 'culture change' (Trompenaars, 1993). They also connect 'success' in terms of certain performance outcomes with greater degrees of autonomy for successful management teams. Conversely, lack of success (or even failure) is dealt with by greater degrees of intervention, or even the wholesale transfer of responsibility to other organisations.

You may already have some experience of attempts in your organisation to examine its own 'culture' and what might be involved in changing it to something more in line with 'the new NHS' or 'joined-up services' or 'partnership' or any of the several terms currently in vogue. To summarise, the key elements of the culture change being sought in health and social care services are listed in Box 1.1.

This is a challenging list and there is no doubt that managers of care services in all sectors and at all levels are seen as being responsible for

---

BOX 1.1 The elements of a changing culture in health and social care

- Focusing on health inequality and social exclusion alongside 'welfare to work', reducing child poverty and increasing levels of skills and education.

- Accountability to the public through trust arrangements and local participation, with less emphasis on formal local democracy and a reduced role for local authorities.

- Emphasising service user consent, access to information, privacy, confidentiality and human rights.

- Transferring power from professionals to service users to the extent (and limit) that they are seen as consumers of services and participants in deciding local priorities.

- Focusing on priorities defined by 'consumers', such as availability and accessibility of services, technical competence, good communication and interpersonal skills, and continuity of care.

- Encouraging or demanding professionals to work 'in partnership' to balance the tensions in policy between short- and long-term plans, prevention and cure, and acute and chronic services.

- Focusing on the 'long term' in the belief that prevention of health and social problems will pay off better than expensive 'cure' programmes.

- Organising services to reflect their function, and overcoming old allegiances to particular forms of organisation (such as social services departments) in the drive towards establishing trusts and partnerships at a local level.

- Current divisions, boundaries and conflicts between professions, professionals and managers, management and labour, health and social care organisations, and the public/voluntary/private sectors are redundant and will not be tolerated.

- Service users should have much more say through consultation processes and the governance of local trust and partnership arrangements than they have in the past.

achieving these changes quickly. This is partly a reflection of public frustration with the performance of public services and partly because any government has to show that its policies are effective within an electoral cycle of one or two Parliaments.

Time and the process of change

To what extent are these plans, and the timetable for them, realistic? Research done by the School of Health and Social Welfare at The Open University involved talking at length to frontline managers of care services about the integration of health and social care (Dimmock, 2002). The responses of one highly experienced manager working in England (involved in delivering services for children with disabilities in a social services department) provide a reasonably representative view. When asked about relationships with other agencies (notably health and education), with respect to changing arrangements for delivering services, he commented as follows.

> There is a danger of us having to relate to several of the new trusts, but nobody really seems to know. We still don't know if the (proposed) partnership trust will include children with disabilities – who do I talk to, how do I make links? There are so many different models about how we could deliver joined-up services – perhaps child development centres, or community-based schools. There are arguments for both of these which tend to be favoured by different professionals in different agencies. I was in a joint planning group last week and there was absolutely no agreement about how to do this. Health wants it centralised into child development centres but we think this will suck in the resources to a building, not get them into communities – there are all sorts of tensions – structures will either make it easier or harder, but it's really down to better communication. The agendas for health, social services and education are so separate ... Even within organisations, like education, we can't solve internal disputes, for example between teachers and educational psychologists. Work with children with disabilities involves so many different agencies. No one professional group seems to be any better than the others in working in a multidisciplinary way. Even when you have the will and groups formed to work across agencies, even when there is really good will, we don't have the time to work out the different beliefs that underlie each group. Change takes a long time, and this is what frustrates governments.
>
> (Dimmock, 2002, p. 5)

This manager also experiences his own agency as less than 'joined up':

> Children's services and adult services within social services act like separate organisations – we can't do this for children who are becoming adults within our (own) organisation.
>
> (Dimmock, 2002, p. 5)

You may have empathised to a greater or lesser extent with this eloquent and comprehensive *cri de cœur* from a committed and experienced manager. It was made just a few months before the formation of a new partnership trust in his area (scheduled for April 2002), which would bring together services for mental health and learning disability from several agencies, including health and social services. If this policy of integration is to succeed, its implementation must address many of the concerns he raises.

Managers who are survivors of the Thatcher revolution (and of previous ones such as the Seebohm reforms of the 1970s) will no doubt raise a sceptical eyebrow or two at this stage. They may experience change as a way of stopping professional staff getting on with the job. This is certainly the experience of the manager referred to above:

> It's not about losing power to another agency, it's about losing your job or not being able to do what makes the job worthwhile – losing your credibility and losing the ability to be human still.
>
> (Dimmock, 2002, p. 10)

Whether New Labour policies (Department of Health, 2000a) of integrating health and social care are any more successful than previous attempts to reorganise services, we shall have to wait and see. Clearly, they must have public support but they also need the support and commitment of the vast army of staff involved in managing and delivering care services. To use an analogy from medical practice, the power, quantity and rate of delivering the medicine to cure the problems of health and social care services may kill the patient in the process. Certainly there are likely to be winners and losers in these changes in terms of the power of organisations and professional groups. What is clear is that the reforms must be judged in terms of improvements for service users, who, it is hoped, will be the real winners in this process of change.

Trust and regulation

At the time of writing, the General Social Care Council for England (GSCC), and the equivalent councils for Northern Ireland, Scotland and Wales, had just completed consultation on draft versions of the standards and values expected of employees and employers (GSCC, 2002a). Although not statutory, these codes, once agreed, will apply to all social care staff in the UK, who will be expected to register with the appropriate council. The numbers are estimated to be close to 1.2 million people in England alone. Only one-third of these people work for local authorities (the rest being employed in the health service and by private and voluntary service providers). Part of the draft code of practice for social care workers states 'As a social care worker you must justify public trust and confidence in social care services' (GSCC, 2002a).

This elicited the following response from Unison (the public services union and the largest single union in the UK), which was quoted in *The Guardian*.

> A spokeswoman for Unison ... says the codes are 'a step in the right direction' but should be more 'plain English'. She says: 'The code is written in social work jargon which may be suitable for social workers, but not for home carers.' Unison would also like more emphasis on the role of the employer in enabling staff to meet the 'very high expectations' of the codes.
>
> ('Guardian Society', 9 January 2002, p. 4)

These codes have emerged as part of a policy to improve the regulation of public services through regimes of inspection, occupational standards, performance targets and a host of guidance, reports and inquiries too numerous to mention. They are all part of the government's policy to 'modernise' public services and to re-establish public trust in order to justify increased resources, particularly for the NHS. What impact is this increasing weight of regulation and inspection having on the role and priorities of managers? One manager we interviewed for the research mentioned earlier felt that the inspection regime they were dealing with 'forces you back into your own little world' and away from the bigger picture of trying to create partnerships with other agencies. Another manager commented on its impact on the training of staff:

> It's increasingly going to make an impact because it will affect how we spend our money on training. So just like any other organisation we are having to get cuter on what I would call workforce planning, which is looking at the sort of work and the shape of our workforce because we've got recruitment and retention problems. People have a sense that regulation is coming in but not quite knowing what that means ... Some service standards have qualifications requirements, so for senior residential staff a social work qualification [is needed]. So what we need is for each area to look into particular provision rather than offer people training and development according to how they might want to do it. We have to be more focused on making sure our particular projects are fit for purpose. It's been very interesting looking at how we deal with the post-qualifying child care award. How you make decisions about who should have the post-qualifying child care award, when there's a government thrust that the qualification should be there. The reality is that quite a lot of people find it difficult to do because it's demanding in terms of time and money. We don't as a voluntary organisation get training and support funds automatically, but equally we're in partnership arrangements, so what should the qualification requirements be? So that's the way it's affecting people, but we don't know whether the requirement for a post-qualifying child care award will then be set against the 'Quality Protects' criteria within a local authority. We just don't know ... We're guessing.
>
> (Dimmock, 2002, p. 5)

You may not be familiar with the particular standards, initiatives and regulations that this manager is referring to (such as Quality Protects, Department of Health, 2001a). However, if you are a manager you may be in a similar situation of trying to make sense of several overlapping areas of policy initiatives, inspection regimes, standards and funding streams that leave you equally bewildered. Do you think that the government trusts organisations and professionals to get on with the job or is there still a long way to go? Do you think that central government is as 'joined up' in its approach to modernising health and social care as it wants managers of care services to be?

Key points

- Government policy is dominated by the integration of health and social care to produce more efficient, user-friendly services.

- Managers are challenged to maintain a particular vision and are expected to achieve cultural change in their organisations quickly.

- The implementation of changes needs the support of staff to meet the government's timescale.

- The new codes and regulations impact on managers' roles and priorities.

1.4 Practice-led management: a model for managing care

The evolution of the managerial role in public services has been well documented by Clarke and Newman (1993). They argue that the weak position of professionals easily gave way to a managerial approach that was designed to conserve the resources of the public purse and enhance the control of policy and practice. Causer and Exworthy (1999) propose an alternative model that moves away from the idea of a simple divide between management and professionals. Instead, it develops a more complex typology that reflects how professional and managerial activities may relate to each other. This typology puts forward three broad roles as follows.

1 The *practising professionals* who may be divided into those who undertake supervisory activities even though they are not described as managers and those whose main function is to 'engage in the day-to-day exercise of professional activities' (Causer and Exworthy, 1999, p. 84).

2 The *managing professionals*, some of whom may combine practice and management and others may be solely managers.

3 The *general managers* who again can be subdivided into those with a relevant professional background and those without one.

The important point stressed by Causer and Exworthy is that most of the subdivisions within the three broad groups 'are characterised by their past or present engagement in professional practice' (p. 84). In other words, the authority to manage professionals is grounded in the credibility of being or having been a practitioner. To what extent do you agree that managers of care services, particularly those on the 'front line', ground their authority in their experience of care practice?

One manager in the health services (a multidisciplinary team providing services for adults with learning difficulties) who was asked whether his job could be done *without* a relevant professional qualification (in his case, nursing) said:

> In theory, yes. Why I answer it like that is partly my own personal bias ... but it would seem evident that at the level I operate at, people tend to run into trouble if they don't understand the business. For several reasons: in terms of leadership as opposed to management it's easier to get a response from people if you have some credibility. Rightly or wrongly, it seems to give you some credibility if you have a clinical background ... You can't operate on a well briefed or well informed perspective [without it]. You need to know. You probably can at the next [managerial] level, but I would be very wary at how far down the line you could take this ... I have some particularly bad experiences of general management.
>
> (Dimmock, 2002, p. 7)

The connection between professional practice and management is at the heart of managing care. A model of *practice-led management* will include:

* promoting social inclusion
* promoting choice
* improving the quality of life
* safeguarding people.

How well does this vision of practice-led management of care services fit with other models? For example, services organised around the assessment of need – often referred to as 'needs-led services' – held a strong ideological position until the end of the 1990s. What about the experience of many people that all this ideological discussion disguises the fact that services are really organised around resources (resource-led services) and the convenience of powerful interest groups that provide those resources (for example, the professions, trade unions and managers)?

Statham (1996) describes a model for planning and implementing change developed by the National Institute for Social Work that includes the values of practice-led management and acknowledges the role of frontline managers in implementing change. This model builds bridges between professional and managerial issues. It supports the role of the frontline manager as a giver of information and expects the manager to have a vision of what outcomes can be achieved with finite resources. It includes:

- involving staff, service users and carers in planning changes before decisions are made, and in their implementation and monitoring of the unexpected consequences of changes;
- being able to identify what should be kept because it is valuable, recognising that change can destroy strengths in the system, and that change does not equate with improvement or better outcomes for users;
- accessing information from the front-line workers, service users and carers as an essential part of planning a needs-led service ... This is the reverse of the usual pattern of information flowing from managers to staff. Listening skills are being emphasised for managers in business and industry and are no less required in community care;
- being skilled in managing the social care task, not only general management, and having responsibilities for leadership and staff development. This involves focusing on the skills required including those of managing practice, conflicts, negotiation, communicating with the public, using front-line information and providing information which supports front-line activity;
- having a vision of what social result is sought from available resources, which provides a framework within which shortcomings in the budget can be negotiated with staff, service users and carers, local providers and politicians;
- identifying the real conflicts that exist and have to be negotiated.

(Statham, 1996, pp. 46–7)

In this vision of practice-led management, managers will try to create a culture that values the views of service users, staff wellbeing, devolved decision making, experience, knowledge, research and the importance of training and professional development. Pearn *et al.* (1997, p. 9) suggest that 'Treating people with dignity is not only intrinsically motivating, it also brings rewards for the organisation.'

Why might this be the case? We think it goes back to our earlier assertion about what motivates people to undertake difficult and often poorly rewarded work in the caring services. If the values of managing care are focused on making the best possible use of all the resources of those involved, people will perform well. If the focus is really on disguising the fact that care services face rising expectations and inadequate resources, improving the quality of services will be impossible. As citizens, people have a right to demand better standards and a responsibility to contribute fairly to their funding. If people are involved in service provision, particularly as managers, they have a responsibility to engage actively with attempts to improve services and, at the same time, to defend the values of care.

Key points

- We argue that practice-led management is an appropriate model for managing care services.

- This model promotes social inclusion and choice, improving the quality of life and safeguarding people.

- Managers need to engage actively in improving services at the same time as defending the values of care.

1.5 Conclusion

Care is an activity that depends on widely shared values for its realisation. Managers of care services need to work closely with their staff and service users to ensure that their organisations listen and respond. They are a pivotal point of communication between organisations and those who use their services. This chapter explored the social and policy context of care and the wider agenda of social inclusion. Managers are at the front line of innovation and change. They are both the keepers and the shapers of the values that underlie the modern welfare state.

Chapter 2
What service users say about services: the implications for managers

Naomi Connelly and Janet Seden

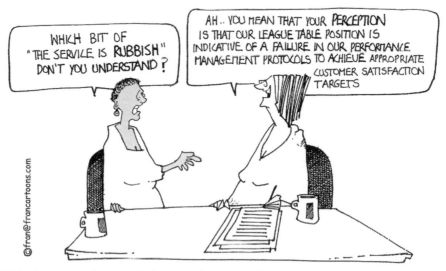

Listening to service users' views can be a complex matter

2.1 Introduction

In one sense we are all service users whether we have used care services in the past or use them now or in the future for ourselves, our families and our friends. Thus the question 'What do service users say about services?' can be interpreted in different ways. We can draw on our own experience, ask individual service users about the services they receive or would like to receive, or look to organisations of service users for information.

There has always been a train of thought that sees some care services as being relevant only to poor and unfortunate people, and that those providing and receiving services are largely separate classes. We want to challenge this view and the implication that the world is divided in such a simple way. Some people are far more reliant on care services than others. This may be just 'the luck of the draw' but it is often because of powerful forces of social exclusion and disadvantage, many of which have continued for generations.

Another set of questions concerns the aims of the consultation processes that are developed to seek out people's views. Why consult in the first place? When will consultation take place and who will control the process? What will happen to the results? Whose aims will be met and when does consultation become tokenistic?

The subject of service users' views is addressed early in this book for a very simple reason. A central purpose of social and health care services is to maintain or increase people's wellbeing and quality of life. Frontline managers, like all workers involved in health and social care, need to keep that objective in mind in their daily work. There is a danger that the challenges of the management task may detach managers from the practice-led context of their work.

Frontline managers have a key role to play in co-ordinating and developing consultation processes. They often instigate action and respond to the results of consultations. Managers also need to balance the views and aims of their organisation or agency, workers and team members, service users, carers and the wider community.

This chapter explores such issues, presenting information about the views of service users, the issues that arise in attempting to ascertain and act on such views, and what has been learned through practical experience. It relates this discussion to the concerns and responsibilities of managers of care services.

In this chapter we look first at service users' views and describe some of what has been learned over recent years. We then explore issues that arise for managers and service users once service users' views are on the agenda. Finally, we move on to consider the practicalities. How can frontline managers make service user involvement work effectively?

The aims of this chapter are to:

- emphasise the critical importance of service users' views in all aspects of social care
- explore the issues which arise for managers in seeking service users' views and experience
- draw attention to the ways in which service users' views can be acted on effectively.

2.2 Policy and practice

Listening to what people say about services has become a key feature of government policies, whether this derives from ideas of service users as 'customers' and 'consumers' of support and care or from ideas about their rights as citizens with a voice in matters that affect their lives. Writing about the service user (referred to as 'survivor') movement in mental health, Campbell (1996) describes how health and social services have opened up to 'consumerist' approaches. He points out that people are seen as *consumers* of welfare, much as they are consumers of newspapers or other commodities. Campbell argues that a more meaningful perception of survivors is as 'citizens'. Some people rarely come into contact with welfare services at all but they feel that, as citizens, they should have the opportunity to express their opinions about the type of services that are provided and funded.

Barnes (1999) states that service user organisations have been 'legitimised' by top-down objectives relating to user involvement but she also notes that 'user groups have experienced tensions in determining the extent to which they should respond to official agendas' (p. 73). In the 1980s and 1990s a developing international theme in debates about child welfare was the child's status as a citizen. Children and young people have a right to have their voices heard and to participate in decisions that affect their lives.

The views of people with learning disabilities are integral to the White Paper *Valuing People* (Department of Health, 2001b). This was drafted in consultation with people who have learning difficulties and it is available in an accessible version as well as on audio-tape and CD. There are equivalent processes in Scotland and Wales (Scottish Executive, 2000; Learning Disability Advisory Group, 2001). Service users' views are also becoming accepted by government as an important element of evidence-based practice and a critical component when assessing the performance of health and social care agencies (Department of Health, 2000b; Scottish Office, 1999). Box 2.1 outlines some key points from the consultation paper *A Quality Strategy for Social Care*.

BOX 2.1 A quality strategy for social care

We must focus on what people want from services. There is now a strong body of evidence pointing to the qualities people value in social services:

- high standards at all levels in service delivery throughout the whole workforce

- responsiveness, speed and convenience of service delivery

- appropriateness – services tailored to individual need, with respect for culture and lifestyle

- services that build on people's abilities and enable them to participate fully in society

- services that involve the user, so that choices are informed and respected

- strong safeguards for those at risk.

(Department of Health, 2000b, p. 6)

Many service user organisations have grown and become more established locally and nationally. Through their work, and the efforts of social care staff and researchers, a substantial amount of knowledge has accumulated about 'what works' in effective service user involvement. Gradual implementation of the Disability Discrimination Act 1995 and the Community Care (Direct Payments) Act 1996 have provided incentives and opportunities for learning from, and acting on, service users' views.

Service user organisations contribute to a growing body of research into care service provision through user-led research initiatives. For example, a research project on what people experiencing mental health difficulties found useful resulted in the widely acclaimed report *Strategies for Living* (Faulkner and Layzell, 2000). The skills of service users as researchers (Rose, 2001; Barnes and Mercer, 1997) and as experts (Beresford, 2000) are informing practice and academic debates.

While some research shows high rates of satisfaction, there are also complaints that people continue to be met with a lack of respect and have to fight for a voice and influence in matters concerning their own lives (Rogers *et al.*, 1993). For managers, this gap between the aspirations of government and the daily realities of service users' experiences raises a particular challenge. It provides a starting point for thinking about what the management task is and what individuals within agencies and organisations can do to effect change. This process will involve developing strategies for the wider influence of service users' views that are an integral part of the way services are organised and delivered.

Key points

- Consultation and involvement with service users is a key component of legislation, policy and guidance relating to service delivery and planning.

- Service users, managers, practitioners and government may hold conflicting and diverse views on how consultation should be implemented.

- Citizenship is a helpful concept to enable wider consultation and involvement.

2.3 Service users' views

Whose views?

Several questions arise about the kind of feedback from users that is most relevant for social care organisations to seek and respond to. What about

people who are unwilling users of social care services? How important is it
that their voices be heard? For example, people may come into contact
with services as a result of formal detention in hospital against their
wishes, under the Mental Health Act 1983. The views of children, adults
and professionals have to be balanced. There are dilemmas in the real
world of practice about compulsion and voluntariness.

Practitioners have to consider children's views and parents' responsibilities along with state thresholds for intervention. For example, when
should families with children living at home be supported? In what
circumstances should a child be removed? Care should be taken to ensure
that skilled direct work enables children to communicate their wishes and
feelings when professional judgements are made about their welfare.
Managers are often very significant people when such balanced decisions
based on complex assessments are made. The practice-led nature of the
management role comes to the fore in situations such as these.

While some service users may have little choice about accepting
services, they will still have valuable insights into the equity and fairness
of the processes they experience. What about those people whose ability
to communicate their views may be quite limited? What about listening to
children? Are they always competent to give their views and who should
decide? How useful are facilitated communication methods, which
workers use to talk with severely disabled children and young people or
older people experiencing dementia? How do managers work constructively with advocates? In finding out what people say about services, a
frontline manager faces a complex range of views.

Although service users and informal carers often have common
concerns and common views, this is by no means always the case.
Therefore, it is important to distinguish between what service users say
and what carers say. In general, this chapter concentrates on service users
but remember that carers are increasingly service users in their own right
and they may have a central role to play in a service user's life. This role
has been recognised in legislation through the Carers (Recognition and
Services) Act 1995 and the Carers and Disabled Children Act 2000. Various
policy documents such as the national strategy for carers – *Caring about
Carers* (Department of Health, 1999c) – further emphasise the importance
of the role of carer.

The research for this book included consultation sessions with groups
of managers and service users. The views presented here are those of the
service users who took part and they echo much other research into what
people want from care services. The consultations were structured around
existing service categories such as learning disability, older people,
children and families: an illustration, perhaps, of the influence of current
models of service planning and delivery on consultation processes. The
participants stressed that life is not neatly packaged in service categories.
For this reason we have not always identified the group from which
individual comments have come. At this point you might like to read the

detailed account of this process and the people who took part, which is in the Appendix.

What views?

Some views from our consultations are shown in Example 2.1, which has comments from people who have used mental health, physical disability, older people's and learning difficulty services, and Example 2.2, which has comments from the users of services for children, young people and families.

EXAMPLE 2.1   Some views from users of adults' services

Treat people as people and not as a problem.

(Rosemary)

Social care managers have got to listen. If they don't listen they don't know what we're saying to them. They've got to listen because we've got to tell them what we want. It's not what managers want, it's what we want ourselves.

(Malcolm)

I think basically from a practical point of view they are having to ration because they don't have the resources to do everything for everybody. What I want to know is who chooses who gets what? We don't have a say in it; you don't have a say in it, do you? ... People who are in the caring professions – and this includes the line managers – should be listening to the person. That's the first thing they should do, listen to them. Find out what's available and then negotiate with them. I'm not expecting just to say I want this, this and this. I *am* expecting them to negotiate with me and I'm still waiting.

(Amanda)

The services kick in at the point of crisis. On the way back you've got places where you can be rehabilitated and gradually get back into society. But there should be places on the way down.

(Richard)

It's independence really, isn't it? It's the biggest thing of the whole situation. Although you need help on occasions, you don't need it all the time. You don't want it thrust down your throat.

(Tommy)

EXAMPLE 2.2 Some views from users of children's services

Whenever I phone to ask what's going on, they tell me that I'm too anxious and I should wait, but the fact that they never phone me doesn't help.
(Parent)

The problem is there is a totally uncoordinated approach to family life with this sort of problem and it's now going to cost them more to put it right ... it's probably the system rather than the people.
(Parent)

Children are not able to influence decisions made about them. Adults who do not know them well often make decisions in large meetings.
(Parent)

Social services ... they were really supportive. I mean, I had to go to court and everything and my social worker came through with me and stuff and supported me through that.
(Young woman)

I met quite a few nice girls at the group as well. They went through the same kind of thing, so you know what you're all going through, so you all have respect for each other.
(Young woman, speaking about a support group)

Social services ... at the start they were very good and then weeks and weeks went by and in the end we wrote a letter of complaint ... because we wanted to know what was happening ... she just didn't keep in touch and when we sent the letter of complaint she sent a letter of apology, so that was the only bit we were unhappy with ... I think what they should do instead of swapping over to different people ... they should keep the child with one person ...
(Parent)

It's certainly been a fight and I wish the professionals would listen to you. You're the child's best advocate, you know their needs more than anyone and sometimes they override that and say 'No, I'm the professional here'.
(Parent)

The messages from these two sets of views are that service users want:

- to be treated with respect and as individuals
- a voice in decisions about the range of services that should be available and which services they receive in particular circumstances
- recognition that while services may be an important or even an essential part of their lives, services are not all of their lives

- acknowledgement that they are reasonable people who understand about resources and other constraints but who think that is a reason for more attention to be paid to their views, not less
- to see signs that the time spent in giving their views has influenced decisions.

Services are organised around specific categories and delivered by a range of qualified and unqualified, paid and unpaid workers. When service users talk about what is important to them as people, they are not as concerned with the profession of the person who provides the care, or the context in which that worker operates, as with the quality and appropriateness of the service (Rogers *et al.*, 1993).

There is no shortage of sources of service users' views. At central government level, Social Services Inspectorate reports include some exploration of service users' and carers' views (for example, Social Services Inspectorate, 2001). Satisfaction surveys are included in the Social Services Joint Reviews carried out by the Inspectorate and the Audit Commission who see a user focus as one of eight key principles in the review process. The user focus is achieved:

> by making the primary focus of the review how well individuals are served by their authority, collecting evidence direct from users and carers, and by using this evidence to inform the management and stakeholder interviews.
>
> (Audit Commission/NHS, 2000–1)

Individual social services departments and voluntary sector and service user organisations have done much research, such as surveys and the use of advisory groups or working parties including service users. People who receive services have also been involved in designing and carrying out training, monitoring and evaluation of those services.

Service users and potential service users from black and ethnic minority communities face additional barriers to involvement and consultation because the service providers lack effective communication skills, under-standing or commitment (Bowes and Dar, 2000; Hatton *et al.*, 1998; Joseph Rowntree Foundation, 1998a; Taylor, 1999). Thus, if discrimination has led to services not being offered in the first place, consultation may reinforce this discrimination by asking only those people who have received the service.

Research studies have played a major role in finding out the views of children and their families about the services they have experienced. Overviews of the researchers' findings, drawing on several large studies, include summaries of views about what was available and the way in which the service was offered. For example, the following main points are from *The Children Act Now*, a review of 24 substantial studies into aspects of the implementation of the Children Act 1989.

- Children value five main qualities in professionals: reliability, practical help, support, time to listen and respond, seeing children's lives in the round.

- The techniques of research can be helpfully used to improve direct work with children.

- A child-centred service demands that adults listen to how children would like services organised and act upon children's views.

(Department of Health, 2001c, p. 95)

What services?

When people are consulted about the services they have received they express strong views not only about access to services but also about what those services are. For example, the shift from a home help service to a personal care service has raised many concerns. The consultations for this book and other research (see, for instance, Sinclair *et al.*, 2000) both indicate that (unknown to managers) workers sometimes go beyond their allotted tasks in order to meet service user-defined needs. A regular, though informal, agreement between care workers and older people may develop. For example, a care plan that includes some form of personal care might in reality entail the care worker doing housework – because that is what is important to the service user. However, housework would not meet most eligibility criteria.

> The manager's understanding of the priorities are not actually the priorities that the people want. That's where it varies: the manager thinks 'Oh, that's what they want', but it's not so. What they want – they might not want to be washed, they might want to have the windows done.
>
> (Barry, service user consultations)

Service users are not usually arguing against professional expertise or discounting the problems of managing complex care systems. Rather, they are insisting that there has to be a much closer relationship between their own understanding of their needs and the social care response. For example, the families who had received services from Homestart – a service provided for families by volunteers – appreciated the difference between this kind of support and local authority social work services:

> [Homestart] seems to be more understanding of situations when you tell them what's going on. They are a lot more sympathetic because a lot of them are a parent themselves.
>
> The volunteer support is supportive to the family. When you ring up you know that your message is going to get through, whereas with social services and health you can't guarantee it.
>
> (Children's consultations)

Service users have specific insights into, and experience of, effective and quality responses from workers and service providers. The style and approach of workers – whether paid or unpaid – may make all the difference to a service user. For example, social workers who are supportive and sensitive and who listen are valued (Aldgate and Bradley, 1999). However, some people may feel reluctant to be critical of what little service they receive for fear that they will lose it altogether. As a result of their experience of the service setting and its delivery, users can play a central role in monitoring and evaluating the quality and effectiveness of services. That will include relationships with workers.

Moving forward?

So far you have read about the development of consultation with service users. Why, then, do service users and their organisations experience a struggle to be heard? What barriers are they encountering?

Service providers may structure consultation around service needs rather than service users' interests. For example, consultation at the planning, delivery and monitoring stages of a new day centre might be informative to service providers as well as a good example of service user involvement at all stages. Conversely, service users might consider that another day centre – no matter how well developed – is not what would best meet their needs.

Another area of contention is the rationale on which service provision is based. Many services stem from paternalistic concepts of 'looking after' less advantaged people. Some disabled people reject notions of vulnerability and personal disadvantage and many people find getting the help they need difficult enough. On the other hand, vulnerability and 'being looked after' can be more positive concepts where children are concerned (but children also want their strengths recognised and to have a voice in what happens to them). How 'care' is defined and the way social problems are defined and prioritised will affect responses to consultations. Medical or individual service models assume that 'the problem' resides in the individual rather than in the attitudes, structures and environments that create barriers to 'ordinary' life.

Are the service planners prepared to listen to such messages? One thing is clear: action of some kind must follow consultation. An area for development may well be more user-controlled services:

> If those who need support in order to live in the community are to exercise choices and have control over how that support is provided then two things need to happen: their preferences about the support they receive have to be expressed and action has to follow based on the expression of these preferences.
>
> (Lindow and Morris, 1995, p. 5)

To respond to the results of consultations, managers need to meet a range of challenges posed by their own organisations as well as service users, and to deal effectively with any tensions that may arise.

Key points

- Social care organisations need to be inclusive in getting feedback from service users and distinguish between what service users and carers say about services.

- Service users want to be respected as individuals and to have a voice in decisions.

- Discrimination can be reinforced by consulting only the people who receive services.

- Service users can play a central role in monitoring and evaluating the quality and effectiveness of services, including relationships with social workers and service providers.

- Action must follow consultations with service users.

2.4 Issues and challenges

It takes time to manage and practise in a way that integrates service users' views into all stages in the social care process and not just in 'one-off' consultation sessions. For example, ascertaining children's and young people's views means taking the time to be with the young people, understanding their interests and their ways of expressing themselves, as well as listening carefully to the significant other people who can help, such as teachers, foster carers and parents. When children and young people are participating in meetings and case conferences about their lives, time for preparation is essential. Management pressure on staff to meet time deadlines can make this more difficult for practitioners and service users.

Are managers ready to work *with* service users rather than *for* them and to be practice led? What about other colleagues, whether frontline staff or more senior managers? Councillors, members or trustees of voluntary organisation management committees and managers or owners of private social care agencies may have anxieties about the shift of power, or the resource requirements, of effective service user involvement. On the other hand, service users may be reluctant to take part in or suspicious of managers' motives. There may be practical difficulties such as deciding method(s) of involvement, timing and who to involve. Once these challenges have been addressed, it may be difficult for all parties to agree appropriate and feasible aims.

Involvement is often developmental and incremental. Managers need to take account of the *process* of involvement when designing consultation and involvement strategies. Time and time again, service users report gaining confidence through access to information and mutual support; and stereotypes on both sides break down when individual managers and individual service users meet on more equal ground. However, clear aims and results are required if people are to be willing to give up their time and maintain commitment (Boaz *et al.*, 1999; Harding and Oldman, 1996; Hemmings and Morris, 1997; Turner, 2000).

Other complicating factors may be managers' concerns that service users' expectations will be unrealistic and unrealisable. They may fear saying the wrong thing, exposing their ignorance or being met with criticism and anger (Harding and Oldman, 1996; Morris, 1994). This is hard to bear even if it is accepted as justifiable. Managers may feel that in their 'in-between' position they have too little power to be able to empower other people. The impact on individual managers in health and social care of working in partnership with other organisations which do not have shared service user involvement strategies may also limit the possibilities. Service users may feel powerless in the face of professional and organisational structures.

Among the most common complaints about consultation are that it is not 'real' – that decisions have been taken before the event – or that the agenda set has excluded important issues. As one person commented in a consultation: 'The head bosses decide so that consultation can be a waste of time.' At the same time, some parameters must usually be set, and set within a realistic context of other decisions that are likely to be under consideration, budgets to be determined, and so on. Service users stress the importance of openness about such matters, as well as a degree of flexibility that can cope with what arises in the course of discussions.

Whose voice?

A manager might want to find 'representative' service users. This quest could pose particular challenges. When planning for individual care, the best 'representative' is the person who will receive the care. When planning the structure of services to be delivered to a diverse range of people, it is important to find service users who represent that range of diversity. However, some service users argue that a search for 'representativeness' is not necessarily helpful. For example, referring to mental health service users, Crepaz-Keay (1996) notes that they are 'a diverse bunch'.

Can a person with one type of impairment represent someone with a different impairment? Does a service user who has learned their way around the social care system cease to be 'typical' of service users and thus 'unrepresentative'? Disabled people often consider that these kinds of question are an attempt to undermine their contributions. They point out that disabled people are likely to be especially cautious about speaking *inappropriately* for others because of their own experience of the 'Does he take sugar?' syndrome.

When considering whose voice should be listened to, many issues arise. How can agencies make sure that all relevant voices are heard, including, for example, very frail and isolated older people, people with dementia and people with learning difficulties who need considerable support to indicate their views? Some women in ethnic minority communities and asylum seekers have little command of English. Who can be said to be their community leader or spokesperson? There is a need for sensitivity to political, religious and gender distinctions within communities.

Managers are presented with several dilemmas here. On the one hand, it is important to include people who have communication difficulties. On the other hand, service user organisations are angered by suggestions that they speak only for a minority. Some people are never asked for their views and have no desire to give them. Others would love to give their opinion but do not know how to become involved. So where is a manager to start when planning consultations with people who use services?

The concern to involve as many service users as possible stems from the recognition of the value and reality of diversity: in particular, diverse interests, diverse experience and diverse ideas. There is also diversity in the methods available to managers for involving service users, from large-scale public meetings to individual home visits; from formal consultation on a specific plan or issue to continuing working parties or 'quality groups', such as those mentioned by Evans and Fisher (1999). However, the method chosen needs to be appropriate for the context of consultation.

Consulting more widely, with local communities for example, may result in conflicting views. As citizens, people express their views by, among other means, the electoral process. Some people may either attend meetings held to discuss service or community development plans or contact local Members of Parliament or councillors. There may be tensions between the views of people as citizens and those of service users. For example, a consultation process may collect evidence from service users of a need for a drop-in facility in a particular locality. Local people who are not intending to use the service may hold opposing views. A public meeting may therefore pose a challenge to a manager who, on the one hand, is responsible for service development and, on the other, is accountable to elected councillors.

In our consultation sessions, service users stressed that personality differences among managers influenced opportunities for expressing views; and that frontline workers often seemed to have a much better grasp than managers of the realities of day-to-day life for disabled people and how they experienced care. Thus, there are issues of 'whose voice?' for the agency side as well as for service users. Another aspect of this is the role of managers and other staff who have been or currently are users of care services. Some may want to play a full part in encouraging dialogue between staff and service users, while others may find the role conflicts too uncomfortable. There is always a danger that their views will be discounted by colleagues because they are seen as being too close to the situation or that, unrealistically, they will be expected to speak for all service users (Joseph Rowntree Foundation, 1998b, c).

The voices of children and young people

The child as a citizen and the rights of children were the focus of attention during the 1990s (Flekkoy, 1991; de Winter, 1997; Knuttson, 1997). This theme of children as citizens with the right to have their voices heard and to participate in the decisions made about their lives is now embedded in legislation in England, Northern Ireland, Scotland and Wales, as is the concept of partnership with their responsible parents and carers. This has considerable practice implications for professionals and their managers in any contact they have with children where they need to take account of their wishes and feelings. It is particularly important in court proceedings and when local authorities look after children.

Young people's views should be considered at all stages of their involvement with services. Practitioners' actions and processes have to be managed in ways that make such consultation with children and their families a reality. This makes safeguarding and promoting children's welfare a complex matter, if one aim is to take account of their wishes and feelings. The *Guidance and Regulations* on family placements for the Children Act 1989 says:

> Children should feel that they have been properly consulted, that their views have been properly considered and that they have participated as partners in the decision-making process. However, they should not be made to feel that the burden of decision-making has fallen totally upon them. Children should not be forced to participate in meetings if they choose not to do so.
>
> (Department of Health, 1991a, pp. 53–4)

Managers and practitioners seeking to achieve this balance will need to review systematically the way skilled direct work enables children to make their wishes and feelings clear. Also, the ways in which interviews and meetings are held need regular review and monitoring. *The Children Act Now* says:

- The Children Act has made a difference to the participation of children in decisions.
- Review meetings should be only part of an ongoing programme of skilled direct work with children.
- Children participate best in meetings when: they are prepared, meetings are small, there is a structured, child-friendly agenda.

- Meetings should be used as vehicles for participatory decision-making and should concentrate on young people's wishes and feelings.

(Department of Health, 2001c, p. 93)

Listening to children and young people requires workers to engage constantly with their views at all stages and levels of interaction with them. Practitioners also need to take account of the possible tensions between the views of children and those of the adults who are involved in their lives. Such differences of perspective and priorities need to be recognised. There may be very good reasons why a child's view differs from that of their carer or social worker. This tension and such differences in views between children, their families, foster carers and other relevant adults require skilled, practice-led management.

To make sure that feedback and evaluation are obtained about what is happening to children, many local authorities have appointed a children's rights officer. In Wales a children's commissioner has been appointed whose role is to take forward and act on issues that children raise. A major role of the manager is to ensure that frontline workers ask children about their views and feelings on a regular basis and to ensure that this information is current. While managers may not be involved directly in this form of consultation, they need to be aware of the professional development needs of staff who work directly with children.

In attempting to cope with all these issues, frontline managers may feel that service user involvement is like tightrope walking or a balancing act, or at least that it adds another ingredient to what is already a demanding role.

Managing service user involvement is challenging and must be part of an ongoing process but there is no need to start from scratch. There is much useful experience on which to build and the next section describes one example.

Key points

- Managers need effective ways of finding out what service users say about services.

- Frontline staff who may be uncertain, or feel deskilled, or have difficulty listening to service users need support from managers.

- At the same time, managers need to find ways of learning from and acting on what frontline staff say about the reality of service users' lives.

- Managers need to achieve results avoiding 'consultation fatigue' and cynicism about change but the results have to be achieved within a context of their overall managerial responsibilities.

2.5 The Wiltshire and Swindon Service Users Network: a practical example

Service user involvement raises issues at many levels and for many people. These issues range from those stemming from the histories and cultures of health and social care agencies, and the people who work in and use those services, to issues of power, accountability and practical matters. The process of involvement will probably be valuable but that is insufficient: it needs clear aims and results for it to be fully effective. Otherwise the involvement is tokenistic and demoralising for the people who take part.

The manager's positive involvement in user consultation will make a major difference to the way it happens. This section draws on the experience of the Wiltshire and Swindon Service Users Network to give a practical example of what can be achieved (Example 2.3).

EXAMPLE 2.3 Achieving involvement

A group of service users and quality managers on the commissioning side of social services was set up to look at ways of improving the quality of home care provision. Users both identified the need to seek views from a wider group of users by means of a survey, and were also involved in making the questionnaire accessible to service users. Distribution of the questionnaire to all users with their home care bill led to a very high response rate. The results were accepted by the home care managers and taken back to the users involved and the Network to discuss dissemination and implementation of the findings. As a direct outcome of this discussion, an integral role for users in evaluating the service was negotiated – local quality groups involving users were to meet regularly with managers, and users acting as trainers were to introduce monitoring of a service which effectively reflected the views and interests of service users. What was critical was users' involvement from the start and a sense of accountability to the users who initiated the evaluation, accompanied by the development of an action plan which recognized the need for the research to be employed for the benefit of service users ...

(Source: Evans and Fisher, 1999, p. 105)

What different forms of individual and group involvement were implemented in this example? Service users – either individually, in joint groups or through the Network – were involved in the following ways:

- initiating the idea of the evaluation
- participating with quality managers in a working group
- suggesting a survey of service users

- helping to devise an accessible questionnaire
- contributing to discussions about dissemination and implementation of findings
- participating in local quality groups
- training
- service monitoring.

Service users were involved in the consultation process at several levels and at various times in the development of the improvements to the home care service. Such a diversity of involvement requires flexibility and commitment from everyone concerned.

The account was written from the service users' viewpoint. Clare Evans, one of the authors, was the founder and first director of the Network. The following were probably some of the critical issues for the managers involved. First, the knowledge that senior management was in agreement with this degree of service user involvement. It would be extremely difficult for an individual manager – or even a group of managers – to introduce this level of involvement into a hostile or an uncommitted context. Second, there was confidence that management colleagues in other sections would support and co-operate in joint working with service users. As noted in Section 2.3, service users have needs that span organisational or service boundaries. Third, the managers involved were willing to give up some degree of personal power. Fourth, this consultation and involvement was part of an ongoing process that was flexible and developed over a period of time and those involved built up trust through previous contact with Network members.

As service user involvement has developed, social care agencies have learned the following important lessons.

- There is a need for *support arrangements* (Lindow, 1996) including *encouragement and training* so that those who have had little opportunity to voice their needs and wants in the past gain sufficient confidence to do so. This can be particularly important in residential settings.
- *Appropriate environments* are also necessary, which can be quite challenging when people with a range of impairments are involved. People with learning difficulties who are members of working groups may require a support worker if they are to make a full contribution.
- *Consultancy fees* should be paid to service users, providing their expertise has become a recognised aspect of involvement arrangements (Evans, 1999).
- Expenses such as travel, childminding and relief for carers should be paid. Any payments should be in a form *acceptable to the individual service user* (McHarron and Nettles, 1999).

- People hoping to move from receipt of services to direct payments may require *support and training to manage self-assessment* (Priestley, 1998).

However, training is required for other people, as well as service users. In a project encouraging participation in commissioning and purchasing (Joseph Rowntree Foundation, 1999), the service users recognised a need for training not only for themselves but also for the commissioners and purchasers. This idea was resisted by the latter group but it has become clear that the major adjustments required for satisfactory service user involvement may require at least as much training and support for managers and practitioners as for service users.

Embedding the changes

McIntosh and Whittaker refer to 'the importance of having service user-involvement so embedded in the service's values and ways of working that it will survive the inevitable bureaucratic ups-and-downs of statutory services' (2000, p. 107). One of the ways in which people have attempted to change the culture of professionals and of organisations is through training. This may be as part of an advisory group on course development or as lecturers and trainers for specific sessions. Davis *et al.* (1999) describe how local groups of people with learning difficulties worked out a programme to teach students on a professional course, and the implications for the students' learning. The Open University course *Learning Disability – Working as Equal People*, which was intended for study by staff, family members and people with learning difficulties, included representatives of People First (an organisation run for and by people with learning difficulties) on the course team and on their own terms.

A training project was set up to provide training for disabled people on their rights under community care legislation and to train disabled people to run courses for care managers (Hemmings and Morris, 1997). The Department of the Psychiatry of Disability at St George's Hospital Medical School in London employs two people with learning difficulties as training advisers (Greig, 2000). Further, Beresford (2000) argues that there needs to be an inclusive approach to social work theorising that incorporates a service user-based body of knowledge, without taking it over and removing the opportunities for service users to have their own discussions about theory.

Diverse situations, diverse approaches

Many steps have been taken, then, to reach out to service users or potential service users, to support service users so that they can make an effective contribution, and to embed learning and involvement. The many suggestions for ways of working include the following.

- Use a diversity of approaches, especially with frail older people (Bauld *et al.*, 2000; Thornton, 2000).
- Be willing to start with small-scale and perhaps obvious methods (Taylor, 1999).
- Consider aiming for small but cumulative changes (Raynes, 1998).
- Increase the information people have about each other and the number of contacts between them (Morris, 1997).
- Make opportunities for service users to talk directly with managers rather than through intermediaries (Bamford *et al.*, 1999; Barnes and Bennett-Emslie, 1997).
- Recognise that service users' views can be flexible, allowing trade-offs between different possibilities (Qureshi and Henwood, 2000).
- Ensure new staff are trained in values as well as procedures, so that progress is not lost (Carpenter and Sbaraini, 1997).
- Share experience and learning (Service User Engagement Project, 2000).

Managers need to be willing to take risks, to try out different ways of working, and to learn from the experience. Experience is there to be built on but there are no 'off-the-shelf' solutions. It cannot be assumed that service user involvement, once achieved, will continue without further effort by managers and workers. Methods need to be found of embedding it into values, policies and procedures and monitoring its effectiveness. Once examples of good practice are identified, managers and workers need to ensure that work continues. Service user involvement is an ongoing process, not a single objective that is achieved before moving on to the next task.

Key points

- Service user involvement is an ongoing process that needs to be embedded in the service's values and ways of working.
- Service user consultations need clear aims and results to be effective.
- Managers' positive involvement in consultations greatly affects how they happen.
- Managers need to take risks and try out different ways of working so that service users can contribute effectively.

2.6 Conclusion

In this chapter we looked at some of the opportunities and challenges for managers in listening to service users' views. We also highlighted some wider implications for service users and managers involved in consultation processes. Consultation is not negotiable: it is part of policy and performance assessment. However, the means of consultation and how they are implemented may have profound effects for everyone taking part. Determination and commitment are essential to bridge the gap between policy guidelines and the practicalities of consultation.

In this chapter we set out to consider three questions.

1   What are the benefits of service user involvement and how can they be achieved most effectively?

2   How far can social care managers respond to service users' views, given the diversity of service users, resource constraints, existing organisational cultures, and political and senior management priorities and pressures?

3   What are the particular opportunities and responsibilities of frontline managers for ensuring service users' views are sought and listened to?

There are plenty of obstacles to meaningful, embedded service user consultation and involvement, not least of which is a tokenistic and mechanistic approach to the process without real commitment. There is no single service user voice, just as there is no single professional voice. Management responses need to be flexible and informed by service users within the context of the service. The involvement of service users in interview processes, for example, may take longer to achieve in a large, public sector bureaucracy than in a service user-controlled project.

In asking for views, managers need to be ready to listen to answers and guard against the risks of stage-managing consultation. Lack of representativeness has been used as an excuse for not acting on, or responding to, challenging views (Crepaz-Keay, 1996). Challenging views may question the fundamental contexts of care services. The neat organisational structures of statutory adult and children's services, for example, are further split into specialisms such as older people, disability and mental health. These artificial divisions do not mesh with the complexity of people's own lives. Someone may be disabled, over 65 and have caring responsibilities. A child may have problems at home or at school and be a young carer. It is the responsibility of managers to ensure that services meet those needs as flexibly as possible.

Informed and practice-led management decisions will be based on an awareness of policy and legislation as well as what is known to be important to service users. A manager needs to reconcile the views of workers, service users, senior managers and carers. There may be tensions between people and practices in achieving responsive and respectful services. This is a matter not of abandoning professional or managerial identities but of defining them in new and innovative ways.

Chapter 3
Managers, managing and managerialism

Barbara Waine and Jeanette Henderson

3.1 Introduction

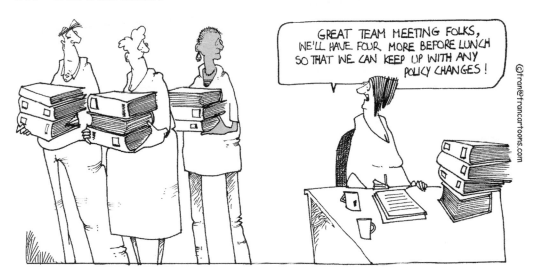

In this chapter we examine the impact of managerialism on the day-to-day life of managers of care services in the changing contexts of management. Managerialism has led to the introduction of methods more familiar to business and industry than care services. Features of managerialist approaches include competition, performance measurement, monitoring and an emphasis on the consumers of services and 'value for money'. The impact of these approaches has been felt by services no matter what their size. A small voluntary sector project, for example a drop-in service for people with mental health difficulties, may need to monitor service user attendance for a funding application. An entire social services department may need to ensure that requests for assessment are met within a stated time. In all organisations, practices and structures will have been shaped by managerialist approaches. In this chapter we provide a critical analysis of managerialism. Other chapters in this book offer contrasting perspectives.

We keep our focus on the frontline manager, while looking in some detail at how the organisation and provision of social care services in the UK have changed since the early 1980s. By frontline manager we mean someone who manages people (whether paid or unpaid, qualified or not) who have direct contact with service users. We introduce two managers who work in different settings: Bronwyn, a manager in a voluntary sector therapeutic project for children and parents in families affected by sexual abuse, and Ted, a manager of a physical disability team in a social services agency.

This focus on individual managers is important. Policy directives and guidance need to be implemented by individuals within organisations. The frontline manager is central to the process of co-ordinating agency responses to policy and balancing agency requirements with staff needs for support, development and training.

After describing the development of managerialism as an approach to the delivery and management of care services, we move on to consider its impact on workers, service users and managers.

The aims of this chapter are to:

- review the role of the frontline manager
- discuss factors which led to the introduction of managerialist approaches in care services
- examine the influence of managerialism on the task of the frontline manager
- draw attention to the impact of managerialism on managers, workers and service users.

3.2 Managers

It's just the amount of change – everything's changing. I think we've all learned so many new skills, but we haven't been able to consolidate them because we've been moving from one new piece of legislation to another. We seem to be performance-managed to death these days, rather than having realistic targets to actually aspire to. [At one team meeting] you're saying this is the way we're going ... and then at the next team meeting you go to it's changed. There's a different target because the department has a different target that it has to meet.

(Manager consultations)

The manager quoted is talking about her experiences of frontline management in a community learning disability team. The pace of change in care services has been overwhelming, and one of a manager's key tasks is managing that change. The features that this manager highlights – targets and performance management – are part of an approach to management in public sector services that is sometimes called 'public sector management', 'new public sector management' or 'managerialism'.

A standards officer in the same agency, part of whose job is to develop ways of implementing performance management measures, argues that these tools (performance measurement and targets) are being misused:

> I'm interested that we see targets and statistics and standards as something that we do for 'up there', not as something we do for ourselves, because I think the management role is really about using those tools.

> If we've got clear expectations of practitioners about what they should be doing, then we don't have to be checking up all the time. We know exactly what they're supposed to be doing in any situation. I think that it's about producing management tools that reduce the workload, rather than adding on extra tasks for us.
>
> (Manager consultations)

Statistics, measurements and evidence are also part of a managerialist approach, but this person is positive about the opportunities they offer to provide a good-quality service as well as to assist managers and workers in their jobs. Indeed, her job title is 'standards officer' – another means of ensuring effectiveness that is part of the managerialist agenda. Other features of managerialism include quasi-markets, quality and partnership. Quasi-markets, performance management and partnership are examined in this chapter, while quality is addressed in Chapter 7.

In most management education the term 'managerialism' is viewed as a derogatory one, used to imply old-fashioned business management or very blinkered approaches to management. 'Public sector management' is used to indicate something different from traditional business management. It is used in management education for a form of management that puts public service first, informed by the values of a public service ethic. 'New public sector management' is more loaded in that it implies modernisation. In the UK this has particular meanings because of specific government policies, but modernisation of public services is an international issue. The term 'new public sector management' is used in many countries to mean something that is value driven and central to the development of society. There is some debate, however, about whether the values of 'public sector management' or the value for money approach of 'new public sector management', or a mixture of both, are key influences in the changes in management approaches used in care services.

In this chapter we use the term 'managerialism' and in doing so acknowledge this debate and present a critique of many aspects of managerialism. By 'managerialism' we mean an overarching set of changes introduced in the UK from the 1980s onwards that involve providing effective services at lower cost through the application of management techniques borrowed from business and industry.

Before we look at the development and features of managerialism, read the accounts of Bronwyn and Ted, two managers who work in different settings yet face similar challenges (Examples 3.1 and 3.2). Ted is a manager of a multi-professional team based in a social services agency and has worked as a social worker, team leader and team manager in adult services for the same local authority for many years. Bronwyn works in a small project that is part of a large, national voluntary organisation that has a regional as well as a national structure.

EXAMPLE 3.1 Ted

We've moved from the old team leader, who was a hands-on, visible manager in relation to a team. Now we've got this team manager role. The job has changed dramatically but the bit that was there in 1991 as a team leader is still there, it hasn't gone away. It is now coming right round full circle because of the volume of standards and expectations on the core task. This is probably one of the fastest, hardest hitting bits of your work in terms of how you write your reports, what you include, what standard it is, how quickly you do it, how efficiently you get it on to the information system.

Senior managers are going to sit at the top end of the department and pull out all the statistics and all the quality measures, to check how you're doing. The impact of new procedures on ensuring standards of care plans and recording has been tremendous. On one side of the coin there's the expectation that you're meeting these targets, but if you're not achieving you don't get a genuine crack of the whip at *why* you're not. That bit seems to be irrelevant. I want to explain to senior managers why we're 20 per cent down on something, and not achieving 95 per cent. It's because I'm three staff down, or this down or that down.

There's the sheer volume of demand and the expectation – not just by the department, a lot of it is government. We can't just say we're going to ignore it. It's law, it's legislation. There's tremendous emphasis on links with health and also links within the Council. It's not uncommon now for me to be part of a housing management committee for the district council. We might be talking about the allocation of property affecting a person with a disability and we're becoming increasingly involved in the culture of the ways of another department, another agency.

It's a huge learning curve. I find it interesting but at the same I'm conscious that I haven't been in the office for two days, and I must see so and so. I only had a brief word with them to shore up something, and I'm not back till tomorrow night. The role of the manager is broadening out so much.

EXAMPLE 3.2 Bronwyn

I've been a team manager for three and a half years working in a voluntary sector project. The project works with children and non-abusing family members where sexual abuse has taken place and offers a therapeutic service to family members. Before I became manager I spent five years as a worker on the same team. Another team member applied for the same management post. I also have a very small caseload, usually with parents.

The team consists of nine full- and part-time workers from a range of backgrounds. Among the staff are teachers, social workers and therapists. I also use sessional workers for specific pieces of work with children or families as and when required. The team members have all got some form of therapeutic qualification and are an extremely lively and creative group to work with. Inevitably, group dynamics are not always easy.

We work from a building that has been refurbished to a very high standard and I'm responsible for all health and safety and the upkeep of this building. This is where the majority of work takes place, although we do a certain amount of 'outreach' work using different venues.

I give staff supervision very high priority. Everyone gets monthly one-to-one supervision and we have a fortnightly group supervision model. I'm available on an ad hoc basis for day-to-day issues that people might have, for example to offload after a difficult session or to discuss child protection concerns and that type of thing.

I manage a large budget that gives me frequent headaches. The system has recently altered to become totally electronic and isn't exactly straight-forward. I rely on my administrator to deal with this on a daily basis, but inevitably the 'buck' stops with me. We also have partner agencies and I represent the project at regular meetings and prepare reports for these.

Overall, I find the work exhilarating, challenging, never a dull moment unless it's compiling statistics and figures, and at times exhausting and draining. Work sometimes seems like a lonely place – I feel like the meat in the sandwich between our organisation and the workers. I value my manager colleagues and we keep in touch – email, phone and the odd drink after work – but nothing regular. Mostly, I'm getting on with the job on my own, dealing with the day-to-day challenges and routines.

As you read through the sections on policy, you might like to refer back to these examples, or to your own experiences, and relate policy developments to management roles. Bronwyn manages people from several different professional backgrounds. Ted manages occupational therapists and social workers, as well as people with no qualifications. The way people have been brought together to manage and deliver social care in increasingly diverse occupational groups has grown from major changes in the way care services are conceptualised and organised. While the need to manage across different professional backgrounds presents many challenges, breaking down professional and agency barriers to service provision is an important aim if you think about the views of users reported in Chapter 2.

> **Key points**
>
> - The pace of change in organisations and in the management of care services has been rapid.
>
> - Changes have included the introduction of performance management and targets.
>
> - There is debate about factors that have influenced these changes and about the terms used to describe them.
>
> - Managerialism is a term often used to refer to changes in the way care services are managed through the introduction of techniques from business and industry.
>
> - Other terms include public sector management and new public sector management.

3.3 Managerialism

The UK Conservative government elected in 1979 argued that the welfare state was too expensive, inefficient, run by bureaucrats and professionals for their own interests and unresponsive to service users. It committed itself to 'rolling back the state', with individual, privatised provision replacing publicly financed and provided welfare services. This entailed individuals providing more for themselves and becoming less reliant on the state. Successive Conservative governments accepted reluctantly that radical disengagement from state finance and provision of welfare services was not possible (Cutler and Waine, 1997). However, they successfully resisted demands to increase spending on welfare, and this presented a problem. The Conservatives had ultimate responsibility for a broad range of welfare services at the same time as restricting the available resources. How could they convince the public that standards of service would be maintained?

The answer was to use resources more effectively and efficiently. By reorganising the delivery of effective services and by applying appropriate management techniques, services could be provided at a lower cost (Pollitt, 1990). This is the key characteristic of managerialism: *getting the greatest benefit from the resources available*. Models of management were borrowed from business, the private sector and industry and applied to public sector services to achieve this aim.

The challenges posed by such managerialist approaches to the hierarchy of professional power and control have been marked. Practice in the medical profession, for example, is subject to more public scrutiny than in the past. Local authorities are required to survey service users to establish their satisfaction with the services they receive. From the 1980s each part of the public sector – the civil service, local government, the NHS, social services, social security and education – experienced structural changes and/or the application of these types of management techniques (Stewart and Walsh, 1992). As these approaches were applied in the public sector, the features outlined in Box 3.1 developed.

BOX 3.1 Key features of managerialism

- Introduction of purchaser–provider split

- Creation of quasi-markets

- Competition between service providers

- Emphasis on consumers of services

- Performance management, with focus on defining objectives, targets and measuring performance

- Performance monitoring

How could these features improve effectiveness and efficiency? A manager in child protection comments:

> It's not all positive, but I remember the state of affairs before manage-rialism. It was a structure in which even the most minor decisions had to be sent 'upstairs' and management was not always professional. My own experience as a fieldworker was that supervision was about casework with little concern for development, training and so on. All the changes brought about by managerialism aren't negative. Some I view as very positive – more flattened managerial structures, enhancing the profile of managerial skills and user feedback.
>
> (Manager consultations)

The key management changes can be grouped under the heading of *performance management*. Performance management incorporates tech-niques from business, to plan, monitor and evaluate activities in a rigorous way and to make comparisons of performance available to the public to encourage best practice. An example here may be the reduction of NHS waiting lists and the comparison of hospitals via league tables. Of the structural changes, the most significant was the introduction of *quasi-markets*. A quasi-market potentially offers more choice for the service user as services may be purchased or commissioned by the public authority from a range of service providers drawn from the statutory, private or voluntary sectors. We will discuss these features in more detail in the next section.

When New Labour came into office in 1997 it inherited a public sector into which managerialism had been firmly installed. The party adopted the language and ideas of its opponents. This involved support for the setting of explicit targets for public services, the monitoring of performance and the use of market mechanisms in the public sector. At the same time New Labour sought to develop its own distinctive brand of public sector managerialism, which can be described as *reformed managerialism* (Cutler and Waine, 2000). This involved two key components:

1 an emphasis on improved and more sophisticated performance measures as a more effective means of improving standards
2 less emphasis on competition – although markets were still accepted – and support for partnership in finance and provision between public and private sectors.

Despite differences in approach, managerialism is now the accepted political orthodoxy of both major political parties in the UK. What has emerged has been described as 'managerialised politics' (Clarke and Newman, 1997, p. 143). This means that the competition between the political parties is about which one can best *manage* the welfare state. Debate and discussion about the social and political purposes of public services, for example issues of distribution and redistribution, have become marginalised (Cutler and Waine, 1997). So, for instance, debate is not about whether eligibility criteria should be applied but about a framing of eligibility criteria that is more restrictive and the best way to implement and manage such measures.

Key points

- A managerialist approach has been promoted by successive governments in the UK.

- The key management changes can be grouped under the heading 'performance management'.

- Debate about the real purposes of public services has been marginalised.

3.4 Managerialism in practice

This section looks in more detail at two aspects of managerialism: quasi-markets and performance management. Performance management appears to have had a profound effect on the work of the manager we heard from at the beginning of this chapter, who spoke about being 'performance-managed to death'. Quasi-markets are less prominent in the accounts we have presented so far.

Quasi-markets

Quasi-markets have features that make them both similar to and different from conventional markets. Central to the quasi-market is the distinction between the roles of the purchaser and the provider. The purchaser, for example the social services or social work authority, is publicly funded. Provider units are drawn from statutory, private or voluntary sectors, and compete for contracts from purchasers. Quasi-markets differ from conventional markets in a number of important respects. In conventional markets profit and financial targets are the main motivation. Although providers compete in quasi-markets, their service delivery objectives may take precedence over meeting financial targets. However, if voluntary sector or private agencies fail to meet their targets the result may be redundancies or the agency may cease to exist.

In conventional markets consumers spend their own money and can exercise real choice if there is genuine competition between suppliers. In quasi-markets consumers are not usually given money to purchase services and often their choice of service is exercised by a proxy, for example a care manager (Le Grand, 1990). An exception to this is the use of direct payment schemes, where payments are made to service users enabling them to purchase directly the support they require (Glendinning *et al.*, 2000).

Quasi-markets were justified on the grounds that they would reproduce the supposed virtues of the market in general; competition would lead to greater efficiency, decentralisation, enhanced consumer choice, diversity of providers and high-quality services. The following are some points to bear in mind.

1 Competition might well *increase* costs. Activities that are marketed must be costed and purchasers billed; if there is a contractual relationship then contracts must be devised, monitored and enforced. These are all costly procedures which might, or might not, be offset by savings as a result of competition (Le Grand, 1990). This contractual process also introduces a financial component into care assessments in the form of scrutiny by finance departments of the care relationship between service user and practitioner.

2 Quasi-markets might encourage decentralisation and a diversity of providers but it does not necessarily follow that there will be a diversity of services (Social Services Committee, 1990). For example, there might be an increase in private sector organisations entering the market. However, because of the higher profit margins that come from, say, the provision of residential services rather than day care, the new entrants would be more likely to offer only residential care. Such a situation would *limit* consumer choice.

3 Conventional markets are often criticised because they lead to inequalities: only those people who can afford goods or services are able to purchase them. This is often the rationale for their replacement by bureaucracies, which allocate resources on the basis of clear and open criteria. Quasi-markets may, though, also lead to inequalities. So, for example, when providers compete they may opt for a narrow provision that results in their attracting users who either improve the organisation's ability to meet performance targets or involve less resource use by the organisation. Examples of the former are schools that seek to attract more able pupils; examples of the latter are residential homes for elderly people that aim to admit more mentally and physically active people.

Performance management

Performance management embodies a number of key techniques from business and industry. Effective organisations need to have clearly defined *objectives* and *outcomes*, and to secure them *explicit targets* must be set. It follows that there must be *performance measures* or *indicators* of the progress achieved, and *performance monitoring* to determine success or failure. In addition, a central assumption of performance management is the idea of *best practice*, which allows star performers to be held up as exemplars, as a means of changing the practice of poor performers. Box 3.2 outlines these terms and gives examples of each.

BOX 3.2 Key terms in performance management

Objectives: *what you want to achieve*

- User involvement in monitoring services

Outcomes: *what you actually achieve*

- User involvement in consultation sessions

Explicit targets: *what you want to achieve broken down into component parts*

- Identify service users who are willing to take part in pilot project

- Work alongside service users to identify any relevant training needs

- Brief staff and projects on user involvement

- Undertake evaluation of three projects by year end

Performance measures or *indicators*: *evidence used to judge how well a person or agency has performed*

- Number of service evaluations undertaken

Performance monitoring: *collecting information to judge performance*

- Service user evaluations of pilot project

Best practice: *a consensus view on what to do to achieve practice improvements*

- Find research reports on similar projects

- Hold joint staff development–service user training session to disseminate results

---

The rationale for performance management is that accountability is strengthened because the public is able to see how service providers are performing (Baggini, 2000). In this way the emphasis on efficiency and effectiveness is reinforced via publicly available inspection reports. It is questionable, however, how much local accountability has shifted to the public arena. Asked about performance measurement, Ted, the manager of a physical disability team whom we introduced earlier, reflected:

> It never felt to me that league tables and performance management made me accountable to the public as a manager, but it did make me accountable to the Department. My other concern is that often performance measures are used in quite a narrow way and around easily measurable areas, for example response times. To really measure 'quality' requires a more in-depth approach. My concern with the 'performance culture' is that it has concentrated too much on the easily measured and the fairly uninteresting and hasn't provided a good basis to improve the quality of services!
>
> (Manager consultations)

It is important to recognise that performance management has generated a substantial critical literature, pointing to a number of conceptual and practical problems. First, organisational objectives and outcomes are usually expressed in very general terms. In social care an objective might be to promote the independence of adults assessed as needing social care, respecting their dignity and furthering their social and economic participation. But what do the terms 'promote independence' and 'respect dignity' mean? How are they to be defined? Whose judgement about outcomes is being used – that of the user, their family or the professional (Riley and Riley, 1998)? Perhaps a measure of performance could be the extent to which managers involve service users in shaping what is to be measured in the first place.

Second, would a favourable outcome be within the control of the provider? For example, an institution providing training may be judged on the employment record of individuals taking its courses, but this outcome will be affected by the state of the national or local labour market. A favourable outcome for a community mental health service may be fewer service users admitted to hospital, but if there are no alternatives to hospital admission, such as crisis services or home treatment services, this outcome will not be achieved. (There is a more detailed discussion about outcomes in Chapter 11.)

Third, there must be measures of whether the outcomes have been achieved. This requires both targets and performance indicators, for example service users moving on from day care. An important feature of such measures of performance is that they are often used in the construction and publication of league tables showing the ranking order of providers. A criticism of league tables is that they do not reflect circumstances accurately, as the manager in Example 3.3 discovered.

EXAMPLE 3.3 Checking the scores

A manager of a mental health team in a local authority was concerned that on league tables issued by the department her team were not meeting the target that all Mental Health Act assessments be undertaken within 24 hours of a request being received. The manager knew that workers in her team responded within at most four hours, yet in the league tables this was not apparent.

After making enquiries it appeared that *records* of assessments were not added to the information system until the assessment was completed, which could take more than 24 hours. So, although the team was meeting the target of assessment within 24 hours, the evidence on which league tables were based – the statistics in the information system – suggested that the team was not achieving all it should.

This manager would have had an additional challenge as a result of the measure designed to ensure better quality of service. She would have needed to deal with the demoralisation her staff were experiencing as well as her own concerns. What the league table also did not show was the quality of the work this team produced and their commitment to finding alternatives for service users to formal detention in hospital.

Another manager, speaking about league tables, commented:

How do you feel when you realise that your team has actually come down the table, rather than gone up? It makes you feel so bad, it makes the team feel bad as well, that they're actually not producing the work that they should.

I just think that has a negative effect rather than a positive effect. I can see why senior managers need that information. Maybe they could talk to the manager individually about the performance of the team. I don't see why it has to be published and circulated to all and sundry. I think that's a negative thing for the department to publish.

(Manager consultations)

So, care is needed when assessing performance indicators and using league tables to ensure the measures are appropriate to the desired outcomes.

One way of bringing together performance measures may be by using *benchmarking*. The term covers a variety of practices that have the goal of improving services. To some people, it means simply the process of comparison, while to others it includes identifying ways of improving services. Effective benchmarking does not necessarily require the production of league tables. However, it needs to be – according to the Audit Commission – supported and driven from the top and must engage commitment and enthusiasm from staff at all levels (Audit Commission, 2000a). Staff should be involved in the process and 'own' any changes introduced.

Inspections and reviews – by external and internal bodies – may also provide evidence of the quality of services. The Audit Commission undertakes joint reviews with the Social Services Inspectorate (SSI). The SSI was set up in 1985 as a professional division within the Department of Health. Inspections and reviews may be experienced by managers as time-consuming and distracting, but it can be argued that it is better to have more information and that this can lead to improvement. The Audit Commission accepts that 'although some benchmarking has produced good results, a substantial proportion has failed thus far to produce tangible benefits' (Audit Commission, 2000b, p. 7).

However, as the report on Bronwyn's project shows, inspection may also validate good practice.

Inspection report

Child protection is clearly very much on the agenda at this project and it was refreshing that, although working with issues of abuse on a daily basis, staff members did not give the impression of being immune to the effects of this. There were high levels of sensitivity, compassion and respect, overtly and appropriately displayed. Together with this was a sense of involvement: the project actively works with people rather than delivering services to them. The children, young people and adults are active partners in whatever work is undertaken and often they become the driving force, determining where it goes. This gives an important and effective dynamic to the work and helps in bringing in fresh ideas and perspectives to the task. Similarly, the project links closely with other agencies and community groups in partnership to provide services for children and raise awareness of child sexual abuse.

This is a project which, as well as offering much needed services to children and their carers in an appropriate and sensitive manner, is also committed to developing the way that these issues are addressed on a number of levels. In terms of service user involvement and working in partnership, it accurately reflects the philosophy of The Children Act and the new Assessment Framework. It is in the forefront of generating ways of helping children and their carers, of spreading awareness and generating training materials. It should be encouraged to develop these separate but intricately linked strands.

> **Key points**
>
> - Quasi-markets are similar to conventional markets in that there are purchasers and providers (buyers and sellers).
>
> - In quasi-markets services are usually chosen by care managers rather than service users.
>
> - Performance management uses techniques from business and industry.
>
> - There must be performance measures or indicators of progress achieved, and performance monitoring to determine success or failure.
>
> - Best practice is a central assumption of performance management.
>
> - There are conceptual and practical difficulties with performance management, especially the use of league tables.

3.5 Developing the managerialist agenda

New Labour did not, as we noted earlier, reject the managerialism of the Conservatives. Key features of Conservative policy – the quasi-market, the use of the independent sector and performance measures – were accepted and embraced. New Labour has also extended and reformed managerialism in social care in several important and distinctive ways.

This extended or reformed managerialist agenda can be found in two key documents on social care: *Modernising Social Services* (Department of Health, 1998a) and *A Quality Strategy for Social Care* (Department of Health, 2000b). In Northern Ireland the reformed managerialist approach was put forward in *Fit for the Future – A New Approach* (DHSSPS, 1999) and in Scotland in *Aiming for Excellence* (Scottish Office, 1999).

Four key themes emerge from these documents:

1 an emphasis on providing 'quality' services
2 the centrality of more rounded performance measurements to the achievement of 'quality' and 'continuous improvement'
3 performance to be evaluated and monitored
4 the strategy for social care to be 'top-down', with government providing the context for the organisation and delivery of social services.

Another important concept these papers emphasised is partnership.

Partnership

The idea of partnership in care services is not new. What is distinctive about New Labour's position on partnership is that it is a central idea in managing the public sector (Ling, 2000). Alongside this is an emphasis on partnerships with service users and the importance of users' views. A straightforward definition of partnership is 'working together'. This can occur at two levels: policy and service delivery. Ted, the manager you met at the beginning of this chapter, spoke about the importance his organisation placed on partnerships with several local organisations and the impact this made on his day-to-day role. In terms of policy, Ted could be involved in one of the Joint Implementation Groups, which are looking at how national policies and guidance might be introduced across several agencies in his locality. As part of his role in managing service delivery Ted works in partnership with the health service manager for physical disabilities in ensuring that their work is complementary.

In 1998 the government published *Getting It Right Together: Compact on Relations Between Government and the Voluntary and Community Sector in England* (Home Office, 1998b). New Labour, as part of its policy of requiring partnership and co-ordinated policies at a local level, committed itself to the development of local *compacts* or agreements between the voluntary and community sector and local authorities. 'Compact' is used in this sense to indicate an agreement between two or more partners. It can also mean 'contract'. The compact *Getting It Right Together* was designed to improve relations and joint working between local authorities and voluntary organisations and shape the way in which these sectors work together. It covers funding, consultation, volunteering, monitoring and evaluation (Craig *et al.*, 1999). This national compact was followed by various local compacts.

Some of the many partnership groupings that are emerging in the areas of health and social care are listed in Box 3.3.

BOX 3.3 Take your partner!

Health authorities have a statutory duty to work with other NHS bodies, local authorities, primary care groups, voluntary organisations and community groups to produce a Health Improvement Programme (HImP). The HImP covers the health needs and requirements of local people and details how these will be met by partnership working.

The NHS Concordat is an agreement between the NHS and two kinds of partners: voluntary organisations and private providers. It enables the NHS to buy services or use facilities in private hospitals and encourage the private and voluntary sector to develop rehabilitation services in addition to provision of nursing and residential homes (Department of Health, 2000a, para. 11.5).

Primary Care Groups (PCGs) have members including local general practitioners, community or practice nurses, a lay member and a representative from social services. PCGs will commission services for a locality.

Primary Care Trusts (PCTs), groups of PCGs who not only commission services but provide community health services, will provide additional opportunities for partnership working.

Care Trusts are partnerships between PCGs and PCTs, plus one or more local authorities, established to deliver services, initially for particular client groups such as older people (Department of Health, 2000a).

Local authority departments such as social services, education, housing, police and probation services may form partnerships.

Voluntary, private and business organisations in a local community may all form partnerships.

Crime Reduction Partnerships include the police, probation service, local authorities and local communities.

Health Action Zone partners may come together in targeted areas where the population has a poor health status to develop and implement a health strategy within the area.

The frontline manager in each of the organisations involved in partnerships will have different degrees of responsibility and decision-making authority. Each of the organisations will have different cultures and histories. The partnerships may have different purposes but each of the arrangements must have the same objective: to provide a high-quality, user-centred service (Department of Health, 2000b, para. 8).

The Health Act 1999 introduced three new flexibilities to the ways in which health and social care organisations could work in partnership:

1 lead commissioning, whereby one agency (health or local authority) takes on responsibility for commissioning a service on behalf of other organisations, for example services for people with learning difficulties

2 pooled budgets, whereby funds are pooled to meet a specific objective, such as the purchase of equipment which could allow a person to remain at home rather than go into residential care

3 integrated provision, whereby services provided by different organisations are brought together in a single management structure, for instance the range of intermediate services for older people. (There is a full discussion of these measures in Edwards, 2000.)

What chance of success will the new partnerships have in achieving better-quality services and closer working links between agencies and organisations? It is too early to give a definitive answer, as it will take time for these partnerships to establish themselves. However, in attempting even to come to an interim judgement, you need to consider the context within which partnerships are being developed. Central to this context is the framework of managerialism. In particular, there is the influence of quasi-markets and performance measurement. The essence of markets is competition, which makes inter-organisational working difficult (Henwood and Hudson, 2000). Performance measures relate to activities within individual organisations. However, an emphasis on targets, and comparisons between these organisations rather than the achievement of broader public sector goals, is being encouraged in an attempt to measure co-operation between agencies. Collaboration and partnership across organisational and professional boundaries is inherently difficult in spite of the expectations of government and frameworks from the Department of Health.

A contrasting view on the potential impacts of partnerships is that comparisons between organisations should not get in the way of partnerships, because the partner agencies will not be in league table competition with each other but with other similar agencies. Moreover, organisations each need their partner agencies in order to improve their league table performance status. District councils, for example, rely heavily on the performance of their local police force and drugs agencies to meet their targets with regard to crime and disorder. An aim of the strategic planning behind such partnerships is to define trans-agency public sector goals and find collaborative means to meet them. For example, the police, Youth Offending Teams and probation services are reviewed and the extent to which they have defined common goals and collaborative means of meeting them is evaluated. In this context performance measurement strengthens partnerships.

Key points

- The New Labour government has developed a reformed managerialism, which places less emphasis on competition and focuses on:

  – more sophisticated performance measures

  – quality services and continuous improvement.

- Partnerships between agencies, organisations and sectors are expected to lead to better-quality services.

- There are tensions inherent in partnerships, the use of league tables and comparisons of agencies and organisations.

3.6 Managerialism and people

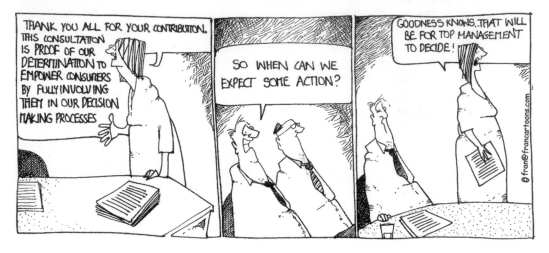

Service users

As Connelly and Seden note in Chapter 2, both *Caring for People* and *Modernising Social Services* placed users at the centre of the reformed systems and structures. The earlier White Paper stated that 'promoting choice and independence underlies all the Government's proposals' (Department of Health and Social Security, 1989, para. 1.8). The latter noted that the proposals for modernisation focus on 'the quality of services experienced by, and outcomes achieved for, individuals and their carers and families' (Department of Health, 1998a, para. 1.7).

The shifts from residential to non-residential alternatives, and within the latter to the use of the independent sector (Government Statistical Service, 1998; Kenny *et al.*, 2000), could be seen as indicators of the success of the new commissioning arrangements. At the strategic or macro level, choice for the user has increased. It follows that choice at the operational or micro level should also have increased. Thus users are expected to make several choices, referred to as the 'what, when and from whom choices' (Hardy *et al.*, 1999, p. 484). Whether service users are aware of the choices available is another question.

A choice of services should be available – residential, nursing home or domiciliary care. In respect of community-based services, choice should be exercised over the composition of care packages – the balance between personal and social care and the times at which this should be provided. There should be choice over the service provider – public, private or voluntary organisations. This choice should take account of any cultural or religious requirements. Some people working in care services question whether, in reality, there is as much choice for service users as implied in government policy statements.

However, services sensitive to local conditions and requirements are also to be delivered through a managerial structure that emphasises tight centralised control and cost containment. Is it possible to have the former with the latter? For example, a residential unit manager may want to meet service users' requests for day outings, and at the same time be expected to remain within budget. What challenges does this pose for the individual practice-led manager? On the one hand, a manager may be consulting service users and staff and striving to structure the service according to their views. On the other, this must be done in the context of financial and organisational constraints. Managers need to be open during consultation processes and negotiations about the constraints that structure service provision.

The workforce

Perhaps by this stage in the chapter you are reeling from the pace of change. This is also likely to be the case for the workforce. There have been shifts in the pattern of service provision. Government is committed to overcoming the old divisions between health and social care and removing the legal obstacles to joint working (Department of Health, 2000a). Such changes can be seen as offering both threats and opportunities to the workforce.

Chapter 8 considers professions in more detail, but it is important to note here a few key points about professionals and professional groups. Professionals have the autonomy to exercise their professional judgement in the best interests of their clients, and often have considerable discretion in the use of resources by deciding, for example, what level of services to provide for an individual client. Professionals work in a world of complexity, uncertainty and ambiguity (Southon and Braithwaite, 1998). Managerialism, with its commitment to targets, performance measures, scrutiny, appraisal and monitoring, represents a clear challenge to professionals. Foster and Wilding (2000) suggest that managerialism has led to professionals being more accountable to taxpayers and service users for what they do and are broadly supportive of the managerial control of welfare professionals. At the same time, they express concern that managerialism can destroy the positive aspects of professionalism: the ability to do high-quality work and provide individualised services for clients.

Public sector managerialism creates tensions for professionals of two major types: tensions for professionals who become managers and tensions between professionals and managers (Farrell and Morris, 1999). Having professional experience does not guarantee that someone will make an effective manager, as this frontline manager in mental health points out:

> What's the difference between being a successful practitioner and being a successful manager? From my point of view they are two completely different roles. I think in organisations I've worked for in the past, we've tended to promote people who were good on-the-ground workers to be managers. It doesn't necessarily follow that they'll be good managers. I have a feeling in my own background that I was a fairly average social worker, and I think I'm better as a manager, but that's not the same for everyone.
>
> (Manager consultations)

Professionals who become managers must take on a new range of duties and tasks – auditing, managing budgets, monitoring contracts, managing change – in addition to their professional tasks. Managers must juggle the different aspects of the management task: the strategic (contributing to departmental policy), the operational (the delivery of services), and the professional (managing and supporting staff) (Henderson and Seden, 2003). A potential problem for managers is the extent to which they can undertake managerial tasks while retaining their professional identity (Farrell and Morris, 1999; see also Chapter 8).

As well as challenges to individual workers, managerialism presents challenges for many groups within care services. For example, residential social workers (other than in children's homes) and home care service workers have found their jobs opened to competition from independent providers. Indeed, there is a trend for some services and the associated workforce to shift from direct local authority provision to contracts with the independent sector (TOPSS, 1999). A key issue here will be the compatibility of wages and working conditions in the new sector with those experienced in local authority employment.

While noting that public sector managerialism can present challenges to the care workforce, it also presents opportunities. Brooks (1999) argues that nursing increasingly bases its claim to professional status on a managerialist discourse. In social care new jobs are created with titles such as 'customer care manager'. Management can thus offer a career progression path parallel to the route of acquiring professional social work skills.

> **Key points**
>
> - Recent government papers have promised more choice for service users.
>
> - In practice, financial and organisational constraints may limit choice.
>
> - Managers may experience tensions between their management role and their professional identity.
>
> - Workers may feel under threat from competition from other providers and from the use of employment contracts.

3.7 Managers revisited

In this section we return to what managers, workers and service users have told us about how they experience the impact of managerialism and changes in frontline management. Managers must attempt to negotiate any tensions between the needs of organisations, service users and workers. Government is concerned with the quality and appropriateness of service provision and measures of performance, as noted throughout this chapter. Expectations placed on managers are clear, but at the same time are underpinned by contradictions and tensions. Managerialism has provided a set of strategies that may help achieve these expectations. Service users are concerned with less easily measured aspects of management practice and may have different views on what makes a responsive manager. Figure 3.1 (overleaf) was drawn by Carlisle People First and illustrates their views of a 'bad' manager.

Workers also have expectations of their managers, often based on policies and government guidance. An editorial in *Community Care* (the weekly magazine for the care sector) about the Victoria Climbié inquiry notes:

> The child protection system is built on the premise that inexperienced members of staff receive regular supervision, support and back-up from their line managers. They can refer up, they can use their managers' experience to gain the often crucial second opinion in a case, and they can expect both advice and direction.
>
> (*Community Care*, 2001, p. 5)

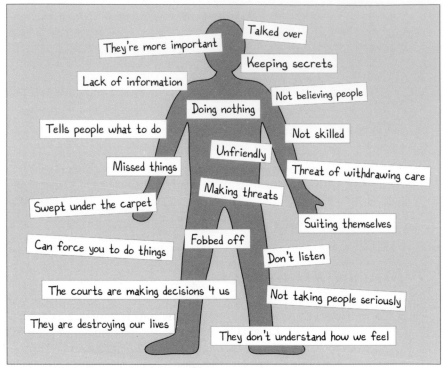

Figure 3.1   **A 'bad' manager**

This support was not given to Lisa Arthurworrey, the social worker involved in the case. The editorial continues:

> This is further evidence that the performance target-ridden approach to managing social services departments can fail to meet the needs of vulnerable clients. An over-emphasis on targets can result in a senior management system focused on achieving success in the eyes of the Department of Health rather than in the eyes of their own front-line staff and, more importantly, users.
>
> (p. 5)

In the consultation process outlined in the Appendix to this book, workers were asked about their expectations and these are summarised in Box 3.4. Workers were keenly aware of the pressures their managers were under and recognised that managers did as much as they could to support staff. However, workers felt that managers were more removed than they should be from the day-to-day elements of the service.

BOX 3.4 Workers' expectations

What do you want from a manager?

- day-to-day access

- support and understanding

- ability to make decisions and stand by them

- to take responsibility

- mutual respect

- to achieve a balance between autonomy and accountability – not leaving you without support

- flexibility

Managers have complex and challenging roles. One voluntary sector manager listed some of her roles:

> I range from being a practitioner, practice teacher, a manager of people, a manager of budgets, a manager of services, a manager of complaints, and responsible for attitudes in the department as well.
>
> (Manager consultations)

So, while aspects of management fit alongside various approaches driven by policy initiatives from central government, managers are also individuals with their own characteristics and approaches. The individual approach of the manager might be equally as important to a service user or worker as a performance measure. Figure 3.2 (overleaf), again by Carlisle People First, illustrates the qualities of a 'good' manager.

However, there are positive and creative aspects to the role of manager. As Ted stresses:

> I might be banging a bit of a drum here, but everyone goes on about the volume of work, variety of tasks, got at from above and below and so on. What about the positives – developing people, being able to make changes, the sense of achievement, feeling able to contribute more? I think we need to promote the positives more so the right people can be recruited to these posts. And think about this – you don't see many managers resigning because of all the negative aspects of the job, do you?
>
> (Manager consultations)

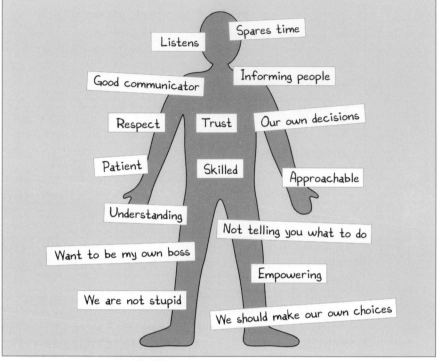

Figure 3.2 **A 'good' manager**

Key points

- Managerialism places clear expectations on managers, but workers and service users may have different expectations.

- Despite the misgivings of many people, there are positive aspects to the managerial role.

3.8 Conclusion

The debates and critiques of managerialism on which much of this chapter is based developed in reaction to a fear that the welfare state was about to be dismantled. The managerialist process has continued and evolved and incorporated more emphasis on accountability, partnership and service user satisfaction. Debate continues about whether there is real commitment to involvement and consultation, as you saw in Chapter 2, and about whether measurement is more important than what is being measured and whether the reality matches the rhetoric.

The reality of a typical day for Bronwyn, recorded in her diary, illustrates many of the points made in this chapter.

BRONWYN'S DIARY

9.00 A consultation/supervision session with member of the clergy who uses project for support and is enabled to do this by her 'superiors' as they provide funding – real recognition of the task that she is doing. I love this side of the work, it is many faceted and always challenging. I am also a member of a committee that looks at the Church's response to Child Protection, a fascinating insight into how another hierarchy conducts its affairs in a way I am unfamiliar with, with a totally familiar subject, quite a juxtaposition at times.

10.30 Back to project for meeting with one of my consultants. Looked at future of our work together and came up with a plan for, hopefully, attracting quite a lot of money to the project. Need to write up discussion and proposal for a service level agreement.

11.30 Local university wanting volunteer projects to do research on outcomes/effectiveness of services. Put my project's name forward as I think it would be helpful to have some academic evaluation of our work. Next task – tell team!

12.00 Read report from Inspection Unit, sent via e-mail. Got quite a buzz, very positive report. It had felt like a gruelling experience, our version of Ofsted, but I know we do excellent work and this confirmed it – told team – arranged to go out for booze and food in near future to celebrate. Plan to start to compile material for a project review. Yes, not only was I inspected, I'm now being reviewed. I also need to complete a business plan, my annual report and all by the end of the next month.

1.00 Team meeting day. The number of referrals has increased at an alarming rate. Spent most of the meeting allocating, making decisions about appropriateness of some, trying to find creative ways of meeting the need for the work. Fortunately the plans drawn up the day before will help towards this. Made date for a team day to discuss new proposals – need to book venue away from office to be able to devote the day to the task without disturbance. Need to arrange equal opps/and child protection yearly refresher courses for team. Team came up with a number of suggestions.

5.00 Phone call to say a funding bid we had put in for a new piece of work had been accepted but the referral criteria were a lot tighter than we'd wanted. Discussed ways we might be able to 'stretch this' but still great news and means we will be working

> alongside colleagues in a specialist health setting undertaking
> innovative work with families where child protection is an issue
> that is very risky.

As Bronwyn's diary shows, the role of a frontline manager is complex and challenging, and the expectations placed on managers are many and varied. In this chapter we have discussed the development of managerialism, often known as public sector management, its underlying philosophy, techniques and application. This diary extract shows some of the effects of changes in day-to-day management. Policy has implications for individuals and so we have looked at its impacts on managers, workers and service users. Have the reforms discussed in this chapter delivered what they promised? Well, Bronwyn and her project workers felt proud and enthusiastic when they received their inspection report and the quality of their work with service users was recognised. Developing partnerships certainly has a high priority for both Ted and Bronwyn. Have reforms liberated resources – both people and financial – so that services can be organised more efficiently? Bronwyn and her workers have put together proposals and applied for funding for innovative work with partners in health settings. The answers to these questions will depend on who is asked. There are no clear-cut answers. Such is the challenge of frontline management.

Chapter 4
Managers and the law

Ann McDonald and Jeanette Henderson

4.1 Introduction

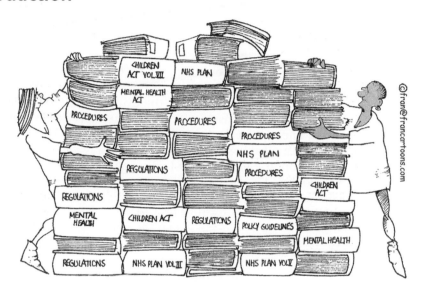

The impact of law on managers in the care services is wide-ranging. Health and safety, child welfare, employment and mental health legislation are just some of the areas of law that direct social care organisations and managers. Some legislation affects the working conditions of people employed in care services; other areas of law drive the work they undertake. By imposing specific duties on agencies and organisations to carry out certain tasks such as assessment and resource allocation, the law makes it illegal not to carry them out. The person most likely to be making initial judgements about these issues – within the context of agency policies and procedures, made at a higher level – is the frontline manager.

The law provides a framework within which the exercise of professional judgement takes place. This is not, of course, the same as providing a single 'right' answer. In the majority of circumstances legislation – particularly in the field of health and social care – provides a choice of more or less intrusive responses to complex social situations. There are times when the policy or values on which the law is based may not always be congruent with practice values. The manager is then faced with dilemmas: how to act within the letter of the law while (as a practice-led manager) respecting diversity and promoting choice for workers and service users alike.

It is necessary for managers to recognise the impact of legal directives in the workplace: on the priority which needs to be given to particular types of work; on the importance of effective staff supervision and guidance; and on the inevitability of challenges to the agency's policies and decisions. Decision making, the efficient and effective use of limited resources, and the auditing and regulation of decisions all take place within a structure, according to legislation, regulation and guidance.

This chapter cannot provide detailed legal guidance. However, managers need to be familiar with primary legislation and are recommended to obtain copies of legal documents relevant to their organisational context. Laws and legal documents are also specific to countries within the UK. In Northern Ireland, for example, mental health legislation is contained in the Mental Health (Northern Ireland) Order 1986. In Scotland in relation to children, the Children (Scotland) Act 1995 applies. You are advised to consult relevant country-specific legislation should you want to know more about legislation in a particular country. If you are faced with a legal concern you should always seek professional advice.

This chapter gives a sense of why law is important to managers. Some legislation, such as that for employment or health and safety, is relevant to all managers, whatever their organisation. Other legislation, such as that for charities, child protection or mental health, is particularly relevant to managers in those specific fields. Managers in *all* settings, however, need to be aware of the range and complexity of law.

The law may be viewed as an impediment to practice. Sometimes it is, but to a much greater extent the law is a crucial tool for what is generally regarded as good practice. The next section asks 'What is the law?' and sets out some key legal terms and concepts. Following this overview of the legal framework of health and social care there is a discussion of management roles and responsibilities in implementing legislation and guidance. Statutory responsibilities and the Human Rights Act 1998 are considered in Sections 4.4 and 4.5 respectively. The chapter then considers duties of care and finally looks at facing challenges – particularly some of the challenges managers face when involved in inquiries and whistle-blowing.

The aims of this chapter are to:

- consider legal issues in the workplace
- raise awareness of dilemmas and conflicts for frontline managers which may be associated with legal issues
- identify key issues of the legal framework of health and social care provision.

4.2 What is the law?

Attitudes towards the law will inevitably be shaped by personal experience. Law may have been experienced as a limitation on freedom of action or as an opportunity for change. In a professional context law may be perceived as directive or regulatory, for example by the way in which it prescribes standards for residential care or places children with foster carers. The law applies to all aspects of an organisation, and many areas of law will impinge on the role of a frontline manager:

- the law giving authorities duties or powers to provide services and making people eligible to receive services
- the law giving authorities powers to intervene in people's private lives, for example child protection law
- employment law, including health and safety legislation and anti-discrimination legislation where it relates to employment
- contract law where services are contracted, including legislation regarding tendering procedures
- the law relating to confidentiality and data protection
- the law relating to civil rights, and particularly the Human Rights Act 1998 and the European Convention on Human Rights on which it is based, and anti-discriminatory legislation where it applies to service users
- the law relating to public financial management
- charities law and/or company law may be important where care managers are not directly employed by local authorities, the NHS or health and social services trusts.

Further complexity enters into the picture where:

- management is exercised under the jurisdiction of the criminal courts as with probation services and youth offending teams or with the forensic sections of the Mental Health Acts for England, Wales and Scotland and the Mental Health (Northern Ireland) Order
- management is within the framework of the civil sections of mental health law concerning detention and discharge from mental hospital or concerning guardianship orders
- management has to take account of the special procedures which apply when juveniles are arrested and detained for a suspected scheduled offence under the Northern Ireland (Emergency Provisions) Act 1991
- the courts are involved with regard to vulnerable people such as children looked after by a local authority or adoption being arranged or, where the English Court of Protection or, in Scotland, the Office of the Public Guardian is involved, with people judged as not legally competent to manage their own affairs.

In addition to the areas just mentioned, like everyone else managers are supposed to abide by the criminal law and to avoid committing civil offences such as defamation or slander. Managers cannot be familiar with all aspects of these areas of legislation. However, it is important that they understand the components which make up a legislative framework, and Box 4.1 summarises components of law found across the UK.

BOX 4.1 Components of law

Statute law is legislation passed by Parliament, for example the Children Act 1989.

Case law refers to rulings made by higher courts that are binding on lower courts. ('Common law' is a term sometimes used to refer to established case law.)

Regulations are made by the Secretary of State for the enforcement of a particular area of policy and carry the full force of law; in Scotland they are made by the appropriate minister in the Scottish Parliament.

Guidance sets out expectations about the way legislation should be implemented to bring about the purpose it was designed to achieve.

Directions can be issued by a Secretary of State in order to place further duties on local authorities.

Policies and procedures are developed by individual agencies and reflect their particular ethos and practices; they must fall within what has been laid down by law.

Codes of practice are advisory and interpret legislation such as the Mental Health Act 1983 and the Mental Health (Scotland) Act 1984; they may be cited as evidence of good practice.

The words of a statute will usually contain qualifying statements which enable subjective judgement to operate. Such terms include 'so far as is reasonably possible', 'if it is in the best interests of ... ' and 'as may be appropriate'.

Subjective wording of this kind implies the need for judgement. In other words, it enables workers to apply the law in practice. So, provided they do not act unreasonably, local authorities will have a measure of discretion in defining who, according to the particular character of their area, is deemed to be a 'child in need' under the Children Act 1989, the Children (Scotland) Act 1995 or the Children (Northern Ireland) Order 1995. Another example is the Mental Health Act 1983, where the definition of 'aftercare services' is a matter for evolving definition through practice and precedent.

Such 'flexible' definitions may pose challenges for managers. For example, adjoining local authorities may interpret 'aftercare services' in different ways. People who attend the same psychiatric hospital but live in different local authority areas may not have the same access to some forms of aftercare services. They may challenge decisions not to provide aftercare that is available in nearby areas. Managers will then need to justify the basis on which their agency definition has been made.

Legislation which contains flexible definitions fits well with the managerial task of defining and setting the parameters of work in accordance with patterns of local demand and available resources. Some terms, however, do have clear definitions, as Box 4.2 illustrates.

BOX 4.2 Definitions

Duty – something an agency must do under the law

Powers – those things an agency may do, but with a discretionary element that allows for choice depending on the circumstances

Responsibility – workers' responsibility to carry out their work in accordance with agency policy and professional values

Remedies – used to enforce rights or ensure powers are properly exercised

---

The law identifies some groups of people as particularly entitled to a service, such as 'children in need' (Children Act 1989) or adults who have been detained in hospital (Mental Health Act 1983). As citizens, everyone has a voice in decision-making processes. The law requires that people should be consulted in a decision to close a residential home for example, or in a review of home care charges (see Chapter 2 for a detailed discussion of user consultation and involvement). Such consultation is part of the legal requirement of 'due process' and emphasises that the way decisions are made can be as important as what those decisions are.

Consultation with service users is fundamental to the National Health Service and Community Care Act 1990. This major piece of legislation contains only nine sections relevant to community care in England and Wales. These sections impose: a duty on local authorities to assess people for community care services (s. 47); a duty to produce community care plans (s. 46); a power to contract with the independent sector to produce a mixed economy of care (s. 42); and a duty to create a system for hearing representations and complaints (s. 50). The reorganisation of the community care system was achieved through these few, but fundamental, sections.

There is nothing in the legislation, however, about the purchaser–provider split or the process of care management. These qualitative changes were introduced through guidance. The key guidance documents in relation to the National Health Service and Community Care Act (Department of Health/Social Services Inspectorate, 1991) are:

- *Care Management and Assessment: Practitioners' Guide*
- *Care Management and Assessment: Managers' Guide.*
- *Care Management and Assessment: Summary of Practice Guidance.*

These publications are essential reading for managers as they describe how the prioritising of referrals can be achieved through the allocation of cases to different levels of assessment, and how the system of care management can be structured.

The Children Act 1989, the Children (Scotland) Act 1995 and the Children (Northern Ireland) Order 1995 were accompanied by volumes of guidance at the outset. Further guidance has been developed in the light of findings from research in the field of child protection and family assessment. Subsequently, materials have been produced to standardise the recording of assessment and planning and this has led to a greater consistency of practice than is the case in adult care. The power to make regulations as contained within the legislation has also been used to standardise the holding of reviews and the monitoring of foster placements, to give just two examples.

An increasingly managerialist state, operating through performance indicators, internal and external audit and inquiry, relies heavily on legislation to help provide predictable and coherent responses to pre-defined situations. However, not all situations may be pre-defined, nor is it possible to anticipate all eventualities, as Example 4.1 illustrates.

EXAMPLE 4.1 Unanticipated events

Terry, who had a history of violent offences, had been in contact with probation services for several years. Following departmental guidance, a comprehensive risk assessment was undertaken involving a range of agencies. The assessment showed that Terry had made good progress and that he presented little risk of reoffending.

Two months after the assessment Terry seriously assaulted an elderly woman. He said the woman reminded him of his grandmother, who had been abusive towards him in the past.

Risk assessment and risk management plans are required increasingly by legislation and guidance. This example shows that, although an agency may comply fully with this requirement, it can never be certain of preventing a serious incident from taking place, especially as a result of unanticipated events. In a similar way, criminal law does not eliminate crime.

Balancing the requirements of law and agency policy

In Example 4.1 the agencies were following guidance that closely echoed legal requirements. The potential for tension between the requirements of law and of agency policy can lead to further dilemmas for managers. Law gives the authority and determines the accountability that are essential for the performance of their managerial task. Yet in their day-to-day role, managers may not be reading or referring directly to any formal sources of law. Instead, within their agency, managers are usually referred to agency policy and procedures manuals. Policies and procedures developed within organisations and agencies should be a distillation and interpretation of the legislation. If or when challenged, the agency's own internal policies will be seen as valid only to the extent that they are consistent with a proper interpretation of statute law, regulations or guidance. For example, in Northern Ireland, as elsewhere in the UK, the courts have occasionally had reason to query the criteria applied by social workers to assess potential foster carers and prospective adopters. To the extent that criteria may stray outside the authority provided by law and incorporate subjective values and lifestyle indicators, they are open to challenge by the court. In a case of conflict, legal interpretation will prevail.

The allocation of places in residential care homes for example, by means of either a waiting list or an allocation panel, is a scenario within which conflicts between legal rights, resources and agency policies may arise. The National Assistance Act 1948 (Choice of Accommodation) Directions 1992 (Department of Health, 1992) enables an individual to seek a placement in what is called 'preferred accommodation'. Service users' choice is limited by agency policy only in as much as the accommodation has to be available on the local authority's usual terms and conditions. If, however, a local authority policy directed that places be filled in its own accommodation or by block contracts, it would be in breach of the duty to allow a choice of accommodation – if suitable accommodation was available in other sectors. So, for example, if Mrs Khan has been assessed as needing residential care and her preferred choice is Sunny View, which meets the local authority standards, terms and conditions and has places available, then the local authority should not require that its own residential care at Willow Trees is given preference.

Managers have a central role in ensuring organisational or agency policies are implemented. Although policies should be consistent with primary legislation, there may be occasions when managers consider that there is conflict between the two. User choice has a major impact in a mixed economy of care. Even though the cost of accommodation must not be more than the authority would usually expect to pay, this is subject to the overriding requirement that the accommodation should meet the user's individually assessed needs. In such a case, the local authority has a duty to provide suitable accommodation, and this legal duty should override any question of resources.

Just this sort of conflict arose in the case of *R. v. Avon County Council ex parte M* [1994] 2 FLR 1006. The local authority wanted to use a local residential home as accommodation for M. However, the applicant – a young man with learning difficulties – was able to establish that only a placement in his preferred (and more expensive) accommodation with the Home Farm Trust would meet his psychological needs. M. was successful in his claim before the authority's complaints review panel and at subsequent judicial review. A judicial review is a process by which the High Court reviews the lawfulness of decisions made by public bodies; in Scotland it is carried out by the Court of Session.

This case gives a clear example of the law and good practice working in harmony for the benefit of service users. The extent to which the majority of service users have real choice, however, is open to debate.

Proceduralism and assessment

When resources are limited, the way in which procedures are followed (*proceduralism*, also known as 'due process') becomes very important in the allocation of whatever resources are on offer. Procedural propriety is an important aspect of decision making and the focus of scrutiny in judicial review. Certain basic principles apply to assessment and to service allocation. The most obvious is that when there is a duty to make a decision, then a decision must be made. That means something more than applying the agency's eligibility criteria to a case. Where there is a duty to make an individual assessment of need, the individual's need must be assessed separately from issues to do with the availability of resources. Assessment is a service in its own right and should be comprehensive, including not just physical but also psychological, social and developmental needs.

The conflict between interpretations of need and resources was explored by the House of Lords in the Gloucestershire case (*R. v. Gloucestershire County Council, ex parte Barry* [1997] 2 WLR 459), summarised in Box 4.3.

BOX 4.3 The Gloucestershire case

The Gloucestershire case challenged the legality of the local authority's decision to withdraw services because of its financial situation. The challenge was based on the argument that an assessment of need led to a duty to make arrangements for the provision of relevant services, such as domestic cleaning and laundry, previously provided under s. 2 of the Chronically Sick and Disabled Persons Act 1970, irrespective of the local authority's resource situation.

1 The House of Lords decided that local authorities can take resources into account both when assessing need and when deciding what provision to make to meet that need. However, any eligibility criteria that local authorities produce must be reasonable and must not be used to fetter discretion in making decisions in individual cases.

2 Services once provided cannot be withdrawn without a proper reassessment of need. Sending a letter to service users withdrawing services is not a reassessment. However, reassessment can be made against any new criteria the local authority has adopted.

3 A breach of s. 2 gives rise to a personal right of action for breach of statutory duty.

Although eligibility criteria are based on principles of distributive justice, so as to balance a local authority's resources against the number of people in need in its area, the application of such general criteria to individual cases necessarily involves a balancing act.

The individual nature of assessment is emphasised by the availability of legal remedies for breach. This emphasises professional accountability.

Sometimes the Gloucestershire case is misinterpreted to assume that resources are the only relevant criterion, but this is not the case. They are relevant only as part of a balancing exercise in which the severity of a person's disability, their quality of life and the limitations on resources are all taken into account. So, local authorities cannot set eligibility criteria so high that obviously vulnerable people are excluded. Nor can they constrain their discretion by making service allocation decisions according to rigid rules; they should make the process flexible enough to accommodate extraordinary needs. Managers regularly take decisions about access to services and may need to justify their decisions to service users and show that this justification was given. This extract from a manager's diary underlines the impact of agency policy.

SURRINDER'S DIARY

I had a review of a child's place at the family centre. I was
feeling a bit apprehensive, because I would be closing the place
and knew the mother would do anything to keep the child at the
family centre. The child no longer met the criteria for a place. I
was very clear that the child had met all the objectives that were
on the referral. Professionals such as health visitors had been
invited but nobody sent any reports or expressed a view about the
place continuing.

The review took place as planned and the nursery officer read
through the child's progress report. The child's mother was given
the opportunity to comment on her view about the service. She
commented on wanting five full sessions, because she had difficulty
in managing his behaviour.

I explained what were the objectives of his place and that there
was no need for the place to continue because it was partly about
respite for her and this could be achieved from other community
provisions.

Offered the mother the complaints form, if she felt I was being
unfair. She declined and said she would contact the number I had
given her regarding child care information.

In my opinion I felt the review was positive because the child's
needs had been fully met, although it probably was not the
outcome his mother wanted.

This section has outlined the scope and complexity of the legislative
framework governing the provision of care services. Knowledge of the law
is essential in order for managers and agencies to develop policies and
procedures to assist the implementation of legislation. There is a delicate
balance to be drawn between the needs of service users, workers, agencies
and legislation. Managers may face dilemmas when presented with
flexible and subjective definitions used in law and need to be able to
justify the decisions they make.

> **Key points**
>
> - The provision of care services is governed by a complex legal framework.
>
> - Knowledge of the law is essential for managers.
>
> - Organisations will develop policies and procedures to assist the implementation of legislation.
>
> - A balance must be struck between the requirements of service users, workers, agencies and legislation.
>
> - Managers may face dilemmas when making judgements that are subjective yet in line with the law.

4.3 The role and responsibilities of the manager

Managers have a pivotal role to play in balancing and responding to the potentially conflicting needs of their agency, the government, service users and workers. The list of areas of law that impact on a manager's daily role (at the beginning of Section 4.2) gives an indication of the at times competing frameworks within which managers operate.

The tensions between resources, rights and needs can lead to dilemmas for managers at strategic, operational and professional levels. Within the organisation, strategic decisions will define broad areas of policy making, set priorities and allocate budgets. The application of strategic decisions on a day-to-day basis in individual cases is made at the operational level where managers interact with workers and allocate work and tasks.

At the professional level, a manager's background, training and values will shape the decision that is made, even in the context of a multidisciplinary team. Interpretations of the legal position will be influenced by the manager's own background and experience, although this may not be a conscious process.

Staff management is crucial to the implementation of law and policy. Many agency policies, for example, specify the amount and type of supervision managers must provide. Different kinds of law are translated from the abstract to the operational through the actions and decisions of individual managers and workers within organisations. A manager may choose to have a policy item on each team meeting agenda or choose to focus on the legal aspects of a case discussion, for example. For legal rights and legal duties to be discharged certain procedures must be in place. Those called upon to administer the law must understand their legal duties. When new laws or procedures are introduced a manager may want to ensure specific and targeted training is available for workers. In Northern Ireland, for example, the High Court has drawn attention to the misguided judgement of social workers who submit court reports with sections headed 'The Paramount Welfare Interests of the Child'. It has pointed out that this is a standard for the court and not for social workers to apply. Management must separate out statutorily assigned operational duties from principles. As well as ensuring that workers understand and implement relevant legislation and guidance appropriately, managers must implement health and safety and employment law. Staff selection and recruitment is an important part of the manager's task, and one that is very clearly regulated. Most organisations ensure that people who take part in shortlisting and interviewing applicants, for example, have attended fair selection training that covers both employment and discrimination legislation.

At a strategic level, managers must be aware of the legal framework within which their organisations operate. The 'constitutions' of public sector organisations are based on the fundamental duties relating to organisation and service provision laid down in the Local Authority Social Services Act 1970 or the National Health Services Act 1977.

Figure 4.1 (opposite) illustrates the cyclical process of disseminating legally based knowledge between managers and practitioners through various levels in an organisation.

Statutes are phrased in terms of target duties in meeting the needs of the generality of the local population. Because both health and social services are locally based, the actual services delivered vary from one part of the country to another. Individual service users cannot directly enforce such target duties; responsibility for their direction and enforcement rests at the organisational and political level. In recent years government may be perceived as increasingly interventionist and directive in filling out the detail of policy.

Figure 4.1 mentions 'unmet need'. There is a particular difficulty with this phrase because it has two meanings. There is a general meaning: all those needs which might be met, but which are not. There is also a specific meaning: all those needs organisations have a legal duty to meet, or have promised to meet in their policy documents, but have not.

The notion that law is clear and predictable is based on a rationalist perspective. From this perspective law is capable of being used to establish precedents for decision making and behaviour. In reality the law is often ambiguous and provides a framework rather than a blueprint for decision making. Adherence to legally required procedures does not guarantee good or safe decision making in situations – such as child protection – where sound judgement is at a premium (Brandon *et al.*, 2001).

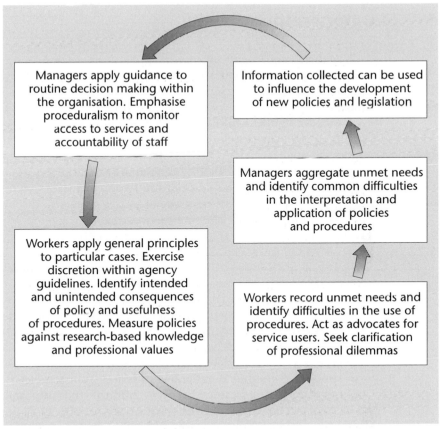

Figure 4.1 **The cycle of knowledge dissemination**

Key points

- Managers in health and care services must resolve the tensions between availability of resources and service users' rights and needs.

- Good staff management is crucial to the implementation of an organisation's policies.

- Adherence to the law, sound judgement and experience are all equally important in decision making.

4.4 Statutory responsibilities

All agencies and organisations have statutory responsibilities and work within legislative frameworks which serve to promote partnerships between and across organisations to a greater or lesser extent. A partnership approach is particularly evident in relation to children. Under Art. 46 (2) of the Children (Northern Ireland) Order 1995 a range of specified agencies (including schools, housing authorities and district councils) are required to comply with a request for assistance from any trust made in respect of a child in need provided the request is compatible with that agency's duties and does not compromise its own functions.

Whether someone is referred to other agencies or whether other agencies contribute to assessments may also be triggered by a legal duty. For example, in s. 47 (3) of the National Health Service and Community Care Act 1990 the social services authority has a duty to invite health and housing authorities to contribute to an assessment where a relevant health or housing need has been identified. In Scotland this provision is in s. 12A (3) (*b*) of the Social Work (Scotland) Act 1968.

The evaluation of risk or whether someone has to be protected may be an explicit statutory duty. For example, there is a duty under the Children Act 1989 to investigate whether a child is suffering or likely to suffer significant harm. Similarly, the Mental Health Act 1983 requires an assessment of whether a patient is suffering from a mental disorder of a nature or degree to warrant their detention in the interests of their own health or welfare, or for the protection of others. Voluntary sector organisations also have responsibilities which are part of statute law. A manager of a crisis telephone service, for example, must ensure that workers understand how their agency expects them to respond to suspicions or allegations of child abuse. Once social services or the police are notified they have a duty to investigate which will override any organisational policy on confidentiality.

The responsibility principle may be a helpful concept to managers in seeking to establish where their agency's legal strategic responsibilities begin and end. So important is this idea of statutory responsibility that a fundamental concept of administrative law has developed around it: the concept of *ultra vires*. So, in judicial review cases an authority will be deemed to be acting *ultra vires* – beyond its powers – and therefore unlawfully if it acts outside the Act of Parliament that lays down its statutory duties. For example, the High Court in Northern Ireland has had reason to criticise a trust's policy to seek freeing orders under Art. 17 of the Adoption (Northern Ireland) Order 1987 for children who are the subject of care orders. The trust's explanation that research demonstrates that long-term foster care is less advantageous than adoption was not the issue for the court. There could not be such a policy because the law requires the needs of each child to be considered individually rather than as the subject of a blanket policy.

Furthermore, administrative discretion in the interpretation of statutory decision-making powers is unlawfully exercised if the decision made is so unreasonable or 'irrational' that no reasonable person or body properly advised would have come to that conclusion. A qualitative measure of reasonableness is thus built into the exercise of decision-making powers.

Within local government the statutory responsibilities assigned to different departments act as internal boundaries of responsibility. Environmental health provides a good example.

Living conditions

Complaints regarding people living in insanitary conditions may come first to social services departments, especially if those people are elderly or mentally ill. Great pressure may be exerted by neighbours or the community to 'do something' about the problem. In fact, the statutory powers of social services authorities in such situations are very limited. If the Mental Health Act 1983 does not apply the local authority has only the provisions of s. 47 of the National Assistance Act 1948. This is phrased in archaic (and ageist) language; it provides for the compulsory removal from home to residential or hospital accommodation, or elsewhere, of persons who are aged or infirm and living in insanitary conditions. This is such a drastic step, with such potential for institutionalisation and loss of autonomy, that it should be considered only in very unusual circumstances and is rarely used.

The British Association of Social Workers has recommended that social workers should only use s. 47 if there is evidence that a person's situation will be improved not only physically, but socially and psychologically, by its use. The continued existence of s. 47 on the statute books after more than 50 years, however, perpetuates the professional dilemma of whether it should be used.

Section 47 of the National Assistance Act gives local authorities no powers to clean accommodation. Those powers are granted under the Public Health Acts and the Environmental Protection Act and would be exercised by the environmental health department (sometimes within the same authority, sometimes not). There are powers of entry by warrant under this legislation, but not for social services. A person's living conditions are an important contribution to their welfare. The conditions may be such that closer co-operation between social services and environmental health departments is indicated. However, public health matters are not the responsibility of a social services department, whose priority is respect for the diverse lifestyles of its service users.

Housing

Boundaries between agencies, organisations or departments may be closely guarded. An example of boundaries being tightly defended to the detriment of social services departments is the provision of housing particularly meeting the needs of homeless families and individuals. Local authorities have a clear gatekeeping role under the Housing Act 1996 in so far as it is their decision who is homeless, who is in priority need and who is not intentionally homeless – all categories of entitlement to the full housing duty under the Act.

There has been a tendency for housing authorities to retreat behind statutory boundaries when refusing to accommodate families deemed to be intentionally homeless. However, social services departments retain a general duty towards children in need in their area under s. 17 of the Children Act 1989. For adults in need of accommodation for reasons of illness or disability, duty stems from Part III of the National Assistance Act 1948. These statutory duties have been interpreted by housing departments so as to require social services departments to finance accommodation for families with children in need or asylum seekers with special needs when their own assessments have disclosed a primary housing need.

These examples from environmental health and housing illustrate the importance to managers of understanding specific and overarching statutory duties in order to know where it is necessary to deny or to accept legal responsibility for the diverse needs their workers may identify at assessment. At a strategic level, negotiation with other agencies is clarified by awareness of the manager's own agency's responsibilities, accepted or potential. None of these agencies' responsibilities extend to keeping all people in all circumstances safe from unforeseeable risks.

Key points

- Organisations have statutory responsibilities, often involving partnerships between them.

- An organisation that oversteps its statutory responsibility is deemed to be acting *ultra vires*.

- Organisations may use discretion in interpreting the law, but resulting decisions must be judged 'reasonable'.

- Within local government statutory responsibility may rest with more than one department.

- Managers must understand the relevant statutory duties in order to know the responsibilities of their agency or department.

4.5 The Human Rights Act 1998

The Human Rights Act 1998 (HRA) may serve to unify some of these competing frameworks. The Act represents an overarching legal regime and requires that all legislation – before and after 1998 – is interpreted in a way compatible with the Act and with the European Convention on Human Rights. The HRA has major implications for controlling the actions of public authorities. Public authorities (not defined in the Act, but including the courts, local authorities, health care bodies and the police among others) will act unlawfully if they contravene the terms of the Act. The Act also provides a sanction against poor practice. A summary of key Articles from the European Convention on Human Rights is given in Box 4.4.

BOX 4.4 The Human Rights Act 1998

(Article 1 is introductory)

Article 2   Right to life

You have the absolute right to have your life protected by law. There are only certain very limited circumstances where it is acceptable for the State to take away someone's life, e.g. if a police officer acts justifiably in self-defence.

Article 3   Prohibition of torture

You have the absolute right not to be tortured or subjected to treatment or punishment which is inhuman or degrading.

Article 4   Prohibition of slavery or forced labour

You have the absolute right not to be treated as a slave or forced to perform certain kinds of labour.

Article 5   Right to liberty and security

You have the right not to be deprived of your liberty – 'arrested or detained' – except in limited cases specified in the Article (e.g. where you are suspected or convicted of committing a crime) and where this is justified by a clear legal procedure.

Article 6   Right to a fair trial

You have the right to a fair and public hearing within a reasonable period of time. This applies to both criminal charges against you, or in sorting out cases concerning your civil rights and obligations. Hearings must be by an independent and impartial tribunal established by law. It is possible to exclude the public from the hearing (though not the judgement) if that is necessary to protect things like national security or public order. If it is a criminal charge you are presumed innocent until proved guilty according to law and have certain guaranteed rights to defend yourself.

Article 7   No punishment without law

You normally have the right not to be found guilty of an offence arising out of actions which at the time you committed them were not criminal. You are also protected against later increases in the possible sentence for an offence.

Article 8   Right to respect for private and family life

You have the right to respect for your private and family life, your home and your correspondence. This right can only be restricted in specified circumstances.

Article 9   Freedom of thought, conscience and religion

You are free to hold a broad range of views, beliefs and thoughts, as well as religious faith. Limitations are permitted only in specified circumstances.

Article 10   Freedom of expression

You have the right to hold opinions and express your views on your own or in a group. This applies even if they are unpopular or disturbing. This right can only be restricted in specified circumstances.

Article 11   Freedom of assembly and association

You have the right to assemble with other people in a peaceful way. You also have the right to associate with other people, which can include the right to form a trade union. These rights may be restricted only in specified circumstances.

Article 12   Right to marry

Men and women have the right to marry and start a family. The national law will still govern how and at what age this can take place.

(Article 13 is not included in the Human Rights Act)

Article 14   Prohibition of discrimination

In the application of Convention rights, you have the right not to be treated differently because of your race, religion, sex, political views or any other status, unless this can be justified objectively. Everyone must have equal access to Convention rights, whatever their status.

(Source: Home Office, 2000b, pp. 3–6)

It is possible to see how Article 3, which prohibits cruel or degrading treatment or punishment, might be applied to repressive regimes in prisons and in psychiatric care. In England and Wales the functioning of Mental Health Act Review Tribunals has been subject to scrutiny under

Article 6, which guarantees a fair hearing in the determination of a person's civil rights. Mental Health Act Review Tribunals consist of three people who hear applications by service users for discharge from formal detention under mental health legislation. However, although the Children Act 1989 has successfully rebuffed challenges based on incompatibility with the Human Rights Act, the Mental Health Act has not. In Scotland Article 6 has been successfully challenged in respect of children appearing before children's hearings (*S. v. The Principal Reporter and the Lord Advocate, 2001*).

Example 4.2 describes the Coughlan case, in which human rights legislation came to the fore and prevented the closure of an NHS residential unit.

EXAMPLE 4.2 The Coughlan case

Pamela Coughlan, a disabled woman, had lived in an NHS residential unit for more than 20 years when her local health authority decided that the resource would have to be closed and patients dispersed elsewhere. Ms Coughlan was referred to the local authority for the provision of accommodation under s. 21 of the National Assistance Act 1948.

Ms Coughlan and other residents successfully challenged the legality of this decision (*R. v. North and East Devon Health Authority, ex parte Coughlan* [1999] 2CCLR 285) on the basis that:

1   The health authority's narrow policy on eligibility for continuing care was *ultra vires* their duty under the NHS and Community Care Act 1990 to provide a 'comprehensive' health service.

2   The local authority's duty under s. 21 of the National Assistance Act 1948 to provide nursing home care was limited to cases where the provision of nursing care was only 'incidental or ancillary' to the provision of residential accommodation. This was not the case here.

3   Ms Coughlan had been promised a 'home for life' by the authority and it was contrary to Article 8 of the European Convention on Human Rights to interfere in this way with her right to family life.

This case illustrates that strategic decision making is constrained by legal powers and duties, and shows the overarching position of human rights legislation. The boundaries between different agency responsibilities are clarified by their legal responsibilities, and it should be possible for agencies to work together in future to ensure that their legal responsibilities work in harmony. As managers from different backgrounds meet more frequently and new partnerships develop, the confrontational use of legislation between agencies is likely to decrease.

> **Key points**
>
> - The Human Rights Act 1998 requires all legislation to be compatible with it and with the European Convention on Human Rights.
>
> - Some Articles can influence the way in which health and care legislation is now interpreted.

4.6 Duties of care

Professional responsibilities towards vulnerable adults and children, and towards the public for their safety, are legally framed in terms of a duty of care. Tension will exist between client empowerment and the protection of the public. Mental health legislation partially acknowledges this by enabling compulsory admission to take place either for the health or welfare of the individual, or for the protection of the public.

Risk assessments based on public protection will bring together agencies outside the normal confines of the Data Protection Act 1998 to develop risk management plans. Actions for breach of statutory duty through non-performance or negligent performance are limited. In *X X (Minors)* v. *Bedfordshire County Council* [1995] 3 A ll ER 353 the House of Lords refused as a matter of public policy to hold a local authority liable for breach of statutory duty in failing to take into its care children who had been known, over a number of years, to have suffered substantial abuse at home. The European Court, however, has recently indicated the need for a change in domestic law by its finding that the UK had failed adequately to protect the children from harm and had failed in their obligation to provide an adequate remedy in breach of Articles 3 and 13 (*Z and others* v. *United Kingdom* [2001] 2 FLR 612).

Protection of vulnerable adults is legally less well developed, as the following example illustrates. There is no legislative equivalent of the Children Act to guide decision making in adult cases.

EXAMPLE 4.3 Difficult decisions

Frances James is the manager of a local authority residential unit for people with learning difficulties. Helen Marple has been resident at the unit for six months since leaving her residential school. Helen is 19 years old. She has no speech, but communicates with staff through gestures, with some use of objects of reference. She is very affectionate towards staff and other residents.

> Frances is aware that Helen was removed from home under a care order at the age of 14 because of neglect. There were also allegations of sexual abuse made at that time. Since Helen was admitted to the unit, her parents, who live nearby, have resumed contact with her and visit twice weekly. They showed no interest in visiting Helen during her time in care. Helen always seems pleased to see them and so far all visits have been confined to the unit.
>
> One day, Helen's father asks if arrangements can be made for Helen to visit their home the following weekend. The family comprises Mr and Mrs Marple and two sons who are in their twenties, neither of whom has visited Helen at the unit. Mr Marple says that a family party is planned and they want Helen to be part of it.

This case illustrates the difficulty of having to make decisions in an area in which there is little legal guidance. Both Helen and her father have rights under the HRA. Because Helen is over 18 there is no statutory framework to define what sort of issues may legitimately be taken into account in determining what is in her best interests. This is a matter of common law in which the courts take the lead. However, the courts have shown that they are willing to protect vulnerable adults where there are identified gaps in the law. There is an obvious tension, however, in the case of Helen with Article 8 of the European Convention and respect for family life.

Transparency in decision making is promoted by the Data Protection Act 1998, which is itself a response to the European Convention's requirement of a right to privacy, previously not well developed in domestic law. Under the Data Protection Act individuals gain rights in terms of both access to files and a statutory basis for the protection of confidentiality. The Act affects how records are written and maintained: under s. 14 an individual can apply for the rectification or destruction of erroneous data. Does this mean information that is inaccurate, or just unproven? If something is unproven it may none the less be accurate. The fact than an application for a care order has been unsuccessful shows that the case is unproven and the threshold for intervention unmet. It does not necessarily follow that the evidence on which that application was based has been shown to be false.

These questions illustrate the tensions between welfare and justice, and the potential conflict between legal rights, duty of care and social work practice (Timms, 1995; King and Trowell, 1992; O'Halloran, 1999). Timms questions whether upholding the rights of adults is necessarily conducive to outcomes which are in the long-term interests of children. In England and Wales the legal process itself recognises this dilemma in so far as the combination in care proceedings of legal representatives, to uphold rights, and the children's guardian (guardian ad litem), to advise on the best interests of the child, seeks to strike a balance between justice and welfare. The invocation of legal proceedings and the involvement of legal advisers, however, is a brief episode often in a much longer-term process which is about safeguarding children and vulnerable people from harm and promoting their welfare.

> **Key points**
>
> - Health and care services have a duty of care to the public.
> - They can face legal action if they do not fulfil their statutory duties.
> - Little legal guidance is available with respect to vulnerable adults.

4.7 Facing challenges

Facing a legal challenge or an inquiry is possibly the most difficult situation a manager in the care services will have to face. Managers need both knowledge and confidence as well as the skills to analyse and deal with the situation and how to survive it. This may involve: dealing with complaints from service users against members of staff or the organisation as a whole; giving evidence to public inquiries; supporting staff who feel they are being treated unfairly; implementing disciplinary procedures. The manager needs to consider all aspects of the situation and attempt to anticipate potential difficulties. Difficulties may stem from organisational structures, policies and procedures that may not be flexible enough to deal with specific situations. Difficulties may be highly personal, and managers need to ensure staff are supported during an inquiry, as illustrated by Example 4.4.

EXAMPLE 4.4 Managing the past and the future

Carl, a mental health service user known by most of a local mental health team, killed himself by jumping off a bridge close to the team office. The team manager was required to provide evidence to the inquiry and produce materials required by the inquiry team. This involved many meetings with senior members of the agency, the managers of other workers involved with Carl and legal advisers.

The manager was also aware of the impact of the inquiry on the whole team, not just the individual worker involved. Extra team meetings were organised to give the team an opportunity to talk openly of their fears and concerns about the inquiry. There was also an opportunity for team members to share their feelings of loss – most of them knew Carl.

> Some time after the event the manager arranged for a staff development session on risk assessment. The session served both to recognise the good practice within the team in risk assessment, and to present up-to-date research into models of risk assessment.

As well as dealing with challenges within teams, managers may deal with challenges related to service provision. Social services departments have specific responsibilities towards children and people with disabilities. These legal duties are often discharged through the use of service providers in the voluntary and private sectors. This is a trend which is also seen increasingly in health, particularly in intermediate care. It is unclear then where legal responsibility lies if things go wrong. The situation is a complex one because it is accepted that statutory agencies may impose quality requirements in contracts that are more stringent than those generally imposed on relevant services by regulations and guidance.

Take residential care for example, where the Registered Homes Act 1984 and regulations impose fairly broad minimum standards. The Care Standards Act 2000 and the Regulation of Care (Scotland) Act 2001 are intended to provide, among other things, a comprehensive system of regulation and inspection of residential and domiciliary services. Penalties for breaching these standards range from criminal prosecution to withdrawal of registration. Specific contractual terms for placements in registered homes may be more precise and more stringent about the quality of the service to be provided. Independent providers may thus find themselves contractually liable in circumstances where no breaches of the regulatory legislation have occurred. However, the authority should not be liable for things done outside the terms of the contract, in the same way that an employer is not liable for the actions of employees which are outside the course of their employment.

Challenges may come from within the organisation as well as from the outside. The Public Interest Disclosure Act 1998–9 seeks to protect employees from discrimination as a result of 'blowing the whistle' on their organisation, or individuals within it, through amendments to employment law. The organisation Public Concern at Work (Ells and Dehn, 2001) runs a free legal helpline for people concerned about serious malpractice in the workplace. It also offers professional and practical help to organisations on how to encourage responsibility and accountability in the workplace, and conducts research and informs developments in public policy.

Where workers reasonably suspect malpractice they will be protected from victimisation if they raise the matter with the employer in good faith. The first stage is the recognition of malpractice. The following case is an example.

EXAMPLE 4.5 What to do?

Phillip Frost is manager of a day centre for older people run by a national charity. Florence Wills is a service user who lives alone and has no family. She is a retired antiques dealer and is known to be quite well-off. Florence has a diagnosis of Alzheimer's disease. She seems particularly fond of Annie Taylor, the deputy manager. Annie is helping Florence put together a life history book.

In the course of their work Florence tells Annie that she now has fewer mementos at home than previously because she has sold quite a few to Phillip over the past year 'at a small discount, because he is so good to me here'. Annie is aware that Florence no longer knows the value of money. She is also aware that Phillip is a major fundraiser for the charity for which they both work.

The Public Interest Disclosure Act 1999 sets out a simple framework to promote responsible whistleblowing by:

- reassuring workers that silence is not the only safe option
- providing strong protection for workers who raise concerns internally
- reinforcing and protecting the right to report concerns to key regulators
- protecting more public disclosures provided that there is a valid reason for going wider and that the particular disclosure was reasonable
- helping to ensure that organisations respond by addressing the message rather than the messenger and resist the temptation to cover up serious malpractice.

(Ells and Dehn, 2001, p. 108)

What should Annie do with the information that Florence has given to her? What support can she expect to receive from the organisation? First of all, there should be clear guidance within agency policy and procedure manuals for staff who find themselves in this type of situation. Some organisations will also run training sessions on dealing with concerns such as those which Annie may have. Annie needs to raise her concerns with her line manager, or the manager above if Phillip is her line manager. She should then be informed of the results of any investigation. This may be a difficult time for all concerned and so the organisation will need support systems that take the needs of everyone into account. For example, if Annie or Phillip are transferred while investigations take place this will have an effect on Florence, who might not be able to continue with her life history book.

Sometimes whistleblowing will occur as a result of an unresolved tension between the agency's interpretation of legislation, or of good practice in its implementation, and staff perspectives on its implementation. For the manager, it is worthwhile anticipating, and in some sense legitimating, this conflict through open discussion of resource constraints, staff training needs and formal legal advice. Managers themselves are not immune from such pressures and will also need access to knowledge, advice, feedback on performance and support throughout any whistle-blowing process.

Legal challenges and reviews

Some conflicts cannot be contained within the privacy of the organisation, and perceived shortcomings will be subject to public scrutiny. Formal means by which individual decisions can be challenged are complaints procedures, applications to the Ombudsman, judicial review and public inquiries. Remedies sought will range from an apology to a change in policy. Such challenges can be reframed positively as opportunities to reflect upon the effectiveness of the organisation in meeting its legal responsibilities.

For example, Part 8 of *Working Together in Child Protection* (Department of Health, 1991b) required case review reports to be produced on child deaths in each area, which were then subject to composite review by the Area Child Protection Committee. Brandon *et al.* (2001) analysed ten such reports submitted to the Welsh Office between April 1966 and December 1998. Specific objectives were to identify recurring themes in the reports, identify action plans arising from reviews and highlight any actions that should be taken to address issues raised by the reports.

Perennial issues following similar reviews in adult and children's services have been the need for greater multidisciplinary co-ordination, problems with professionals' assessment skills, thresholds of concern and the inadequacy of recording. It is worth remembering, however, that reviews will also highlight areas of good practice in very difficult situations. The impact on staff of going through this process is well recognised:

> The dual notions of culpability and accountability for decision-making are at the crux of the review process. This inevitably entails scrutinising the competence of all personnel connected with the case directly and indirectly. Although most Review Reports highlight where mistakes were made, they generally avoid any clear allocation of individual blame.

> Nevertheless it is imperative to recognise the potential impact that a child's death and the process of review has on individual professionals. Staff need to be supported throughout and reassured that instead of a negative and critical assessment of the work undertaken, positive outcomes can be achieved.
>
> (Brandon *et al.*, 2001, p. 9)

The report concludes that the role of procedures is limited and that competent multidisciplinary work has to be firmly grounded in competent and confident practice in one's own profession. Access to new knowledge from research and the ability to interpret and critically appraise the usefulness of various studies are seen as essential to this process. A similar analysis of inquiries relating to mental health was undertaken by Reith (1998).

Helping workers to make sense of the mass of material collected in any individual case is an important managerial task. Ironically, the implementation and maintenance of procedure-driven practice is often a response to such inquiries. Such methods of working may lead to defensive practice and this in turn prevents workers from moving beyond the basic task of information collection. They are not then able to reach a level of analysis where they may identify patterns in events and behaviour and the implications for a child. The best response thus appears to be the use of reflective practice to inform actions.

What is it like to be a manager caught up in an inquiry? What support can be offered? Sound legal advice will be needed on what to expect in terms of both substantive questions to be asked and the procedure that will be followed. An ability to articulate their own agency's legal responsibilities and procedures, including recording, should not just be a response to an inquiry, but should, as argued above, be inherent in the responsibilities of managers to set out the agenda for their work.

Key points

- Managers need to respond appropriately to complaints, inquiries and whistleblowing.

- Time for reflection on practices, processes and procedures is essential.

- When voluntary and private service providers are used, it is not always clear where responsibility lies.

- Managers must have a thorough knowledge of their organisation's responsibilities and procedures.

4.8 Conclusion

This chapter has identified some of the key components of the legal framework as it applies to health and social care services. It has been argued that implementation of law presents managers and practitioners alike with challenges and dilemmas in seeking to ensure equitable services within resource constraints while meeting legal requirements. There are few clear-cut answers in law, and managers must live with uncertainty, but the law provides an essential foundation on which to build effective professional and management practice.

The fact that services operate within a legal and increasingly structured framework does not detract from the fundamental need for managers to be supervisors of professional good practice as well as monitors of procedural compliance. Although the law can guide action and emphasises the importance of clarity in decision making, it rarely resolves professional dilemmas about the proper allocation of resources, the use of partnership or compulsory action, or the proper objectives of intervention. Legal challenges should not be seen as threats to autonomy, but as opportunities to reassess the interrelationship between strategic, operational and professional goals. Managers in health and social care are centrally placed as interpreters – between the devil and the deep blue sea perhaps – of these different areas of concern.

Adherence to principles of good practice supports reflective practitioners. The opportunity to pursue good practice may, however, be jeopardised by structural constraints within and outside the organisation. The fulfilment of statutory duties depends on adequate resources and sufficient staffing. Challenges to the organisation necessitate a reappraisal of strategy, operational policies and professional competence. Fulfilment of externally imposed duties thus requires the organisation to reappraise itself and examine causes and effects of actions. Legislation does not make decisions: it provides the framework within which managers and practitioners make decisions.

Part 2 The Contexts of Care

Introduction

There are many answers to the question 'What is the context of care?' A hospital or nursing home, a drop-in centre or playgroup, a hostel or group house, a pavement or front room are a few of the environments where care is offered. They are all places – some are buildings, others are locations – where people may experience care services. Other answers to this question would focus on contrasts between faceless and regimented or flexible and responsive statutory services or local projects. Organisations and agencies are not bounded by place: they have cultures, histories and structures that also influence the people who work in them and the form of care provided.

Quality forms a link between these contexts. Quality can be accessible and well-decorated buildings, as well as respectful and responsive care provision. The contexts of quality, however, may also be open to debate. Who defines quality and what it involves? Service users? Managers? Government? The contexts in which care is received, delivered and managed are influenced by many factors. Part 2 looks in turn at organisations, caring environments and quality: three interconnected aspects of context.

In Chapter 5 'Managers and their organisations', Seden examines the influence of the organisational context, looking at the structures and cultures of organisations providing social care. The extent of a manager's power and influence is related to organisational structure and shaped by organisational culture. Here Seden argues that an understanding of the ways in which organisations function can help managers to be more effective in carrying out their roles and tasks. Practice-led managers use their knowledge and experience of the front line to influence the approach taken in their team or unit. They also look for opportunities to have an effect further up the management chain and across organisations.

Although a context might be solid – like a building – it has different meanings for the people who use it. The impact of physical space is the focus for Chapter 6 'Managing environments' by Peace and Reynolds, who note that any one environment may be multifunctional. Taking an innovative approach to management, they argue that a residential care home, for example, may simultaneously be a place for living for the residents, working for staff and managers and visiting for relatives and other professionals. The atmosphere in a care home makes a critical difference to the experience of service users who live there. The authors review how the environmental factors that influence care may be managed and how the careful design and use of space can contribute to improved quality of life in the management of care. Peace and Reynolds also consider relationships between people, places and quality, recognising the impact of the manager on caring environments. A focus on practice here emphasises the role of the manager in drawing out debates over values and best practice to help care workers feel supported and confident about the care they provide.

Quality is perhaps the most abstract of the contexts discussed in this part, yet it is the one that is most often quantified and measured. In Chapter 7 'Quality matters', Walker, Murray and Atkinson look at quality and how to promote it across various contexts and at different levels. They cover not only the inspectorial end of quality assurance (standard setting, inspection and regulation) but also the developmental aspects of quality and the practicalities of implementing it on the ground. How can agencies and their workers, charged with 'implementing quality', turn the experience into a useful and empowering one? Care staff can find the language of quality and its 'business' connotations alienating; service users may find this too, perhaps to an even greater degree. The authors draw on views about quality from managers in different settings and note different aspects: the quality of life of the people who use their services; the quality of the experience of using the service; and the quality of the workforce and how valued and valuing people are in their work. Formal reviews, inspections or audits often underpin the evaluation of quality. Managers may have their own more informal measures: for instance personal feedback from service users and the community, or staff retention rates and what staff who leave go on to do. Who checks that the frontline manager is right about the people who use services, and what constitutes good quality from their point of view? Practice-led managers draw on their own experience of good practice in order to be reflective (and responsive). The outcome of the service for the service users is the most important aspect of quality, which links with managing for good outcomes, the subject of Chapter 11.

Chapter 5
Managers and their organisations

Janet Seden

5.1 Introduction

Organisations matter to managers of care services because they are the context or environment for everything the managers do. The importance of this is shown in the exchange of correspondence between two managers in *Community Care* magazine in Examples 5.1 and 5.2. A correspondent, who wished to remain anonymous, wrote under the title 'Sick organisations create stress' (Example 5.1).

EXAMPLE 5.1 Stress in the front line

Your article on early retirement ('Under the Weather', 24 August) raises some interesting points, notably the variation between different local authorities in rates of ill-health retirement.

What the article fails to recognise is the impact of sick organisations on their employees. Social work is a responsible and sensitive occupation, undertaken with vulnerable clients. It requires organisational structures which promote support. Most fundamentally it requires managers who can be reflective and who do not persecute and blame their front line staff.

Over two years I saw rational management break down leading to high stress levels among the front line staff. This stemmed in particular from the appointment of certain personalities into positions of responsibility who could not manage their own anxiety but persecuted others instead. The ruthless pursuit of structural change and the implementation of new processes – often dictated by government policy – creates a dangerous climate as work tensions filter through to clients in the form of haphazard and brusque practice.

I was on the receiving end of such practices and left to pursue my career elsewhere. I and other colleagues retired through ill-health and all of us are now working successfully in healthier organisations. Our efforts to raise our concerns about the bullying in our social services department with councillors, occupational health officers and management were met with a conspiracy of silence.

Sadly, it is not the weakest in the organisation who are likely to leave in these circumstances but the healthiest and strongest who refuse to submit. Therefore there is a serious loss of the ablest staff.

Those over 50 may gladly seize the opportunity to leave organisations which are then depleted of their experience and their often more balanced approach to caseload. It is noteworthy that politicians, lawyers and doctors are often valued as being at their most capable at this age. Why then does local government see no value in the skills and experience of its older employees?

If the consequence of sick organisational structures is the ill-health retirement of front line staff who recover after leaving, then the answer is to address the root cause and not to victimise stressed front line employees.

(Source: *Community Care*, 21 September 2000, p. 16)

Three weeks later, Jane Buckley, another manager, responded as shown in Example 5.2.

EXAMPLE 5.2 Managing with humanity

The letter on the impact of stress on the social work profession (Letters, 21 September) touched on my feelings enormously.

... I have seen colleagues both survive and crumble from experiences such as those outlined in that letter.

However, for those of us who survive, and stay, there are often more positive experiences. Those who opt for management roles are able to retain their social work values and ethics, along with a sense of their humanity. There are managers who do juggle and balance the pressures of constant and often superficial changes in order to support the frontline case holders. Those managers often take their share of the stress and are sensitive and caring to their staff's bad times.

So, although that letter made valid points, perhaps it would be more constructive for the profession to flag up the 'good guys' as well as those with less integrity.

(Source: *Community Care*, 12 October 2000, pp. 16–17)

These letters highlight an important aspect of organisational life: the need for organisational structures that support and organisational cultures that enable. Without them it is difficult for managers and their staff to maintain their ability to provide services for people and care for staff. It may be less a matter of some managers not having integrity and more the degree of understanding the manager holds of the organisation and the individual's ability to operate in an ambiguous and fast-changing environment. The most destructive individuals are often those most in need of help. These letters also show that the impact of organisational changes applied insensitively can sometimes make managing a daunting experience for frontline managers.

It is essential to know how an employing organisation works in order to get things done. Therefore, first I shall consider some aspects of the structure and culture of the organisations in which social care managers work. As the power and influence of managers are closely related to structure and culture, this is discussed next. Finally, some aspects of working across agency boundaries in partnership are considered.

There is a substantial academic literature about organisations. Much of this is generic theory but there have been some applications specifically to social care.

The aims of this chapter are to:

- explore some understandings of the organisational context in which managers work
- consider ways of being effective in an organisation when in the role of manager
- introduce concepts that are relevant to working across organisational boundaries.

First, here are some thoughts about what is meant by 'organisation' and 'organisational theory'.

5.2 What is an organisation?

Theorists about organisations first focused their attention on identifying the best organisational structure for the workplace (Taylor, 1911). There followed a literature which acknowledged the importance of good human relationships in organisations for achieving an environment where motivated workers produced better outcomes (Mayo, 1933). More recent writing has recognised the complexity of organisational structures (Mintzberg, 1981, 1992, 1994; Brody, 1993; Hales, 1993; Handy, 1993, 1995; Morgan, 1997; Kakabadse et al., 1998; Arnold et al., 1998).

These authors offer a variety of organisational structural models and explanations for the way organisations and the people within them behave. It seems no one now doubts the complexity of the subject if studied in depth. Morgan (1997) suggests that if you truly want to understand an organisation, it is much wiser to start from the premise that organisations are complex, ambiguous and paradoxical. Similarly, the management theorist Charles Handy says:

> I came to the study of people in organizations expecting certainty and absolute knowledge in the behavioural sciences. I anticipated that I would find laws governing the behaviour of people and of organisations as sure and immutable as the laws of the physical sciences. I was disappointed. I found concepts and ideas abounding. I found, too often, ponderous confirmation of the obvious and weighty investigation of

trivia. But the underlying unalterable laws were not there, organizations remained only patchily efficient, and the most exciting of the ideas did not always work.

(Handy, 1993, p. 13)

Handy acknowledges that understanding your organisation might not be simple. There are many variables at work, and theories about organisational design do not always fit neatly with people's experiences. However, he is enthusiastic in his continued study of the ways in which organisations work and suggests that, while an organisation is constructed of many variables, the manager who understands these will be able:

- To identify the key variables in any situation;
- To predict the probable outcomes of any changes in the variables;
- To select the ones [the manager] can and should influence.

(Handy, 1993, p. 17)

Morgan (1997) similarly suggests that the key to managerial competence is the ability to read and understand what is happening in the organisation. In summary, organisations are many things at once. They are complex and they involve structures, cultures, roles and tasks. They are multifaceted and they are paradoxical. Trying to understand your own organisation and those of other professionals, too, is a complex but exciting task. If managers want to be more effective in a management role they will need to understand not only their organisations but also those of their partner agencies.

There are many ways to define an organisation, as the literature on organisations shows. For the purposes of this chapter, our working definition of an organisation is that given in Box 5.1.

BOX 5.1 Organisation – a working definition

An organisation can be described as a way of arranging a set of people and resources together to achieve certain goals.

The system that results will have both formal ways of doing things (rules and structure) and informal ways of acting and behaving (culture). The people in the organisation will have varying degrees of power and control to make decisions, use resources and carry out tasks. These elements – structure, culture, human and material resources – work together to create the workplace environment. An organisation is experienced as a living, dynamic and interactive place. This is shaped in turn by its relationship to external factors such as other organisations, the clientele, law, social policy and public opinion.

These key elements – structure, culture, power and the organisation's relationship to external factors – are the four main considerations in this chapter.

Key points

- Organisations are complex, ambiguous and paradoxical.

- Managers need to understand their organisation and those of their partner agencies to be effective.

- An organisation can be defined as a way of arranging a set of people and resources together to achieve certain goals.

5.3 Organisations in social care

Traditionally, organisations in health and social care have been based on a bureaucratic model of a hierarchical organisational structure. Each post carries specific responsibilities and the person occupying it should have the relevant skills. As shown in Figure 5.1, the basic shape of many organisations is pyramidal, consisting of roles, usually represented as little boxes, occupied by individuals, with the head at the top, middle managers in between and frontline managers and their staff at the bottom. The bigger the organisation gets, the taller the pyramid becomes, which is why some of the reorganisations of the late 20th century sought to cut out layers of middle managers.

Weber (1947) identified seven main characteristics of bureaucracies, which are listed in Box 5.2 (overleaf).

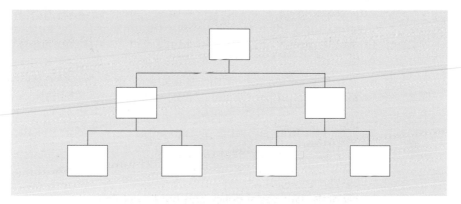

Figure 5.1 **A hierarchical organisational structure**

> ## BOX 5.2 Characteristics of pure bureaucracies
>
> 1 A division of labour in which authority and responsibility is clearly defined for each member, and is officially sanctioned.
>
> 2 Offices or positions are organized into a hierarchy of authority resulting in a chain of command.
>
> 3 All organizational members are to be selected on the basis of technical qualifications through formal examinations or by virtue of training and education.
>
> 4 Officials are to be appointed, not elected.
>
> 5 Administrators work for fixed salaries and are career officers.
>
> 6 The administrative official does not own the administered unit but is a salaried official.
>
> 7 The administrator is subject to strict rules, discipline, and controls regarding the official duties.
>
> (Source: Weber, 1947, cited by Handy, 1999, p. 129)

Social services departments, benefits agencies, hospitals, national voluntary agencies and many other organisations involved in social care use variously modified forms of a bureaucratic model. There are many advantages to a well-run bureaucracy. Clear rules and procedures help the people who implement them and make processes visibly fair. They may provide a single point of access that makes it easier for people wanting services to make contact. Workers know what is expected of them in order to gain promotion: they can expect staff development opportunities in the course of their career because this is also to the organisation's advantage. There are limitations to the bureaucratic model in social care: Coulshed and Mullender (2001, pp. 30–1) identify the following.

- It is best suited to routine, stable and unchanging tasks – the focus in social care on people inevitably means unpredictability and a need for flexibility.

- The question of professional autonomy – for instance for social workers – means that some bring an expectation of the authority to make specialised and complex decisions. A hybrid term of 'bureau-professionalism' is sometimes applied to the social work context, although there is debate about whether managerialism has superseded this model by imposing centralised control.

- There are many competing stakeholders beyond the immediate employing organisation – including professional organisations, employers' organisations, service users and carers, and partner organisations.

- The increasing diversity of activities and clientele requires greater complexity in the shape of the organisation. Social services departments may sprout side-shoots in the form of specialist teams, or workers are placed in integrated teams with health care trusts – creating complexity of managerial supervision and accountability.

There is an increasing array of different types of organisational structure that do not conform to a bureaucratic model, or that have little pockets of activity that are differently organised. For instance, is a residential care home, where residents need to feel 'at home', best conceptualised as a bureaucracy? Or do the residents form part of the organisation, perhaps organising some of its functions themselves? The larger organisation responsible for its management may well be a bureaucracy, but a registered manager may operate a different kind of structure within the home.

In the voluntary sector there are organisational types that are very different from mainstream models: some where managers as such do not exist. Camphill communities in Scotland, for people with learning disabilities, were established to create and maintain an environment where the economic, social and spiritual lives of the community complemented each other. At the outset, all those working in Camphill communities did so not as a job in the usual sense of the word but as a way of life. A community of co-workers was created who shared all the work that had to be done – teaching, caring, household tasks, gardening, and so on. Everyone who lived and worked in the communities was seen and treated as a 'co-equal' with the result that there was no hierarchical management structure.

Other collaborative or collective ways of working, established for instance in women's refuges or by organisations run by service users, similarly may lack visible managers or rotate the management roles. This can cause difficulties for outsiders looking for a point of liaison and influence. A non-hierarchical organisation still needs to have ways of organising to take decisions, and to co-ordinate and allocate activities, but it may involve more people or a more diverse cross-section of people in these managerial processes.

Changing organisations

All health and social care managers are likely to experience change and flux in how their organisations are structured in the course of their careers. For example, a manager about to retire from children's services may have experienced both specialist children's departments and generic field teams. They may have seen commissioner and provider arrangements replace directly managed services in their own organisation; children's homes created and closed; and services reshaped with the move to strengthen assessment, fostering and adoption services. Adult services' workers will have seen a major shift away from institutional care towards more flexible and networked community arrangements. Organisational structures have been affected by the aims and objectives held by government at any given point in time. Managers find themselves responding and being positioned, as Clarke and Newman (1997) suggest, by tensions between central control and the dispersal of power.

Many managers experience this tension as a practice dilemma. Managers' roles in social care can change with organisational shifts. While this is a challenge for frontline managers (Henderson and Seden, 2000), some managers can identify strategies for coping with the interface between the demands of strategic organisational change and the operational practice task. One manager we interviewed said:

> I can see the importance of change and you learn from it. It is important that change builds on the assets of the past and it is important to acknowledge the value of what people have done. I can remember in restructuring when a number of new male managers came to the family centre I was in then and said 'You need to change'. It remains an example of how not to treat staff ... I felt awful and remember how I felt. It is important to acknowledge feelings and to help people by valuing what they have achieved: from that and their strengths change can come. People need time to look at what they are afraid of and to go through change with their feelings acknowledged. The psychological part of managing change is important, so is vision and the ability to analyse how goals might be achieved.
>
> ('Under-eights' project manager)

Other managers interviewed by Henderson and Seden also identify the importance of taking staff with you, timing the way information is given and making sure that where new skills are needed training is given. Fast change is often a feature of the organisations that provide social care.

Fit for purpose?

Organisational theorists say there is a range of ways of structuring organisations to get things done, and a variety of ways of viewing their functions, but that there is no one best way of organising the workplace. This is best expressed by Mintzberg (1981), who says that what is most important about any organisation is not whether it is based on the latest theoretical model but, rather, whether it is the best 'fit' for its aims and objectives. Managers of care services will want to know which structures are useful for the task of organising social care and which are best left to car manufacturing or some other production process.

Mismatches between an agency's goals and its structure can cause tensions for managers, workers and service users alike. You might have experienced this while trying to find a service for yourself or a relative. Or perhaps you wished you had the power to change the way agencies manage social care. For example, the dominance of professional bureaucracies in the social care field in the 1970s and 1980s created some particular dilemmas for the professionals working within them. Such organisations have a hierarchical (top-down) line management structure, fixed rules and procedures for worker activity and often several layers of management between practitioner and chief executive. They are designed to manage and promote the personal welfare of citizens and establish mechanisms whereby eligibility for services is assessed, so that resources are shared out equitably. Formal procedures and systems of accountability have to exist, through committee structures and layers of management to elected political bodies. The core activities of these service organisations are still the relationships between staff and clients, although many staff never meet the service users.

Hasenfeld (1983) suggests that clients and frontline workers may lack power in professional bureaucracies because the organisation of the agency mediates the series of transactions by which resources and services are exchanged. This power advantage which large organisations have enables them to exercise considerable control over the lives of recipients of their services. The service users of such large organisations have argued that even frontline managers are too far removed from the impact of their decisions (service user consultations).

The bureaucratic structure usually contains mechanisms to challenge decisions but these may seem so complex that workers lose confidence in their effectiveness. There may be consultation with workers but little organisational flexibility to incorporate workers' views. This may result in an informal network of consensus between workers and clients which can subvert or side-step formal procedures and replace them with informal ones. Lipsky (1980) describes social workers in large public agencies as 'street-level bureaucrats' because often they make flexible decisions in practice that are not altogether in line with published policy:

> the decisions of street-level bureaucrats, the routines they establish, and the devices they invent to cope with uncertainties and work pressures, effectively *become* the public policies they carry out. I argue that public policy is not best understood as made in legislatures or top-floor suites of high-ranking administrators, because in important ways it is actually made in the crowded offices and daily encounters of street-level workers. I point out that policy conflict is not only expressed as the contention of interest groups but is also located in the struggles between individual workers and citizens who challenge or submit to client processing.
>
> ... At best, street-level bureaucrats invent benign modes of mass processing that more or less permit them to deal with the public fairly, appropriately, and successfully. At worst, they give in to favoritism, stereotyping and routinizing – all of which serve private or agency purposes.
>
> (Lipsky, 1980, p. xii)

Lipsky and Hasenfeld both illustrate the way in which large bureaucratic organisations structure the delivery of services to the public. They analyse how formal structures are influenced by informal arrangements that develop between the public, practitioners and frontline managers, who interpret rules and exercise discretion in decision making within written policies and procedures. Thus working practices develop 'between the lines' of written procedures, as described in Example 5.3 – an informal arrangement in home care that is not unusual (see Chapter 1).

EXAMPLE 5.3 The home care worker's assessment

Some home care workers will not stick rigidly to care plans designed to meet the needs assessed by social workers. Consider the following example.

Mrs Lewis has been assessed as needing help to get up, get dressed and have breakfast each morning. The time allowed for this is 30 minutes. Mrs Lewis does find it very difficult indeed to get up and get ready but what she wants is to have her windows cleaned and bits of housework done. The local authority does not provide such a service. Mrs Lewis sets her alarm clock very early and takes about two hours to get up. When the home care worker arrives she does as Mrs Lewis asks and tidies the house. A clean and tidy house has always been a priority for Mrs Lewis. The worker provides what Mrs Lewis says she wants, not what she is assessed as needing. The social worker is aware that this is happening.

(Source: service user consultations)

Large structured organisations may leave managers facing in two directions at the same time. On the one hand, they are responsible for mediating rules and procedures designed to produce routine transactions. On the other hand, they are professionally supervising caseworkers who, together with their clients, may ask for discretion and a more flexible response. In large bureaucracies, frontline managers form the link between the public, the practitioners and the layers of strategic management to whom they are accountable. Balancing these demands is a challenging task, as this manager commented:

> It is a dilemma – because you want to provide the best service you possibly can for [the service user], particularly that person who's got the need at that particular time. You are often pulled between getting an operational plan or your team plan developed and sent up to your senior manager or actually dealing with that particular problem. You (and I think a lot of managers do this) put the client first and then usually do the other work at home or at the weekend. Because you can't choose between one or the other, you've got to do both. And it's sort of balancing both of those things.
>
> (Manager consultations)

However, large, formally structured organisations also offer benefits for users, workers and managers alike. The explicit formal rules make role accountabilities clear. Arguably, this makes the use of resources visible and fairer. The mission statement will reflect governmental intentions and the agency can be monitored and evaluated against its own systems. The check that this can put on individual discretion and partiality means that service users are (in theory at least) advised what their rights are and, therefore, can know better when and how to complain about a service or appeal about a decision. Kitchener *et al.* (2000) argue that, following scandals in social care, a more bureaucratic approach has been seen as a way of regulating and monitoring the quality of care, protecting service users from the whims of discretion and abuse. However, their data illustrate that such managerial control has been implemented unevenly in social services departments, because of practitioners' preferences for autonomy.

It is sometimes difficult for an individual to influence the structure of a large organisation based on role (except by subversion). Consequently, the delivery of services can seem inflexible. Burton (1998) predicts that managers who have personal authority, values and principles at the core of their management activity will at some time find themselves in conflict with their organisations. Within large and seemingly inflexible organisations, there are often sub-groups and teams, which operate on other models, where the manager can be more influential. Also, cultural norms grow up where the rules are subtly changed in line with the values and beliefs of the practitioners about their role with service users. Individuals can be very influential in shaping the cultures of their organisations. The manager who has a remit from the agency to direct work and allocate resources has power as well as influence to shape the culture of the workplace. The manager's influence on culture is the topic of the next section.

Key points

- Many social care organisations have characteristics of bureaucracies, including a hierarchical structure, clear-cut roles and an emphasis on rules and procedures. There are advantages as well as disadvantages to this.

- Managers need to give and get support at times of organisational change.

- The interpretation of rules and procedures can give managers opportunities to exercise some discretion. This can create dilemmas but it also offers managers a source of influence on the culture of their organisations.

5.4 The culture of organisations

Structure and culture in organisations are two linked concepts. Embedded in the structure of an organisation there is usually a mission statement or set of policy directives about the values of the organisation. Culture can be defined as the underlying values, beliefs and principles that underpin an organisation's management system. In other words, it is the way things are done: the behaviours, the patterns of delivering services that exist in any organisation, agency, office or team. While structure influences culture, it is observable that just as families are all different, so the culture of one social care team or group will include key differences from that in another team or group in the same organisation. The culture will have developed from the shared experiences and traditions of the way the group has established its norms. New staff are often socialised into this culture through explicit or implicit rituals: for example, team lunches or reminders about celebrating team members' birthdays.

This section now draws on the work of Charles Handy (1995, 1999) and Gareth Morgan (1997). These authors were chosen because they have extensively studied the structures and cultures of organisations as well as

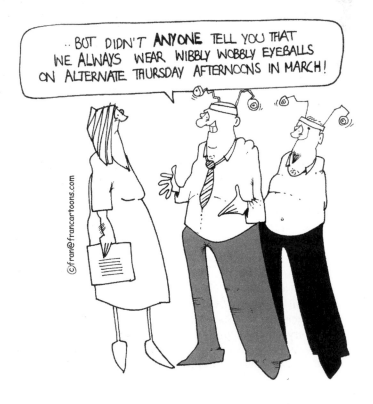

the behaviours of workers within them. Both authors have made a substantial contribution to the way organisations may be understood.

Handy's four organisational cultures

Handy describes four organisational ideas or beliefs about the best way to 'organise things and get something done, about the right way to treat people and the right way to behave' (1995, p. 145). He calls these four cultures *power*, *role*, *task* and *person*. They are summarised in Box 5.3.

BOX 5.3 Handy's organisational cultures

The power culture

This kind of organisational culture is represented as a spider's web with the key to the organisation being at the centre. Lines of responsibility stretch out from the centre and lines of trust link them. This type of organisation is centred on a leader and a group of like-minded people. The advantages of such organisations, which work on trust, is that they can respond immediately to change because there are very short lines of communication to the centre. This kind of organisation can thrive only if the group is small (fewer than 20) and the person at the centre is making sound judgements. If the 'spider' at the centre of the web is weak or corrupt or makes poor appointments, the organisation can fail. This kind of structure is seen in smaller entrepreneurial social care agencies and can be recognised as the pattern of some social care teams in both field and residential care, the team leader being the 'spider' at the heart of the web.

The role culture

The structure here is a pyramid, with the roles set out in job boxes as in Figure 5.1 (Handy avoids the term 'bureaucracy' since it now has a pejorative tone). This logical and orderly plan provides the roles and responsibilities needed to do the agency's work. It is a common structure for public agencies. Individuals occupy a prescribed role. If the arrangement is not delivering the outcomes that are wanted, the structure will be changed to meet new priorities and the role of individuals reordered. These kinds of organisations are formally managed through procedures. It is an arrangement that offers predictability and certainty and is suitable for stable and unchanging tasks. The weakness is that it is not a flexible arrangement for responding quickly to change or exceptions to its rules. If the design is correct for the work, this can be a very efficient way of fulfilling administrative tasks. Managers who have worked in social services departments, schools, hospitals or benefits agencies will be familiar with this kind of structure.

The task culture

This is depicted as a net. The organisational idea is that of recruiting a team with certain abilities to suit a particular task. Each task gets the team and resources that are appropriate to what the organisation plans to achieve. This kind of co-operative group of professionals without much hierarchy works by planning and reviewing, and remaining open to new ideas and ways of doing things. A task organisation can be expensive because it needs to employ experts. Task cultures can be seen in projects and specialist teams within role organisations.

The person culture

While the other three models put organisational mission and purpose first and fit individuals into a grouping to carry it out, the person organisation brings individuals with talent into a group to work together. These groupings are rather loose coalitions of people with similar skills who work together, for example a GP practice or a social care consultancy. Often there will be minimal formal role organisation and equality of status. This organisational culture allows for individuals to work in their own way and at their own pace in ways which might not work well for the complex organisational responsibilities of a hospital, school or social services department.

(Source: adapted from Handy, 1999, pp. 183–91)

Handy also says that organisations can be a mix of the four cultures. For example, role organisations can contain teams based on the other models. For individual managers, depending on their personal style and preferences, some of these work environments are better than others. For example, a power organisation could feel very unstructured to someone more used to role organisations and vice versa.

Although Handy refers to role *culture* you will have noted from the description that it is also a structure – bureaucracy. Bureaucracies have layers of management with clearly worked-out job and person specifications. Each person knows who they are accountable to and what are the limits of their authority. However, by focusing on the elements that can be thought of as cultural, Handy highlights that within any one organisation there can be different kinds of culture. So while an organisation may be a bureaucracy, it may have some parts that conform more to a role culture alongside specialist teams, which can be seen as task cultures, and sometimes projects, which may be power cultures. Residential units may be based on a power culture but also have aspects of a role culture, especially if they are part of a large network of homes run by a social services department or large voluntary agency. Voluntary sector projects are often power or task cultures at a local level, even if they are managed by a national organisation based on a role culture. Network organisations can fit in with Handy's idea of a task or person culture. Management groups can often seem like person cultures.

Images of organisation

Morgan (1997) also suggests ways of looking at organisational design but he uses a series of metaphors to do so. Metaphor, he says, stretches the imagination to aid understanding but also has its limits. In a metaphor the items compared have only some aspects in common. The metaphor of the organisation as a machine, for instance, with a system of interlocking parts, is a common one. Another image is of the organisation as an organism: a living thing that can be born, grow, develop, decline and die. This metaphor brings out the importance of adapting to the environment. More disturbing metaphors are those of psychic prison, or instruments of domination, where workers are disempowered or limited in some way by organisational culture. Morgan's suggestions (1997, pp. 6–8) can help managers think creatively about organisational shapes and functions.

The manager's relationship with organisational culture

Managers' relationship with structure is positional: that is, their authority comes from the terms of their appointment. A manager's relationship with the culture of an organisation might be much more personal and influential. A new manager may discover that there is already a positive culture that guarantees a good start. For example, a family centre manager commented:

> I inherited a good culture, with team meetings where moans can be aired ... and there is a lot of openness ... most of the staff know to come to me if they aren't happy about something or have ideas ... they know I will respond.

(Manager consultations)

This manager made her own mark on the culture she initially encountered by fulfilling the trust that staff placed in her. It is important that managers work to create and model a positive staff culture. In some day centres such openness and dialogue include service users, as the extract in Example 5.4 (overleaf) illustrates. Rohhss is a support worker with Carlisle People First, and the other speakers are members of this organisation, which is run for and by people with learning disabilities. You were introduced in Chapter 3 to some of the group's work on the qualities of a good and not so good manager.

EXAMPLE 5.4 Views on the manager from People First

Rohhss: Does anyone know why she was a good manager?

Andy: Because she got people out on trips and got people doing different things.

Lou: And what was it she said? If you want to have days off, you can stay at home?

Rohhss: So she was more into talking to people and listening to what people were saying?

Elizabeth: Yes, people's problems.

Lou: She did. I can remember when I used to do facilitation work. Once a month we used to have a meeting with the manager. When we used to talk with her things were done. Then when she left and you talked to the manager, things were not done.

(Source: service user consultations)

The manager referred to by Lou was demonstrating a practice-led approach that recognises the importance of learning directly from service users.

A review of 11 research studies of residential care for children summarises their findings (Department of Health, 1998b). These show the importance of managers in establishing a positive culture for good outcomes for young people. Whitaker *et al.* (1998) suggest that positive culture comes from having a manager who is clear about the children's needs without stereotyping; keeps in touch with staff problems; supports staff, without compromising their corporate responsibilities; communicates opinions; takes care over admissions; and keeps staff up to date and positive. Berridge and Brodie (1998) suggest that a manager's ability to express a clear theoretical or therapeutic orientation or clear working methods is beneficial for the quality of care that children and young people experience. They also argue that managers need to create a staff culture that is in keeping with the objectives of residential living by creating a healthy environment for both the children and the staff.

The failure to promote a positive culture contributes to a climate where abuse is possible. Cultures can also be enabling or disabling in residential care for adults. A residential or nursing home is a complex organisation. Working, living and visiting spaces are all organised in this one setting. Peace (2000) reviews the nature of institutional abuse and some studies that have examined the nature and frequency of abusive behaviour in residential care homes. She suggests some points for managers to practise that would contribute to a climate of openness and awareness in care environments: these are shown in Box 5.4. Chapter 6 develops the discussion on the importance of managing the care environment.

BOX 5.4 Points for practice

- Has your agency/service developed policies and procedures to protect vulnerable adults from abuse?

- Has your staff team examined the way you work and how you would define abuse in your setting?

- Is everyone – residents, relatives, staff – involved in discussing the aims and objectives of the home?

- If you work in an institutional setting would you call all areas of practice acceptable? Are there any that are unacceptable? What can you do about this?

- Do staff support and help each other in their day-to-day work? Can you learn from one another's experiences? Do you have systems of appraisal and staff development?

- Is there a system for recording information on abusive practice?

- Some of the people you care for may be at risk of abuse from other residents. Do you know how to intervene to safeguard residents who find themselves at risk?

(Source: Peace, 2000, p. 32)

Brody (1993) stresses that managers set the tone in their organisations through the way they lead. Setting the tone can be done in frontline managing, too, even when the manager's power over structures, policies and procedures is limited. Brody also suggests that culture can be influenced to become not just the way things are done but also the right way to do things in an agency. In other words, the manager creates a climate where values guide the work of the organisation. Box 5.5 (overleaf) summarises the values that Brody considers important.

Of course, values are not simply communicated through written statements: the ways in which jobs are advertised and interviews are undertaken, and the processes of induction, training, supervision, appraisal and staff meetings, all say something about values. Brody concludes that:

> managers are mindful that the organization's culture has a strong influence on staff behavior and performance. Cultural values are entrenched as traditional ways of thinking and doing and are developed over a long time period. Effective managers can influence the shape and strength of staff values by stressing job ownership, by emphasizing the importance of meeting the needs of service consumers, and by making certain work quality encompasses both service delivery and outcome ...
>
> (Brody, 1993, p. 34)

BOX 5.5 Setting the tone

Job ownership

Employees are encouraged to care about their work and the way it is done. Managers create a climate where employees are expected to support each other in complex tasks. Managers aim to model and build relationships of trust between workers and foster the desire to build a better service.

The primacy of the consumer

The organisation is friendly towards its service users by answering telephone calls and letters promptly, and conveying respect in its interactions with service users. It treats users as genuine partners by engaging them in activities that evaluate and develop services.

Work quality as central

Quality is a complex idea but Brody frames it in terms of consumer satisfaction. Are consumers made to feel welcome? Are their negative feelings and views attended to? Do they feel there is a high level of concern for their welfare?

Communicating the organisation's values

Managers are responsible for making sure that the values statement is communicated, shared, owned and practised through the agency.

(Source: adapted from Brody, 1993, pp. 25–33)

Key points

- There are often different cultures within the same organisation, sometimes operating despite the predominant structure and its cultural implications.

- Managers can do much to set a positive tone and influence the culture in their working environment.

5.5 The manager's power and influence

The formal structure of the workplace shapes a manager's roles, tasks and responsibilities towards others. It defines their territory or sphere of influence. In particular, it defines their legitimate authority and power. This includes both permissions and limitations. In this section we consider the sources and uses of the manager's power.

Social care has a large practice literature on 'empowerment' (see, for instance, Bray and Preston Shoot, 1995; Humphries, 1996), which generally means the transfer of power from an advantaged group to a more disadvantaged one and a focus on what social care users say they want. Managers have to acknowledge that they do have powers – more at least than their staff or service users – and they should therefore act in ways that are empowering. They have the power of role and position. They are likely to have power or some control over human and physical resources. They can also, however, be the recipients of the power and authority of senior managers, management committees, commissioning agencies or inspectorial bodies. This can make their position feel ambiguous and uncertain. Frontline managers often feel that no one listens to them:

Managers don't feel listened to.

Middle managers keep consulting with and asking managers, but don't seem to listen to the response.

(Manager consultations)

It has been suggested that power can only be understood if there is careful analysis of its extent and limitations. Kakabadse *et al.* (1988) suggest that power has five aspects.

1   It is a firm base from which to act.
2   The organisation has given the individual a role and resources.
3   There is the potential to achieve or succeed.
4   The organisation has values and norms within which the individual acts.
5   The individual has to think about how it is best used.

These aspects are all relevant for managers. There are various strategies or levers that the individual (and the organisation more widely) uses in the exercise of power, which are listed in Box 5.6 (overleaf).

Although Kakabadse and his colleagues refer to race and gender as attributes of personal power, they are all too often made relevant in access to the other potential power levers. Managers in social care organisations will recognise these different aspects of their power. Even people without a clear management role, working perhaps in task cultures or co-operative organisational structures, will have some of these sources of power. A lack of management structure does not mean that no one has power: there are still established ways of getting things done and people with more or less information or skills in the most co-operative of ventures. How a manager uses power will strongly influence the way staff work and the culture of the organisation. It is the misuse of power by managers that concerns the writers of the letters in Examples 5.1 and 5.2.

BOX 5.6 Levers of power

Reward power

The ability to influence the rewards others have, such as bonus payments or holidays.

Coercive power

The authority to hire and fire and discipline others.

Legitimate power

The authority to appraise, supervise and organise workload.

Personal power

The power gained by personal characteristics: attributes such as race and gender may be relevant here.

Expert power

The power of skills, knowledge and professional qualifications.

Information power

Knowing facts and deciding to what extent to share or disclose them. This may be agency or personal information.

Connection power

Making contacts and building networks at conferences, meetings, support groups and unions.

(Source: adapted from Kakabadse *et al.*, 1988, pp. 215–25)

However, power is not a one-way transaction: it operates up, down and across the lines of responsibility in an agency. The politics of power can be complex in organisations. Having legitimate power does not mean a manager can always use it effectively if staff cannot be persuaded or influenced to do what is expected. People without much apparent power can exercise 'negative power' illegitimately to stop or block something – for instance, a team clerk has little power to initiate but can misdirect or mislay important documents (Handy, 1999).

As a manager, you may not always feel as though you have any power. If a senior manager uses their power oppressively, and the staff use theirs negatively, the role of the frontline manager can truly be 'between a rock and a hard place'. None the less, most managers usually exercise their power within the remit that the organisation defines as their role. This tends to allow them to delegate responsibilities and allocate resources. Managers have the power of their personal ability to lead and influence others. They also have to earn authority through the exercise of expert power as they supervise the professional elements of the work. This kind of power is often the most effective because it is given by others as they recognise their manager's authority to lead and influence. People from other agencies and staff can use their power to block, so that managers cannot simply rely on legitimate, information and coercive powers. They need to be able to compromise and analyse the way their power can be used positively for the users, staff and agency. Power, therefore, has structural, cultural and personal components.

Key points

- Managers should act in ways that are empowering.

- There are five aspects of power that are relevant for managers.

- The levers used in exercising power are: reward, coercive, legitimate, personal, expert, information and connection.

- Power has structural, cultural and personal components.

5.6 Working across organisational boundaries

The shape of social care organisations has traditionally put boundaries around managers' sphere of influence. However, developments to make social care services more accessible and logical for their users since the 1990s mean that managers increasingly have to think about the way their organisation relates to others, in terms of partnerships, co-operation and collaboration. Managers now have responsibilities within the boundaries of their own workplace and also within new organisational arrangements, networks and partnerships. This means that managers need a clear understanding of their own organisational remit and that of others and the way in which such structures and culture impact on each other. As one manager said:

> It's not uncommon now for me to be part of a housing management committee, for the district council, because we're talking about the allocation of property affecting a person with a disability and all of a sudden you're moving – not out of social services because we represent social services – but we're becoming increasingly involved in the culture of the ways of another department, another agency. There's a huge learning curve.
>
> (Manager consultations)

The only safe assumption is that social care managers will continue to operate in a changing world as successive political initiatives shape the patterns of social care delivery. For the foreseeable future, social care will probably be delivered through arrangements between differently resourced agencies in a 'mixed economy' of welfare. Hardy *et al.* (1992) draw attention to the kinds of barriers that make inter-organisational co-ordination and collaboration complex, and they are listed in Box 5.7.

BOX 5.7 Five categories of barriers to inter-organisational co-ordination

Structural

- Fragmentation of service responsibilities across inter-agency boundaries

- Fragmentation of service responsibilities within agency boundaries

- Inter-organisational complexity

- Non-coterminosity of boundaries

Procedural

- Differences in planning horizons and cycles

- Differences in budgetary cycles and procedures

Financial

- Differences in funding mechanisms and bases

- Differences in the stocks and flows of [financial] resources

Professional

- Differences in ideologies and values

- Professional self-interest

- Threats to job security

- Conflicting views about user interests and roles

Status and legitimacy

- Organisational self-interest

- Concern for threats to autonomy and domain

- Differences in legitimacy between elected and appointed agencies
      (Source: Hardy *et al.*, 1992, cited by Hudson *et al.*, 1999, p. 241)

Barriers no doubt still exist but the government's encouragement of closer working between health and social care is leading to initiatives in joint commissioning, integrated care trusts, and the separation of commissioning and providing functions, which may help smooth the way. Structural, procedural and financial barriers are perhaps the easiest to identify in any particular situation but will require detailed negotiation at a high level to resolve. The other barriers – professional and status and legitimacy – may be subtler and will need managers with good interpersonal skills if they are to be resolved. There are structural and cultural as well as power issues to be understood and engaged with when managers seek to work in partnership with other organisations. As government agendas and service users' views are also an essential part of the picture, it can be quite a balancing act to manage all the differing interests.

Sometimes the disparate interests are combined into one large organisation. However, as the brief discussion in Section 5.3 of the bureaucracies of the 1970s and 1980s shows, these struggles can still go on among sub-groups between people with differing cultural or power perspectives within large structures. Alternatively, bridging structures are created between agencies that serve the same stakeholders: for example, Youth Offending Teams, created as a task organisation to co-ordinate a multi-agency response to a particular group – young offenders. Issues of power and difference still need to be addressed in such settings and relationships can be complex, as Example 5.5 suggests.

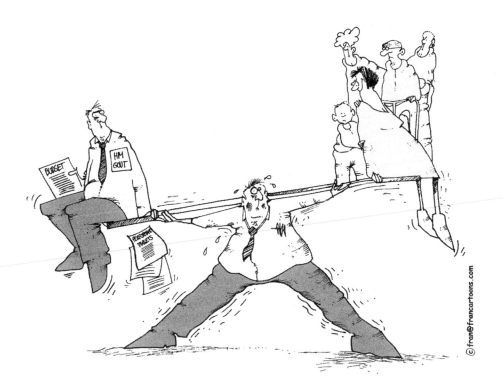

BALANCING ACT

EXAMPLE 5.5 Colleague, competitor or service user?

The manager of a local branch of Age Concern works with people from other local voluntary agencies both as colleagues and as competitors bidding for the same resources. His agency is a supplier of services to the primary care trust and the social services department; it is also represented on the joint commissioning committee. A member of his management committee also serves on the management committee of other local voluntary agencies and she is a carer who uses Age Concern's services. Relationships are complex with many potential conflicts of interest.

Martin and Henderson (2001) suggest that mapping can help you to understand how your service sits in the wider environment. This is increasingly important as organisations develop partnerships together: 'Your organisation does not exist in isolation: it is part of a large and complex network of patients, service users and their carers, suppliers, competitors, regulators and so on' (p. 75). The economy, social trends and technological innovations also have an impact on your organisation. Mapping can lead to planning and the identification of ways of building bridges and influencing other organisations. Box 5.8 shows the different types of environment that are influential.

BOX 5.8 The three environments

There is a dynamic relationship between these three environments.

- The *internal environment* is composed of the staff, resources and facilities within the organisation. These components can be *controlled* – to a large extent, at least – by the organisation's managers. The internal environment is, however, influenced by the near and far environments, which the organisation is unable to control.

- The *near environment* includes patients, service users and carers, contractors, suppliers and competitors. It also includes local politicians, other organisations that are partners in service delivery and local pressure groups. These components of the environment are all close to the organisation and they interact with it in a variety of ways. They cannot be controlled by the organisation, but they can be *influenced*.

- The components of the *far environment* are those factors that can neither be controlled nor influenced from within the organisation. They include a wide range of social, technological, economic, environmental and political factors. Every organisation has to *respond* to the impact of these external factors. Some respond more thoughtfully, quickly and successfully than others.

(Source: Martin and Henderson, 2001, p. 76)

Each of the three environments presents a different kind of task for managers. The internal environment can be controlled the most immediately because a manager has the authority, power and the resources of the agency as a mandate to act. Most managers in social care find themselves working just as closely with the near environment, which will include a variety of stakeholders over whom managers have less legitimate power and whose resources may be controlled by someone else. Managers need to negotiate their influence and agree forms of action which take account of other stakeholders' perspectives. This requires the ability to network and hold an 'image of connectedness' (James, 1994a, p. 104) across organisational boundaries, perhaps in spite of suspicions lingering from the days of competitive tendering. The far environment can seem the most threatening because that is where the individual manager has the least power and control over events. Government may pass new laws or issue new directives that affect what a manager does. The way business is done may change: for example, information technology has made an enormous difference to most workplaces. Managers find themselves responding to and implementing such changes, which are often closed to influence and unpredictable in their scope and effect.

Martin and Henderson's three-stage model of the environment shows that no organisation is independent. In social care, resources depend on political decisions at national and local level. The delivery of care to service users is dependent on the availability and skills of staff as well as the expressed needs of service users. Martin and Henderson, therefore, suggest that the issue of influencing the near environment (stakeholders) might be approached by recognising the need to share resources. Using the 'resource dependence' approach described by Pfeffer and Salancik (1978), which is outlined in Box 5.9 (overleaf), Martin and Henderson argue that organisations have to interact with others in their environment. All organisations experience similar difficulties obtaining resources, so those working geographically close to each other or providing similar services are often interdependent.

Much external management beyond an agency's boundary is about strategies which maximise resources to deliver services. The role of the frontline manager is increasingly in negotiating across organisations to broker arrangements for services that are delivered in partnership arrangements. Managers need the power and influence to make sure services are what users need, and to release appropriate resources. As James (1994a, p. 7) suggests, 'the empowering manager is the one who creates the conditions under which innovation can happen'. It has been argued here that this can only be so if managers have a sufficient understanding of the organisation and of its relationship with the environment.

BOX 5.9 Balancing dependencies

Pfeffer and Salancik suggested that there are four ways in which an organisation might balance its dependencies.

- *Adapt to the conditions.* This could be done by reducing levels of service, restricting use of resources, slowing down the speed of response to demand or influencing the types of demand made on its services. For example, a small hospital might reduce the number of different services offered, and specialise in treating a particular condition or a particular group of people (for example, admitting only older people or only children).

- *Alter the interdependencies.* This could be done by merging with another organisation that controls some of the needed resources. It could be done by growing and providing a wider range of services, so that the organisation is not dependent on providing only one type of service. For example, a small community-based home care service might link with a community health service to provide care for people who need support at home when they leave hospital.

- *Negotiate the environment.* This could be done by creating partnerships with other organisations to deliver services jointly or to share resources. One way in which this is increasingly happening at the present time is by developing links between social services and health services, sometimes including contributions from the voluntary sector.

- *Change the environment by political action.* This could be done by influencing decision makers to change the conditions in which the organisation operates. An example would be lobbying local Members of Parliament in an effort to prevent the closure of a hospital or to try to obtain subsidies or special financial allowances when the demand for a service increases unexpectedly (as often occurs for health and social care organisations in harsh winters).

(Source: Martin and Henderson, 2001, p. 85)

Key points

- Managers need to understand how their organisation co-operates and collaborates with others in the current mixed economy of welfare.

- There are five barriers to inter-organisational co-ordination: structural, procedural, financial, professional, and status and legitimacy.

- Mapping places an organisation within the wider environment and helps it to build bridges between and influence other organisations.

- The three influential environments – internal, near and far – present different tasks for managers.

- Managers increasingly have to negotiate across organisational boundaries to maximise resources for service delivery.

5.7 Conclusion

In this chapter you have considered the structure and culture of organisations and the way these impact on the manager's role. The chapter made selective use of organisational theory and developed some major concepts that may be helpful to managers. The models presented offer a broad means of understanding the ways in which organisations function and how managers can attempt to influence practices, improve services and increase input from service users. Thus, using power and influence does not have to be negative process.

The discussion on inter-organisational working shows how the drive to partnership can have beneficial outcomes for managers and service users, both in streamlining and improving services and in facilitating better working with a range of organisations. However, this way of working also demonstrates problems with the concepts of structure and culture, illustrating how organisational structures are not fixed and that hybrid types can be created by organisations collaborating with each other. These may develop their own culture and ways of working, which could be very different from the parent organisation's. This, in turn, raises interesting challenges and possible tensions to balance.

Chapter 6
Managing environments

Sheila Peace and Jill Reynolds

6.1 Introduction

How do managers think about the environment in which they work? The environment is complex and meets many needs. It can be bounded in place, space, time and behaviour. If you work in social care, you may leave your home and go to an office-based setting that was designed for a certain task where people understand the rules, manners and behaviours of the organisation. Here you can 'read the signs' and understand your part. However, this is far from always the case. Sometimes you might spend part of a day in an office and part in a different group service centre, such as a family centre. Alternatively, you might move to someone else's domestic situation, for instance on a fieldwork visit. Here you are perceived in a formal rather than an informal way but the setting is totally informal and conveys different messages. You may be part of a residential service and work night shifts, and time may be a particular factor in how you perceive your role.

For many social care employees there are everyday changes from places that are domestic to those that are non-domestic; from private to more public spaces; from those where people may be part of a group to those where they are very individual; and from situations of formality to informality. Settings, situations and types of space may be shifting. The impact of these changing contexts on the role of managers forms the basis of this chapter.

The ambiguity of social care adds to the complexity already identified. In any situation people's behaviour will be part of its construction, and what they construct will be sensed in terms of the apparent climate or culture that pervades – the atmosphere that exists. Yet, despite the geographic metaphors, the environment is more than the place or space: it is a setting for experience that Lewin (1936) calls the 'lifespace'. The setting will feel owned (or not owned) and there will be different forms of attachment to places. The design and use made of the physical space available for working and being needs to be thought of in relation to the primary purpose of the caring organisation. Our focus is on the impact that managers can have on the development of the organisational atmosphere of a setting, and how they can recognise the diversity of people with very different needs as workers, service users and visitors. We also look at how environmental quality can be developed, and the tensions that exist in situations where a manager may work at a distance from the other employees: overseeing services but with different levels of intervention.

The intellectual background to this chapter is in the fields of environmental and social psychology, sociology, anthropology and human geography. Concepts such as *territory*, *privacy* and *boundaries* are introduced, as they can underpin the ability to develop environmental quality.

First, we shall look at the multifaceted milieu that any care environment can be. As central examples in this chapter we use care homes, drawing on the work of one of this chapter's authors concerning residential care homes for older people (Willcocks *et al.*, 1987; Peace *et al.*, 1997; Peace, 1998). While care homes have distinctive features, we are really using them as an example to focus attention on issues that are common to other contexts of care, which you can learn from and apply to your own context. Notions of space, setting and identity are rarely covered in management and organisational research, and so we shall discover new knowledge together with you in this chapter.

The aims of this chapter are to:

- demonstrate how any one environment may be multifaceted
- discuss what is meant by 'atmosphere' and the manager's role in how this is developed and understood
- review the scope for the careful design and use of space to contribute to improved quality of life in the management of care
- consider the issues of supervision of workers by managers who are at a distance from the working environment
- discuss the tensions between environmental quality and standards of care.

6.2 The many faces of the environment

Within any setting, people's experiences vary as they will be present for different reasons; their control or power over their situation will differ, and this may give them different levels of access to a range of spaces or areas. One person's experience may be very different from another's, as shown in Example 6.1.

EXAMPLE 6.1 Rights of passage

Sitting in one of three seats near the main entrance to Swift Lodge, Mrs Jenkins can see many 'comings and goings'. The foyer is square in shape with chairs along parts of two walls, offices at two sides and a corridor forming the fourth that also has an entrance to a lift. There is a porch area attached where some people, mostly male residents, like to go to smoke.

Mrs Jenkins has just had her hair done in the hairdressing-room opposite her and has decided to stay sitting here until it is time to go to the dining-room for lunch. Just next to the front door is the administrator's office and this is linked to another office used by Mrs Jones, the head of the home (now called a registered manager), and other senior staff. The only people going along the corridor so far have been members of staff but two visitors have arrived. One is a visiting GP, who has come to see resident Bill Smart, and the other is Sue Gilmour, who has come to see her Aunt Gladys.

The situation described here could be set in many residential homes for older people and immediately makes you begin to relate the people to the place. For the residents it is their *living environment* – preferably a place where they feel 'at home' through being able to control how they interact with others in both public and private areas. However, in this scenario the entrance hall is also a reception and a waiting area, and people are coming in and going out. It is therefore a fairly public area and it may have similarities with reception areas in a range of services. As Mrs Jenkins knows, this is a place of activity; she is inquisitive and likes to see 'what is going on'. She comes to this spot at other times without a specific reason as, for her, it is a place of connections between home and community, past and present, which tells us something about her attachment to the place. Figure 6.1 (overleaf) is a rough diagram showing the layout of the reception area.

Other residents may not be drawn to the entrance hall unless they have a specific reason: an appointment with the hairdresser or a need to see a particular member of staff or to see a visitor leave the building. Some people may not like sitting in close proximity to members of staff, feeling uncomfortable. Gender and cultural differences can also affect where men and women feel it is appropriate to sit. Mrs Jenkins did not want to sit with the men who were smoking in the entrance porch. Others may find this part of the building is difficult to reach or too distant from other activities and they are dependent on a staff member's help. Access to different parts of buildings can vary depending on the mobility, visual and aural ability and motivation of the individual. The design of the building may be crucial: the number of stairs; the ease of manoeuvrability for a wheelchair user to change floors by lift; the gradients of hallways and exterior pathways – all aspects of creating an enabling environment.

The reception area, as a public place where visitors are received, is slightly detached from the daily life of the home where everyday events occur. It is a threshold, a point of entry that is a 'public' *boundary* between inside and outside. However, there are other less public boundaries. When staff come to work not all of them enter through the front door. There is an entrance through a door by the kitchen to the side of the home. Swift Lodge is a *working environment* for the staff and their access can change during the day and night: on-call sleep-in arrangements still occur here.

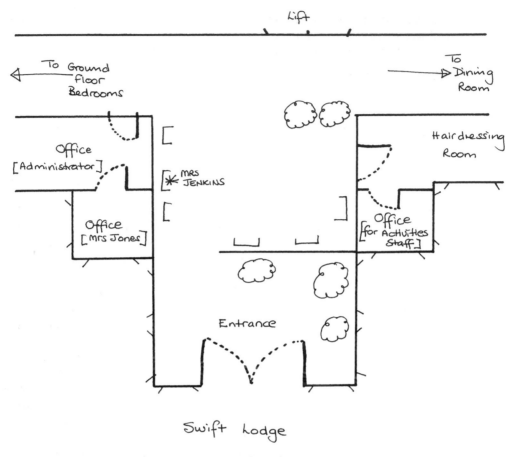

Figure 6.1 **Layout of the reception at Swift Lodge**

These boundaries tell us something about the status and power of different people.

The offices at the entrance are places where there should always be an administrative officer and some senior staff at different times of the day. The administrator, or care staff member, often acts as receptionist in that they offer a welcome and give information and directions. They also provide a link between people and may facilitate access by using their inside knowledge of what is going on and who is doing what at any point in time. To other people this might be seen as 'delaying tactics' but it may enable the system to run more smoothly or prevent conflict. At Swift Lodge the *visiting environment* involves people with various kinds of access. For many residents, visitors are family and may have been close informal carers when the person was living in their own home. If known, they may often just walk in and out. However, they may be more distant relatives and less frequent visitors, unsure of procedures. Consequently, visitors can be seen as informal or as formal and more official. The latter may be different practitioners – health, chiropody, hairdressing – and some may be part of the local community. They may also come in and go out at different times of the day or night.

So already this example has given us a place that is:

- a living environment
- a working environment
- a visiting environment.

This combination of activities is common to many places in which care occurs and has to be managed. When you consider an entrance hall, its importance as a boundary is obvious, but in looking at the three kinds of environment outlined above, the boundaries may be less clear. The degree to which different care environments involve people in different ways will vary but this example helps to identify the complexity.

Obviously, there are other parts of a residential home that are private places, such as residents' bed-sitting-rooms. These are very much part of the living environment and could be called *intimate spaces*. However, they are also places that can be used for visiting and working. So an understanding of who has control over this space will reflect the values underpinning the culture in this home and be an important guide to behaviour. However, working space such as the more public offices may also need a level of privacy and confidentiality, depending on the activities carried out within them or the information held there. So *function* is important in determining the nature of space. Functions can also change momentarily as people and places interact, and the power that some people may have – because of their role, status and the values they impose – can influence the atmosphere. For instance, the pleasure of eating, albeit at a slow pace for some people, may be destroyed by a staff member who wants to clear the dishes in a hurry. Our example uses a 24-hour environment and so each of these elements may be constantly changing because of the density of people and variations in need and response.

It is important to recognise the multifunctional nature of organisations, as different aspects may need to be managed in different ways. At Swift Lodge the management of care staff as employees will need to be considered differently from the management of the residents' day, although the two intertwine. How this is handled should be reflected in how the overall culture relates to different people's needs. If the balance is tipped in favour of social control by staff then the experiences of service users may be endangered. In addition, there are the transitional needs of visitors, who may have very different levels of attachment to the person visited – from a lifetime's history to a recent meeting. The complexity evolves.

This picture demonstrates that a *situational* approach to management is crucial. There is no simple formula for resolving matters. Managers need to keep central the purpose of the service they are managing while balancing the needs of the various people involved so that they complement each other. How this is done creates the culture that pervades the situation. Before we examine different situations for managers in influencing the environment, some of the basic concepts of this discussion – territory, privacy, space and their impact on behaviour – need further explanation.

Key points

- There are divisions between public space and private space.

- There are issues about levels of privacy.

- The boundaries between these spaces are often invisible but do exist.

- The time of day will affect the use of space.

6.3 Understanding territory and privacy

In care work the working environment can vary greatly depending on who you are and how close you are to offering a direct service. For people involved in a managerial or supervisory role, the context of work may vary between *formal* and *informal*, in terms of duties or functions that will affect perceived levels of professionalism, and *public* and *private*, in terms of the degree of privacy. These contextual changes can be charted within a *territorial net* – see Figure 6.2.

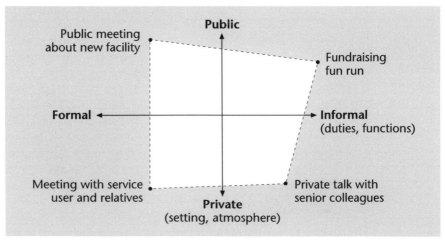

Figure 6.2 **The territorial net**

The variety of managerial roles or functions can be located on this diagram: from listening to a service user and their family, which might be formal but managed privately, to presenting a public relations briefing, which might be formal and very public, to having an informal, private chat with a senior colleague. Within any one day a manager may move between them. This variation highlights how multiple constructions of culture and role inform different reactions to space, identity and setting. By exploring this framework, it becomes easier to see how different forms of *territory* are established for different tasks.

How is territory defined within the working environment? Does everyone need a space that is theirs at work: a so-called *defensible space* which they can demarcate in some way even in open-plan offices (Sommer, 1969; Veitch and Arkkelin, 1995)? Also, does a person in a managerial role have a right to their own territory – is it a part of the power of the position or to enable privacy for others? Does it reflect a certain dominance? On the whole, many organisational environments maintain levels of territorial separation between people of different status or with different functions.

Research has shown similarities with natural environments, where confined areas can lead to dispute, and the importance therefore of individual territory (Veitch and Arkkelin, 1995). In the working environment many people share office space and, even if schedules differ, how space is allocated and set out is still an issue. It says something about roles

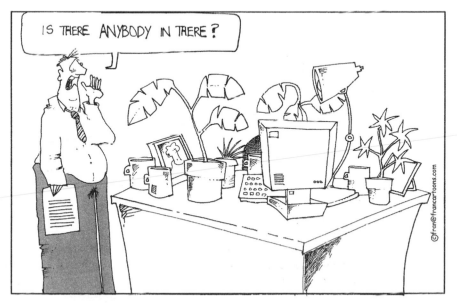

Most people need a working territory that they can personalise

and affects the interaction between people. An office may be open plan and noise may carry or it may have separate rooms for smaller numbers or individuals. The office desk is marked out with books, files, arrangements of furniture and the position of light to create a personalised area. The ownership and personalisation of space can be important to all employees – it reflects their identity. A sense of ownership also allows for changes of use, and for times of privacy when individuals may engage in isolated, one-to-one or small group tasks. In this way *privacy* becomes one aspect of territory but it depends on the level of control that the owner has over space as to how it is used. The concept of privacy is an important issue throughout this chapter but what is really meant by privacy?

Privacy often relates to forms of behaviour that people want to engage in either alone or with chosen others. The content of the behaviour may be seen as very personal, individual or even secret. In this case the person does not want the public interest of others – they avoid public attention. Privacy can also relate to disruption or interruption. The task may require close attention and confidentiality because of the information being passed between people and how that information needs to be stored. There will be a need for protected time, space and sound. Of course, while thinking of the values attached to privacy, it is also possible to see how privacy can entrap people in close contact with others and give opportunities for abuse – physical, sexual or psychological.

These ideas surrounding territory and privacy are also found in the writings of the Canadian sociologist Erving Goffman (1922–1982), who used the techniques of dramaturgical role performance in his analysis of the way people behave. The notion is that people stage-manage the impression they want others to receive of them (Goffman, 1961, 1969) through their personal front, or manner, which can be influenced by situations as well as affect how situations are defined. Goffman describes many instances of how people understand situations and their position within them either as individuals or as part of teams. He looked at how people try to control situations and, of particular relevance here, he considered the impact of place on behaviour. Box 6.1 sets out some of Goffman's useful concepts of performance.

We shall return to some of these ideas later in this chapter but, regarding the discussion of privacy, the concept of the regions of performance – 'front regions' and 'back regions' – is especially helpful. The 'back region' becomes a place where people may 'drop their front' and stop maintaining a performance that they will have to resurrect elsewhere. In discussing these ideas, Goffman talks of the way in which different impressions are given in different spaces: for example, the value often attached to the living-room in a domestic home; or activities 'behind the counter' at a reception desk. As the following extract shows, regions may change their character, depending on the behaviour of the occupant.

BOX 6.1 Concepts derived from Goffman's dramaturgical approach

- **Rule following** is found in social interactions – what the actors should and should not do.

- **Role distance** – when you detach or distance yourself from the normative expected role.

- **Self-presentation** – trying to fit the expectations of those to whom you perform.

- **Front and back regions** of performance – how different places affect performance.

- **Audience segregation** – where interactions with different people take place separately, allowing for contradictions to occur.

(Source: adapted from Goffman, 1961, 1969)

However, while there is a tendency for a region to become identified as the front region or back region of a performance with which it is regularly associated, still there are many regions which function at one time and in one sense as a front region and at another time and in another sense as a back region. Thus the private office of an executive is certainly the front region where his status in the organization is intensively expressed by means of the quality of his office furnishings. And yet it is here that he can take his jacket off, loosen his tie, keep a bottle of liquor handy, and act in a chummy and even boisterous way with fellow executives of his own rank ...

(Goffman, 1969, p. 127)

In this way an individual may change the nature of a space simply by acting differently.

Key points

- Managers use space differently according to the public or private, formal or informal nature of their work.

- Most people need a working territory that they can personalise or use for private matters.

- As well as physical demarcation, people use more subtle changes of behaviour to define how space is to be used.

6.4 Working environments – whose territory?

Power and control

In order to look more closely at how concepts of territory and privacy might work in social care settings, we shall continue with examples of residential care for older people, and make links to other areas of care. The question becomes whose territory dominates the value base within the care setting and how is balance achieved? The following account of one woman's experience in a nursing home is shocking.

> Whenever friends visited – and they did most days – she told them of the indignities she now experienced. Never before had she considered eating breakfast whilst emptying her bowels, but that became the norm with a care assistant who told her that she did not have enough time to get all the jobs done without adopting this time-saving routine, placing Betty on a bedpan while feeding her. When Betty resisted, the care assistant became yet more determined and handled her roughly, her actions accompanied by harsh words.
>
> (Bright, 1999, p. 193)

This account is reported in a research study on the quality of care in homes for older people. It might seem an isolated example of an untrained care assistant but the researcher argues that such appalling practice is not that unusual and has been documented in other studies (for instance Jenkins, 1997, cited in Bright, 1999). The reported behaviour flouts all ordinary conventions of privacy as well as dignity. You may wonder how it is possible for such a thing to happen in any establishment aimed at providing care. There are three possibilities.

1 It did not happen – Betty made up a complaint in order to cause trouble for a member of staff she did not like.

2 It did happen – the care assistant was largely unobserved in terms of how she went about her work, effectively having privacy to institute regimes that suited her.

3 It did happen – other people knew about it but did not take action.

Clough (1999, p. 216) points out that a climate that fosters abuse is more likely under particular conditions, which include when staff members are working alone without oversight or supervision from others, and when work is private, away from other residents. Goffman's notion of a 'back region' might be extended to performances that happen in care settings 'out of sight' – in this case, away from the scrutiny of managers or other workers and residents. However, often when there are unacceptable activities many people are implicated through their awareness and failure to take action. In such cases, the 'back region' is constructed by the tacit agreement of everyone concerned to ignore events, in other words 'out of sight, out of mind'.

In Chapter 5 you were given definitions of culture, which included 'the way things are done', the behaviours, the pattern of delivering services, and the underlying values and beliefs of an organisation, a team or an office. Where one environment is being used by different people for different purposes, with contrasting traditions or ideas of what they want from it, there will be not one coherent identifiable culture but many. Questions of who 'owns' the territory are fundamentally questions about how shared space is to be used.

Lewis and Gunaratnam (2000) look at a different kind of issue for personal space and privacy – *noise*. In research on hospice care, nurses reported concern about the mourning rituals of people from West Africa. These could be construed by other dying patients and their visiting friends and relatives as noise that was offensive to them and invaded their own sense of privacy or quiet intimacy. Whose need to pursue their preferred cultural behaviour should predominate? Is there a role for staff in 'managing' these tensions?

Issues of power and control emerge in several forms here. Where different ethnic groups are involved there may be a tendency to assume that the behaviour of those in the dominant white culture is the 'norm' and that anything different is 'other' and not to be encouraged. It is a short step from such an assumption to a racist response that fails to give appropriate care to people from ethnic minority groups.

Power relations between staff and residents emerge in other forms. As well as the imbalance of power that physical dependence implies, the values that inform caring activities may further undermine the power of residents. Core objectives of care provision, such as control, containment or protection, may conflict with the residents' rights to territory, personal space and privacy. Burton (1998) proposes that clarifying the primary task is the first act of management at every level. This may not be straightforward – flushing out and debating competing views is part of the process, but some of the more covert objectives and values that create and reinforce dependency may not be easily accessed or voiced.

Clough (1999) acknowledges the tendency in residential care to push complexity away and avoid recognising the tensions. He calls for management to create a forum in which people can recognise the complexity of the task, define the purpose and be free to air their concerns. The balance of power and issues of partnership are central to developing independent living in a range of settings. If you try to apply the idea of being *practice-led* to this discussion of the use of power and contested territory, you may wonder 'whose practice?' In care homes it is the manager's job to try to ensure that residents' privacy and independence are respected. The foundation for this will be through a common understanding by care staff of the standards they work to. However, there are also practical decisions in residential care that managers need to make with their staff team on a case-by-case basis. These invariably bring with them issues of values and, again, it is the manager's job to help the staff team to develop an approach that addresses competing perspectives on what is right.

Managerial space

What about managers' needs for territory of their own and privacy? As you read through Example 6.2, consider which kind of management tasks might require privacy for Bronwyn.

EXAMPLE 6.2 The manager without an office

Bronwyn, who you may recall from Chapter 3, is the team manager of an all-female team for a therapeutic service for children and families, run by a major voluntary agency. Here are her comments about her working environment.

> We took over an old property on three floors which the agency split between two projects. We have the top two floors and, since the other project moved, we now have two new workers associated with our project who are using the downstairs space. The team room is shared by all of us – myself, project workers, administrative and secretarial staff. Nine of us in all, although usually no more than seven people are in at a time. It has been very helpful sharing the office space: it means that I'm always aware of what is going on and, when a crisis is going on, I get early warning of it. I enjoy the repartee of us all being in together, and I think it adds to our sense of team cohesion. The team members say that they like me being so accessible to them and aware and involved in the work.
>
> However, there are some difficulties about always being so available to others, and I am now thinking that I will move into offices downstairs, together with the administrator and secretary. They can find it hard to get on with their work when there is a lot going on around all the time. The workers who are currently down there would be better in the team room.

Bronwyn noted the following points about working in the team room.

- While it was good knowing what was going on, it could deflect her from work of her own that needed doing. Increasingly, she was taking organisational tasks home or doing them in her own time.

- She could get caught up in work that was going on – if it was a crisis, she might become enmeshed by being involved in it all, and less able to bring a fresh or more detached view.

- Some calls needed privacy, perhaps when she was talking to another manager in the group and needed to talk about matters confidential to them.

- Feeling always 'on show' was not easy – a taxing telephone call might mean she did not feel confident about being overheard. While she could go to another room to make calls, this then drew attention to her need for privacy.

- On the other hand, moving downstairs would make her less accessible to team members and the physical space might create a barrier.

(Source: manager consultations)

Privacy serves two basic functions according to Veitch and Arkkelin (1995, p. 279).

1 The achievement of a self-identity
2 The management of interactions between the self and the social environment

The first function is important to allow people to drop their social mask and to free them from concerns about how they look to others. Bronwyn raises this in her preference for privacy for some telephone calls when she was not confident about what she had to say. Privacy also allows time to reflect on experiences and to formulate strategies. The use of private space for any of these purposes links with the management of performance described by Goffman (see Box 6.1).

The second function, which for the purposes of this discussion could be the working environment, is also important in helping with the first: self-identity. Altman (1975) was among the first to emphasise the importance of privacy and he draws attention to its complexity. Too much privacy may be as unpleasant as too little. It is important for managers to have some control or regulation over which people they are available to and when. It also requires negotiation with other people. Thus Bronwyn both wants the opportunity to focus on her own tasks and is concerned that other people may be deterred from asking for advice or help when needed and that she may lose the sense of involvement she gets by being on hand.

As an alternative to physical boundaries through separate offices, people can use behaviour to regulate contact. In other words, the way you behave may lead other people to understand that you want to be on your own: what has been called an 'opening' or a 'closing' of the self (Altman, 1975; Veitch and Arkkelin, 1995). In this way managers can be selective about who has access to them, which can have a range of effects. For instance, when a manager sits alone in the garden for ten minutes, or joins a group of residents for coffee, or writes a report at the dining-room table, she conveys different messages about her need for privacy. By considering some managerial roles which vary in their need for interactions with individuals or groups, it is possible to see how privacy can be more or less important, and how both the design of the building and the philosophical underpinning of the staff group can affect its use. Where the environment becomes more complex and staff, service users and others intermix, private space for one-to-one or small group work can become crucial.

An enabling environment for all

Design is an important factor in improving people's wellbeing. Yet, for much of the 20th century, care service workers and users were rarely asked for their views on the design of their environments (Sommer, 1969; Willcocks *et al.*, 1987). Design and advances in technology can be enabling, and the rights of people with disabilities to accessibility to and within buildings are being recognised. As a result of the Disability Discrimination Act 1995 and the Disability Discrimination (Services and Premises) Regulations 1999, duties to make reasonable adjustments to the design and construction of buildings and fixtures and fittings will be introduced in 2004. Of course, some of the best ideas regarding the design and use of space can work for everybody. Detailed advice on the physical settings that work best for people with dementia is a useful example. For instance, arranging chairs around coffee tables to create a more natural feel encourages interaction; using signs and pictures on doors means they can be easily identified; different decoration schemes for corridors facilitate orientation; dead ends or areas that present confusing choices can be avoided; varying the levels and types of lighting can reflect changes in the season and time of day; and furnishing spaces such as landings, alcoves and entrance halls may give people additional choice of sitting places which aid stimulation (Clarke *et al.*, 1996, pp. 17–8).

The principles of design for people with dementia that are emerging as an international consensus are:

- design should compensate for disability;
- design should maximise independence;
- design should enhance self-esteem and confidence;
- design should demonstrate care for staff;
- design should be orienting and understandable;
- design should reinforce personal identity;
- design should welcome relatives and the local community;
- design should allow control of stimuli.

(Judd *et al.*, 1997, quoted in Marshall, 2001, p. 130)

Few people would disagree with these principles. There is a recognition here of the need to cater to the different uses of care environments by residents, visitors and workers. It is not only in relation to dementia that design underpins the care task. Burton points out the importance in questions of design of returning to the primary task – that is, the reason for the organisation's existence – and the questions it prompts:

What is this building for? Which needs will be met by this room or that piece of furniture? What are we trying to say to people by the way we arrange the front door and entrance?

(Burton, 1998, p. 151)

Burton draws attention to the kitchen as a focal point for its symbolic emotional value as the heart of many care homes, whether for adults or children, providing more than mere physical nourishment. Yet kitchens have often been off-limits for older people, predominantly women, living in residential homes, perhaps for hygiene or safety reasons. What does this choice of space tell us about care, familiarity, risk taking and underlying gender issues? Many managers will be aware of the role that the design of their building plays in facilitating the kind of service they are trying to give. In some services it often means trying to balance different requirements, some of which may conflict (those of health and safety with those of being natural, for instance) – as well as the cultural needs of different individuals, staff and residents – for the kind of environment that best suits them.

Joanna, a manager for a disabled children's respite care home, commented wryly:

> I am responsible for the training development of the staff team, support for the staff team, recruitment and other staffing issues, and also for the building. So I would put it down to three things: it's the young people

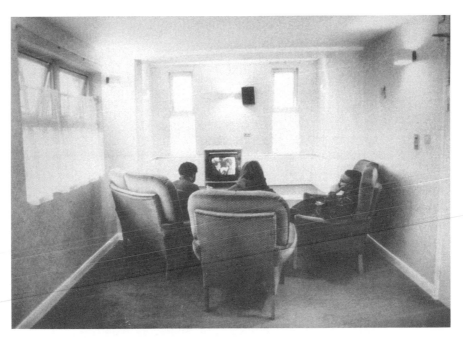

Design is an important factor in improving people's wellbeing
(Source: Brendan Wilson)

and their issues, it's staffing issues and the bricks and mortar that go with it as a residential manager. You don't get training on building regulations; you learn that as you go along.

(Manager consultations)

The environment becomes the backdrop against which all occurs.

Key points

- The way in which space is used underlines the power relations between managers, workers and service users.

- Managers need some control over the balance between accessibility and privacy.

- The design of care environments has an important role in facilitating the service offered.

6.5 Managing at a distance

So far in this chapter we have been looking at the managerial role, boundaries and the environment when people work closely together, often in an interdependent way. Although there are many situations where this is the case, frequently managers do not work on the site where the care takes place but they may visit it. A home care manager, for instance, will probably visit people requiring home care in order to assess the situation but may not need to enter their homes again. Managers of fieldwork teams may visit service users only when a problem has arisen. We shall look at issues for managing at a distance through an example concerning the external management of children's homes.

Richard Whipp and his colleagues found a wide variation of management practices both within and between authorities. This was particularly true of the relationship between line management and the control of homes, with differences between managerial approaches, as the extract in Box 6.2 identifies.

This brief sketch of different management systems and styles highlights many issues and tensions for managers working at a distance, and the people who are managed by them. We look now at those identified in Box 6.2.

BOX 6.2 External line managers of children's homes

There were marked differences in the span of control of line managers, a fact which influenced the amount of time and effort managers were able to devote to supervision. Differences in management style were also noted, with some managers adopting a 'hands-on' approach – *maintaining regular contact* with homes and intervention in operational matters – and others, a more 'hands-off' style. Depending on the context, a 'hands-off' approach was viewed either as positive, allowing the officer in charge *much greater autonomy*, or negative, resulting in the greater isolation of the home from the department. Not surprisingly, the credibility of line managers with home staff was found to be greatly enhanced if they had *previous experience in residential care*. In about half the cases, a problem of children's homes *becoming increasingly isolated* was recognised, with some attempts made to *draw unit managers into wider decision-making processes* through joint training sessions, placement meetings, multi-functional project groups and strategic workshops. In some local authorities, a *delegation of responsibility for budgets* from line manager to officer in charge had occurred. While not always liked, this move had the advantage of allowing officers much greater flexibility to link spending decisions more closely to the particular needs of the resident group, for example, in the allocation of over-time hours and the purchasing of food and materials.

(Source: Whipp *et al.*, 1998, p. 87, emphasis added)

- *Practice experience.* Managers have more credibility if they have experience of the kind of work that the people they are managing are doing. This is important where management of a residential home is concerned. The unit is a whole system in itself and requires understanding of the culture of the home. What about home care workers? Should their managers have experience of their work and, if not, what can they do? Home care workers often face stressful and difficult situations of their own: for instance the death of a client, high levels of dependence which require commitment and reliability, handling people's finances and exposure to accusations of theft (Bradley and Sutherland, 1995). Managers often have to manage people doing jobs for which as managers they lack experience of or expertise in the skills involved, and this can be a source of anxiety. What are the possibilities for them? Getting to understand the job from the workers' point of view is important, perhaps by spending time with them while they are doing the job. Consultancy from outside experts or mentors may be another resource for workers whose manager is not experienced in their field, as well as 'learning from each other' through peer support.

- *Regular contact.* This is linked with managers who might intervene in operational matters. However, regular contact can also guard against the dangers of isolation and Burton (1998) gives an example of a service manager who spends much time in the homes he is responsible for, and acts as a conduit to senior management, explaining the needs of the residential establishments. This approach can also be applied in day care or fieldwork settings and we might think of it as being practice-led. The line manager will need to be sensitive to issues of territory and boundaries.

- *Recognition of the need for autonomy.* People who work at a distance from their managers need clarity about what their remit is and what authority they have. Without a degree of autonomy to respond to situations as they arise, they can feel undermined and ineffective.

- *Recognising isolation.* A less desirable aspect of autonomy is the isolation that may be involved in work done at a distance from managers. A study of stress experienced by home care workers considers the isolation of their work and the possibilities for staff support networks (Bradley and Sutherland, 1995). The authors point out that this would require a clear commitment by the organisation to make time available for it, since work overload is also a frequently cited source of stress. Support through telephone contact and the use of mobile phones are other ways to help combat isolation. Visits to people's own homes can raise personal safety issues for both visitor and visited. Managers have responsibilities regarding training and awareness of boundaries for staff working in isolation.

- *Engagement in joint decision making.* This is a way of integrating frontline managers into the wider purposes of the organisation, and of making sure that considerations about their work are taken into account when planning policy and strategy. Activities that might be called 'training' are the vehicle for this, with perhaps some involvement in strategic discussions. It sounds good – but there are some tensions. How much time do managers have for organisational meetings? Does more activity on this front draw them away from their detailed involvement in their unit's practice and give them new organisational duties?

- *Devolution of budgets.* While this can be a mixed blessing, bringing additional administrative work, many budget decisions are better made at the point where their impact will be felt, providing there really is some flexibility about how money will be used.

In this section we have drawn attention to some of the tensions that distance involves for managers and the people who are managed. One way of dealing with concerns over the quality of work is to increase control and tell people what to do. Another is to spend more time with the workers and service users in order to get a clearer picture of how they see things, and why certain kinds of decisions are taken. A third way is to work on the quality assurance systems, which is the approach discussed next.

> **Key points**
>
> - There is a delicate balance for managers at a distance from the site of care practice. Too much intervention can be undermining; too little contact can seem like indifference.
>
> - Support for isolated workers from peers or through involving them in wider organisational developments can compete for time with the main focus of their work.

6.6 Living environments – environmental quality and managing standards

Residential homes are regulated services and are inspected to ensure compliance with statutory regulations. Managers are part of this regulation – they need to be registered with the appropriate regulatory body. Does regulation have an impact on the quality of care provided, the quality of the environment and the quality of life experienced? How is this achieved and what compromises are made in order to bring about change? There are issues for individuals and organisations responsible for running the business, and there may be particular issues for operational managers who are not in a position to change some aspects of the environment, such as the building or the level of staffing (Rouse, 1999).

Before looking at the environmental aspects of quality of life within residential care for older people, it is important to understand the structures and guidance offered through regulation. At the turn of the century the regulation of services has been moving through a period of change. As a result of the Care Standards Act 2000, a regionally based Commission for Care Standards has evolved in England to replace the former registration and inspection system run by local authorities and health services. A devolved structure has been developed and from April 2002 regulation is undertaken in England through the National Care Standards Commission; in Scotland through the Scottish Commission for the Regulation of Care; in Wales through the Care Standards Inspectorate for Wales; and in Northern Ireland at the time of writing (May 2002) there is a wide range of agencies with a regulatory role. The Commissions and other regulatory bodies have responsibility for regulating a range of services for children, adults and private and voluntary health care agencies. Also note that at the time of writing it was announced that the new National Care Standards Commission will merge with the Social Services Inspectorate (SSI) to form the Commission for Social Care Inspection, which will be in operation from 2004 (Brown, 2002).

Registration to operate a service under the Care Standards Act 2000 builds on former legislation, and registration is based on tests of fitness. Registration may be refused where a person is deemed not to be fit and where the facilities and certain procedures are deemed unfit. After registration, fitness is also to the fore as failure in any one of these areas may be deemed an offence. While not outlined in detail, it has been commented that the 'requirements for *good* management are implicit rather than explicit in the Regulations' (Department of Health, 1999b, p. 62).

Alongside the Act and the Regulations, *national minimum standards* for all services have been developed by groups of experts in order to guide the work of the Commissions (some services are still in that process at the time of writing). In relation to residential care for adults, the national minimum standards in England and Wales were the first set to be developed through an advisory group led by the Centre for Policy on Ageing. The standards are intended from their inception to provide 'core requirements' – a minimum level of resource that can provide the basis of quality. Box 6.3 shows the areas covered by minimum standards for care homes.

BOX 6.3 Minimum standards for care homes

The areas covered include:

- choice of home

- health and personal care

- daily life and social activities

- complaints and protection

- environment

- staffing

- management and administration.

(Source: Department of Health, 2001d, p. viii)

However, the introduction of what might appear to be quite modest requirements has an immediate impact on how many homes can continue to operate. A controversial issue for homeowners and for operational managers has been the specification of room size and the availability of choice of single rooms (McCurry, 2001). Changes in the basic building structure have immediate cost implications in terms of both the cost of alterations and the potential to recoup this outlay, and the ability of the home to avoid going into deficit if it cannot take the same number of residents as a result. Example 6.3 describes the actions that the registered manager at Swift Lodge is taking in order to meet standards.

EXAMPLE 6.3 Juggling the room allocation

In the long term, Rita Jones (the registered manager at Swift Lodge) anticipates that the voluntary body that owns the home will build another wing of rooms that meet, or exceed, the standards. In the short term, she is having alterations made to several of the larger rooms to provide en suite bathrooms. These rooms will be allocated on the basis of need. However, there are three shallow stairs to the corridor where the converted rooms are, so the residents of these rooms will have to be able, unaided, either to use the stair-lift she is having installed or to climb the steps. This places an immediate limitation on the sort of need that might have priority.

Two rooms that were previously used as residents' bedrooms do not now meet the standards, and Rita is thinking that, unless they can get permission to continue to use them temporarily, she will convert them to a guest bedroom and a staff room.

The overall number of resident places that Rita can offer is reduced. Her manager expects her to keep the maximum number of places occupied by residents – whether they pay entirely for themselves or have additional top-up monies from the local authority – in order to show there is sufficient income to justify keeping the home open. So far, Rita has never had to leave a room unoccupied for long and has always been able to meet her financial targets. She is wondering whether she can continue to do this given the current limitations on how she can use rooms.

(Source: manager consultations)

After much debate and lobbying on both sides, from homeowners and from the Coalition for Quality in Care (a campaigning group made up of some 50 expert bodies), implementation of some standards was deferred or the requirements were weakened (Department of Health, 2001d, 2002a). From 2003, new care homes are expected to be built with single rooms of a minimum of 12 square metres. There is some flexibility for existing provision that does not meet these standards but is otherwise of good quality.

As a living environment, the importance of having a single bed-sitting-room has been commented on by residents from the days of overcrowded workhouses and later the growth of local authority homes, right up to the times of the current diversity of settings (Willcocks et al., 1987). More recently, ideas about the value of private space have moved on to a recognition of the importance of spatial control that offers the opportunity for people to be themselves at different times of the day, in different moods, alone or with others, surrounded by objects that reflect something about them. Recent research within Methodist homes for older people shows that where rooms exceed 20 square metres people can personalise them, differentiate spatial areas and maintain the self more easily:

> Whilst most residents managed to create a living environment in rooms which averaged around 20 square metres (with toilet/wash room), many admitted that this was rather restrictive. In the light of recent debates around minimum spatial allocations in residential and nursing home settings for older people, where a minimum of 12 square metres is recommended for the future (Department of Health, 1999b), it is salutary to see what these residents experienced as a workable and realistic minimum. That 20 square metres were regarded as just adequate is further supported by the finding that about a third of informants said that they wished they had brought more or other items of furniture. Sometimes this had not been possible because there was simply not the space; sometimes it was a regrettable miscalculation as to what space was available and what items would fit in ...
>
> (Kellaher, 2000, p. 14)

Once standards of a certain quality are achieved, the question of which issues are most important to service users may change. The attitudes and behaviour of the people involved enable the living environment to be used to the full. How can managers develop the atmosphere of their service to improve environmental wellbeing? They will want the right of individual residents to privacy to be well understood by all parties. An important way may be through a recognition of everyday routines and the different ways in which people may approach them. The tensions between individual needs within the collective setting have to be acknowledged and it will be the managerial role to take responsibility for understanding the ways and routines of different people and the conflicts that may arise through a range of interactions.

Key points

- Minimum standards provide a means of raising the overall quality of care provision.

- The introduction of standards may be problematic for some care providers and nevertheless may fail to meet service users' needs.

6.7 Visiting environments – crossing the boundaries

As we commented in the discussion of the environment at Swift Lodge, many working environments are multifunctional and are visiting environments as well as settings for living or working. Returning to Goffman's consideration of behaviour within areas termed the 'front' and 'back' regions, he argues that there may also be a need to control the 'front' region in the way it is presented to outsiders, especially when they appear unexpectedly. It is here that connections can be made with the different forms of environment that were identified earlier and which lead us to look at the impact on the managerial context in more detail:

> when we shift our consideration from the front or back region to the outside we tend also to shift our point of reference from one performance to another. Given a particular ongoing performance as a point of reference, those who are outside will be persons for whom the performers actually or potentially put on a show, but a show ... different from, or all too similar to, the one in progress. When outsiders unexpectedly enter the front or the back region of a particular performance-in-progress, the consequence of their inopportune presence can often best be studied not in terms of its effects upon the performance-in-progress but rather in terms of its effects upon a different performance, namely, the one which the performers or the audience would ordinarily present before the outsiders at a time and place when the outsiders would be the anticipated audience.
>
> (Goffman, 1969, pp. 135–6)

You will probably need to read this passage several times as you think about the different types of performance that are referred to here and apply the idea to different contexts. For whom is the show being put on, and who are the performers and who are the outsiders or visitors? The outsiders to a home for older people are varied: other professional workers; inspectors; the family and friends of the service user; potential service users; and tradespeople. For managers who are managing the work of someone at a distance, they themselves may be the visitor – for instance, as a line manager of a residential home – or both manager and worker may be visitors to the home of someone receiving home care. They will be operating on a different part of their 'territorial net'. The emphasis changes according to your reading of the presentation by those in charge of the environment. Decisions have to be made about which performances should be played along with, which ones may need challenging or rescripting, and how this can be done in a way that respects ownership of the territory.

What kind of presentations need to be managed in a visiting environment? Does it make a difference whether the visit is planned or unplanned? Registered managers need to be ready for either – a feature of inspection visits is that some will be made without prior warning. This points to the need for a clear understanding of standards, and agreement between manager and staff on how these are met, so that everyone feels confident that they are going about their work in the best possible way at all times. In our original discussion of Swift Lodge, we considered the welcome that would be given, and the role of the reception area and its staff in facilitating the visit through communication to all parties.

As with inspectors, line managers or home care assistants, other visitors may have a 'job' to do on their visit. Relatives may have a demanding conversation ahead of them, perhaps sorting out important issues to do with financial or personal decisions, or responding to a change in the health or wellbeing of their family member. Some family centres make space available for access visits by parents to their children. What kind of planning and preparation can the manager do to make sure that intimate encounters are given the privacy and the space that they need, and that staff respond appropriately to the unexpected as well as planned arrangements?

Rita Jones at Swift Lodge comments that her time can often be taken up by a son or a daughter wanting urgently to discuss a resident's situation. She does not regard this as an interruption that should be rescheduled at a time convenient to herself: visitors have often travelled long distances, and she believes it is important to respond to them when they need to deal with, or avert, a problem. However, consider again Goffman's insights in Box 6.1 – the concept of audience segregation may be relevant here. A manager may feel that it is important to take a relative to a private place where they are not overheard by staff or residents. Sometimes it can be important to tell two different versions of the same story, each containing more or less detail. Variation in performance can be crucial to the visiting environment.

Key points

- Working environments can also have important functions for visitors.

- The performance of managers and other workers is likely to vary according to whether they are an outsider or an insider.

- Managers need to be able to respond with sensitivity to the demands of different people using the same environment for distinctive purposes.

6.8 Conclusion

In this chapter we explored the manager's role in relation to the different and complex settings in which social care takes place. What can managers do to facilitate the use of space, territory and privacy by different people, with different aims and preferences, interacting in any one social care environment? This aspect of managerial competence is not one that is routinely considered in social care and, in reading this chapter, you have taken part in some new ways of putting together knowledge.

Although not every social care environment serves as many different purposes as residential care homes, they are all likely to be multifaceted. Some environments are affected by the changes in use of a room or a building throughout the day. We suggested that managers need an awareness of these different functions and meanings. In particular, they can usefully analyse the public/private and formal/informal nature of what takes place in the care environment, and the implications for this of the degree of privacy and territorial ownership required by the people using it.

The notion of territory carries with it the potential for competition and dispute. We considered issues of power and control over how space is used. The provision of services is underpinned by values, not all of which will be openly acknowledged. The manager has a role in drawing out values more explicitly, debating those that are contested with staff and, where possible, service users, so that some understanding and agreement can be reached about how people's needs for privacy, self-expression and choice can best be met. The accomplishment of what might be thought of as 'ground rules' includes consideration of the management and facilitation of visitors and other outsiders who may need to use the care space for different purposes.

Thoughts on the main purpose of a building, and the environment and atmosphere that need to be created, make a good starting point for considering the use of design. There are major implications here in making places accessible for people with disabilities, and in considering the meaning of different kinds of building for the people using it, but not all design issues carry heavy costs.

When the territory where care is taking place is not shared by the manager, so that managing is at a distance, managers need to find a balance with those they are managing that takes into account the need for autonomy; reduces feelings of isolation as well as fears of insufficient accountability; and engages those who work at a distance in creating a vision of aims and ethos that the organisation can support without distracting them from their primary task of providing good care.

Increasingly, managers will be aiming to meet standards, many of which have a direct impact on the kind of environment considered suitable for the care task. As ideas about what is considered to be the minimum baseline change and additional improvements are sought, managers will often find themselves juggling what is required and what is feasible in terms of finance, income and fixed costs. These discussions link closely with the subject of the next chapter on quality in social care.

Chapter 7
Quality matters

Steve Walker, Barbara Murray and Dorothy Atkinson

7.1 Introduction

Quality matters. It has become an increasingly important influence on the purchases people make and the services they use. So much so that advertisers often focus on quality to sell products: 'If only everything in life was as reliable as a Volkswagen!' In health and social care, where services have a direct impact on people's lives, quality has a far greater significance. It matters in terms of the quality of the service delivered and the quality of life experienced. Consequently, managers in health and social care find themselves increasingly involved in having to 'think', 'do' and 'measure' quality, and are faced with what can often feel like a bewildering number of quality initiatives. Recent examples from the Department of Health include Quality Protects (1998c), National Service Frameworks (1999d) and Quality Strategy (2000b).

Although quality is so high on the health and social care agenda, it remains an elusive concept to define and a mystery to be unravelled (Pattison, 1997; Donabedian, 1980). Quality implies excellence, or at least the pursuit of excellence – but what does that mean in practice? According to Coulshed and Mullender (2001), it means providing services that are fit for their purpose, but doing so at a reasonable cost and with due regard for ensuring informed choice on the part of the people using them. In the consultation document *A Quality Strategy for Social Care* (Department of Health, 2000b) quality is not actually defined. However, it is described as a process of changing and improving (modernising) services, so that they are accessible and consistent, and are delivered by a competent workforce to meet the needs of those who use them. In health and social care the two aspects of quality are interlinked; how good a service is can be understood by how well it supports the quality of life of those who use it (Burton and Kellaway, 1998).

Although quality is supposed to be everyone's concern these days, it is the responsibility of managers to deliver it. In this chapter we look at definitions of quality and the different perspectives of various stakeholders on what it means in practice. We review the origins of quality and trace how it has developed in the health and social care field. We consider current perceptions of quality and examine the various strategies used in recent years to promote it. We explore approaches to implementing quality and, finally, consider how it may be evaluated.

The aims of this chapter are to:

- explore the concept of 'quality' and its various meanings
- understand the different perspectives on quality of various stakeholders
- trace the origins and development of quality in health and social care
- review current ideas and debates about quality
- consider and compare key approaches to implementing quality
- identify ways in which quality may be evaluated.

7.2 Exploring quality in health and social care

Although quality is hard to define and remains elusive in abstract terms, nevertheless it is possible to tease out what it means in practice. Just as people know a poor-quality service when they see and experience it, so they can recognise a high-quality one from first-hand experience. This first-hand experience, according to some commentators, is what determines quality. On this basis, quality derives from knowing who uses your service, understanding what they would like from you, and being able to respond appropriately to their requirements (Martin and Henderson, 2001). This is a view expressed in the management literature, by Peters for example, who consistently argues that successful organisations must stay close to their customers to ensure that they meet their needs (Peters and Waterman, 1988). This is echoed in the social work field: 'The ultimate test of quality will always be what users and their families think of the services we provide' (Coulshed and Mullender, 2001, p. 60).

Quality becomes particularly important in health and social care services where the people using them – the 'customers' – are at least temporarily disadvantaged and vulnerable through adverse circumstances. This means that people with relatively little power are in contact in their day-to-day lives with organisations that are correspondingly powerful. The imbalance of power between, for example, learning disability services and the people with learning difficulties who use them, means that quality itself is vulnerable to:

- financial pressures
- the interests of others, especially staff and families
- a drift from high standards over time
- the societal position of disabled people (relatively low status and priority).

(Adapted from Burton and Kellaway, 1998, p. 225)

There are at least two perspectives on the quality of services: the views of those who provide the services and the views of those people who receive them. To explore the meaning of quality both sets of views must be taken into account. We put the question 'What does quality mean to you?' to managers in a variety of health and social care settings. Some of their replies are shown in Example 7.1.

EXAMPLE 7.1 What does quality mean?

'Quality means that we are trying to achieve the best we can in whatever we do, and that's part of our whole philosophy, that really goes through everything we do. So it's quality of life we're interested in, the quality of life of our residents, and that includes their physical and emotional wellbeing and whatever spiritual striving they have. So we're looking at ourselves and each other, and very specifically our residents as well, as whole human beings where every aspect of their and our humanity has to be addressed in our daily life.'

(Manager of a village community for people with learning difficulties)

'Quality for me is an open, honest, respectful and well-practised service. It's a well-informed practice, so if you're offering a service to young people it has to be a genuine, understanding, supportive and open service. So quality means to me that young people are getting a good-quality service, and for the workers, quality in their work is that they actually believe what they are doing. So they're honest, open, respectful and they value each other. They feel valued, and so we get good-quality work.'

(Manager of a children's centre)

'I think a quality organisation is one that values the people within it. Quality initiatives are extremely current at the moment in all areas of health and social care, and this organisation has in the past couple of months achieved Investor in People accreditation. It's been an extremely positive experience for us.'

(Regional office manager of a mental health voluntary organisation)

(Source: manager consultations)

In this instance the managers are from the voluntary sector. They describe quality in terms of:

- the *quality of life* of the people who use their service, and how good that is
- the *quality of the experience* of using the service, and how open, honest and respectful the service is to those on the receiving end
- the *quality of the workforce*, and how valued and valuing people are in their work.

It is interesting that managers here define quality as referring to how people are treated while they are using a service and what outcomes – or quality of life – they derive from it. Similarly, the document *A Quality Strategy for Social Care* (Department of Health, 2000b) states: 'We must focus on what people want from services'. According to a 'body of evidence', they want high-quality services, meaning services that:

- meet high standards
- are responsive
- are appropriate
- build on people's abilities and enable them to participate fully in society
- involve the user so that choices are informed
- offer strong safeguards for those at risk.

(Adapted from Department of Health, 2000b, p. 6)

There is no doubt that quality is high on the agenda nowadays – but why? The next section traces some of the origins of current interest in quality.

Key points

- Quality is an elusive concept in abstract terms, and is best defined in terms of people's experiences.

- Quality, in service terms, refers to the quality of life, the quality of experience, and the quality of the workforce.

- A high-quality service is responsive, enabling and inclusive.

7.3 Origins of quality in health and social care

Where did the notion of 'quality' in health and social care come from? The way in which it is viewed by practitioners and managers can be traced back to the circumstances that surrounded the introduction of quality management into the social care field in the 1980s. This is not to suggest that there was no concept of, or interest in, quality before then, but rather that in the 1980s the concept of quality, the way in which it was characterised and understood, altered quite radically. Until then, social care had adopted what Pollitt (1997) termed a *professional* approach to quality. A professional approach meant ensuring that 'services are technically of a high standard in terms of prevailing professional aspirations' (Pollitt, 1997, p. 34). In this sense, quality belongs to, and is defined by, the profession, normally through senior members of the profession or groups of experts.

Professional approaches to quality are concerned with inputs and processes rather than with the outcomes of the service for the people who use it. The manner in which the service is provided becomes the primary concern. Typically, in professional approaches, quality is assessed through the production of professional standards or competences against which the performance of an individual professional is measured by means of some form of inspection or peer review. A key benefit of such approaches is that quality is more likely to be embedded in the core values and based on the technical competences of the profession. As a result, notions of quality are more likely to be 'owned' by those working in the profession than if they were externally produced and 'handed down'.

However, there are a number of potential weaknesses inherent in professional approaches. Quality, from this perspective, becomes an essentially introspective process that takes place within the profession and from which the user of the service is excluded. Quality assurance, therefore, can 'degenerate into a situation of cosy connoisseuralism in which senior members of a profession or expert group exercise great influence without having to justify their judgements in terms of transparent or evidence based criteria' (Pollitt, 1997, p. 34). Further, although the profession may define standards, it is usually left to individual professionals to ensure that their practice adheres to those standards. The assumption is that there is no need to establish systems to ensure that changes are implemented, as professional staff are considered to be so well motivated that they need no incentive or sanctions to embrace best professional practice.

It was against the background of this professional approach that quality became an increasingly high-profile activity in social care in the 1980s. Wistow (1991) and Hardy and Wistow (1997) identified five key influences that underpinned the development of quality in social care. First, there was a growing body of evidence from research and inquiry reports of poor performance in social care. A series of scandals, particularly in relation to child protection and residential care, had raised concerns among both politicians and the public that previous policy guidance had not been translated into improved practice. Second, there was a climate of budget reductions that meant it was no longer possible to improve quality by increasing the level of services. As a result, the emphasis of quality shifted to improving services through greater efficiency and cost effectiveness.

The third influence was the rise of an increasingly powerful consumerist movement. In the health and social care field this took the form of specific interest groups such as disabled people, mental health survivors, carers and 'looked-after' young people. These groups challenged the notion that the professionals always knew best and lobbied for service users to play an active role in the design, delivery and evaluation of services. The fourth influence was an increasing consensus between professionals and service user groups that the outcomes of social care should be 'towards enhancing the quality of individuals' lifestyles and their experience of service delivery' (Hardy and Wistow, 1997, p. 175). The final influence identified by Wistow was the change in management culture within social care.

These factors need to be located within the political context that existed in the 1980s, as it exerted a profound influence on the way in which quality developed and is currently perceived in health and social care. The then Conservative government viewed public services as monopolistic, restrictive of individual choice and freedom, and limiting the ability of the free market to operate. From that perspective they could be viewed as representing the antithesis of the values at the heart of the Thatcher government. As a result, a key government objective was to transform the nature of public services.

The planned transformation of public services, it was argued, could only be achieved if there were a similar transformation in management. Setting the scene for this process of change was the assertion 'Efficient management is the key to the (national) revival ... And the management ethos must run right through our national life – private and public companies, nationalised industries, local government, the National Health Services' (Heseltine, 1980, quoted in Pollitt, 1986). Existing management within the public sector, drawn mainly from within the professional groups, was considered too reactive and preoccupied with inputs and processes to push through the radical changes necessary.

Quality was a key issue used by the Conservative government to legitimise its agenda for radical changes to the way in which health and social care was structured, managed and delivered. However, quality was also the tool used to effect these changes. If the public sector did not have the necessary knowledge, skills or experience to provide high-quality services, then these would have to be imported. The government looked to the private sector, where quality was enjoying a renaissance. Peters and Waterman, in their book *In Search of Excellence* (1988), argued that it was the development of a culture of quality within an organisation, where quality was recognised as the responsibility of each individual, that provided the basis of the achievements of the USA's most successful companies. Success could be achieved, it was argued, through the pursuit of quality. The White Paper *Caring for People: Community Care in the Next Decade and Beyond* (Department of Health and Social Security, 1989) reflected this view, identifying for the first time in the personal social services the notion of quality control as a way of achieving a 'high standard of care' (James, 1992, p. 38).

> **Key points**
>
> - Before the 1980s quality was defined by professionals in terms of inputs and processes.
>
> - The professional view of quality was challenged at all levels, from government to service users.
>
> - The drive to improve services led to the introduction of quality control.

7.4 Development of the concept of quality

The introduction of private sector concepts and practice changed the focus of quality in health and social care. Unlike the professional model, with its emphasis on inputs, the business model of quality is concerned with outputs. To be successful, in this view, an organisation has to provide customers with what they want. In fact, more than this, the organisation should aim to surpass its customers' expectations. Competition should be encouraged, it is argued, as this improves quality. Increasing the amount of choice available to consumers forces organisations to increase the quality of their products and services in order to attract and keep customers. A key feature of the Thatcher government's approach to public services was to introduce or increase competition. In social care the role of local authorities was shifted from a 'monopolistic role to an enabler, purchaser and occasional provider role within a mixed economy of provision' (James, 1992, p. 41).

It could be argued that the business model of quality was brought in and imposed on managers and practitioners who were, in the main, unready for such a shift in ethos. Indeed, it could also be argued that the field of health and social care is unsuited to such an approach because of the nature of public services. Put simply, the rationale for improving quality in business is to increase customers and profits. How far can this approach be applied in health and social care settings? While there may be a drive to increase customers in some private residential homes in order to increase profits, much health and social care is provided free of charge or at a subsidised cost. Furthermore, it is not just the direct consumers of services who take a keen interest in health and social care: their families, future users, wider society and politicians at both local and national level are all potential stakeholders.

As inspection was already well established within social care, some agencies responded to the new climate by using inspection as the basis for their approach. However, inspection is concerned with quality control *not* quality assurance. Quality control involves monitoring services against agreed standards. This means using statistical and other routinely gathered information to check that services are doing what they say they are doing. According to a key Social Services Inspectorate document, quality control is concerned with 'processes of verification [based on] systematic monitoring, including statistical and other management information, recurring and one-off audits and inspection activity designed to establish whether standards are being achieved' (Social Services Inspectorate, 1991a, p. 30).

Quality control is essentially top-down and reactive. Its focus is on actual and potential defects. Consequently, it is often perceived by practitioners as a negative experience. Quality control approaches do not identify the extent to which practice has exceeded standards, only where they have not been met or reached. A quality control approach to quality, therefore, can only improve quality to the level of the standards set. It has no mechanism for the ongoing improvement and development of services.

Quality assurance, on the other hand, is more proactive in that it involves putting measures into place in advance. It is also a more 'bottom-up' approach in that it tends to involve staff more in the process of delivering a better-quality service to the people who use it (Coulshed and Mullender, 2001). To meet the demands of the new quality agenda, many organisations in health and social care established what they called 'Quality Assurance' sections. However, in practice this often involved little more than changing the name of the Registration and Inspection Unit, which reinforced the view that quality assurance was a form of quality control. Not only was quality equated with inspection in these organisations, but also it was perceived as being detached from everyday practice. Quality was seen as the responsibility of the Quality Assurance unit. It did not involve frontline practitioners and managers, other than through their co-operating with inspections by the Quality Assurance unit and ensuring that standards were met.

Equating quality assurance with quality control results in an approach to quality that is dominated by the achievement of standards and performance indicators, which become the only criteria for success. The drawback of this approach is that it pays no attention to how performance indicators are achieved. It is easy to see, therefore, how this approach to quality can be viewed by practitioners, and experienced by users, as unrelated to and unhelpful in practice. Some aspects of care, although not directly measurable, are nevertheless very important. Some qualitative issues, for example, are difficult to capture through performance indicators, which are generally quantitative in nature:

> So often it is the style of the way that services are delivered rather than the service itself which provides a quality service ... the home carer who gets you up in the morning can do this in an empowering way which enables you to face the effort of the day positively or in a way which means that you are dressed and ready but not psychologically ready.
> (Wiltshire and Swindon Service Users Network, quoted in Beresford et al., 1997, p. 77)

Quality assurance is concerned with pursuing good-quality services. This means taking a systematic approach to service delivery: documenting processes, ensuring well-supported and trained staff, and reviewing practice. It demands a culture shift so that the notion of quality is embedded in services:

> Quality assurance is used to refer to those processes which aim to ensure that concern for quality is designed and built into services. It implies commitment on the part of local authority social services committee members and senior managers to a systematic approach to the pursuit of quality and will be demonstrated by an explicit statement of policy, setting out agency expectations and standards. Systematic and comprehensive arrangements to ensure that the required standards are achieved will be evident throughout organisational procedures and will include processes for verification and feedback.
>
> (Social Services Inspectorate, 1991a, p. 30)

Quality assurance is not just about the assessment of quality. It includes the mechanisms the organisation has in place to promote quality, such as mission statements, policy documents and procedures, such as training and appraisal, to ensure that staff have the necessary skills and expertise to meet the required standards. The differences between quality control, quality assurance and Total Quality Management (discussed later in this chapter) are outlined in Table 7.1.

Table 7.1 **Three different approaches to quality**

Characteristics	*Quality control*	*Quality assurance*	*Total Quality Management*
Works through	Standards	Systems	People
Purpose	Uniformity to standards	Efficiency of systems	Improve outcomes for users
Responsibility	Inspectorate or Qe unit	Each division or each unit	Everyone, but led by the manager
View of quality	Absence of defect	Preventive	Opportunity
Primary concern	Detection of error	Co-ordination	Impact
Popular forms of expression	Inspection	Quality assurance systems	Total quality management Continuous quality improvement Quality improvement process Quality improvement teams/ quality circles

(Source: James, 1994b, p. 202)

The way quality assurance is currently perceived within social care was also influenced by the financial climate that existed in the public services in the 1980s. Quality management was being promoted at a time when most organisations were experiencing reductions in the level of expenditure. Consequently, many authorities used quality assurance 'primarily as a means of financial constraint' (Social Services Inspectorate, 1991b). Quality assurance thus became a way of identifying service areas where capacity could be increased in order to allow cutbacks in other areas or services. Unfortunately, identifying greater efficiencies in one area of a service did not result in a reallocation of resources; rather, those resources were simply lost. Therefore, for many practitioners quality assurance became associated with service reductions.

> **Key points**
>
> - Private sector concepts of customers and competition were introduced to public services to drive up quality.
>
> - Quality control mechanisms were introduced to monitor services against certain standards and performance indicators.
>
> - Quality assurance has become a more helpful, and acceptable, approach to achieving high-quality services: it promotes quality rather than imposing it.

7.5 Current perceptions of quality

Quality in social care is not a simple or straightforward concept. Its origins are somewhat mixed, a point made by James (1992, p. 38): 'From the beginning financial, ideological and political imperatives were to be wrapped together in what was later to emerge as quality'. Quality emerged from the 1980s as one of the key issues around which the future of social care would be debated. This debate has become increasingly polarised. On one side is the development of standards and the establishment of professional competences, and their enforcement, through the establishment of the General Social Care Council (and its counterparts in Scotland, Wales and Northern Ireland). This is seen as the means by which professional standards will improve and, thus, public confidence will be restored. On the other side of the debate the managerial approach to quality has been viewed as a mechanism for limiting the professional freedom of the individual practitioner.

The view of quality as constraint is articulated by Parton:

> The increased emphasis on management, evaluation, monitoring and constraining professionals to write things down, is itself a form of government of them, and more crucially, of those with whom they are working. It forces them to think about what they are doing and hence makes them accountable to certain norms.
>
> (Parton, 1994, p. 96)

The issues for Parton and others are how and by whom these norms are established and what is the potential for them to be hijacked to meet political agendas. The view of quality as cost cutting is also viewed with concern:

> Consequently it is perfectly possible for commentators to see the NHS and Community Care Act, for example, both as a clear attempt to rein in the costs of social care and reduce the state to a residual role – and an attempt to make services more flexible and responsive to the differing circumstances and preferences of individuals.
>
> (Beresford *et al.*, 1997, p. 66)

This debate is not simply an academic issue; it is one that must be understood by frontline managers. The way in which individuals and teams understand and approach issues of quality will be influenced by the debate, even if this is not always articulated.

Key points

- There is a debate around the notion of quality.

- Is quality a means of ensuring high standards of care or of restricting the autonomy of the practitioner?

- Is quality a means of ensuring a flexible and responsive service or of cutting costs?

7.6 Developments in promoting quality

In recent years two key bodies were responsible for promoting quality in social care: the Audit Commission and the Social Services Inspectorate. As well as their separate programmes of work, since 1996 the two bodies have undertaken Joint Reviews. Subsequently, the Quality Protects programme was launched in 1998, and in 2000 Best Value was introduced as a mechanism for ensuring quality services. This section will consider each of these developments in turn.

Audit Commission

The Audit Commission was established through the Local Government Finance Act 1982. Its role was to assess public services against the criteria of the 'three Es': economy, efficiency and effectiveness. Its initial approach was to use its technical expertise in quantitative analysis – an approach that aims to look objectively at a service in order to measure its performance in some way. This could be by comparing it with other services, for example. The 1986 Audit Commission report *Making a Reality of Community Care* used simple comparative statistics and performance indicators to highlight the perverse financial incentives that existed within service provision for older people. Put simply, several factors in place at the time meant that it was actually cheaper to place older people in residential settings than to support them in their own homes. Clearly, this did not make sense at any level, and the report proved influential in bringing about the sweeping changes that occurred in community care in subsequent years.

Performance indicators became one of the key tools used by the Audit Commission for systematic analysis of services. Performance indicators identify key areas where information about the service performance of an organisation should be gathered. They also identify a level of performance that the organisation should meet. Typically, they measure such things as referral rates, response times, waiting lists and the like. These can then be evaluated against costs, resources, staffing levels and other inputs. In this way performance indicators allow the performance of local authorities to be both monitored and compared, and consequently remain a key quality tool in social care.

The use of performance indicators and similar tools for systematically evaluating performance was promoted by the Audit Commission for two reasons. At one level, this method was effective as a means of externally auditing and comparing services. At another level, it proved to be a mechanism that local authorities could use internally to promote and support change. Local authorities were encouraged to use the national performance indicators as a baseline from which they could develop their own range of indicators based on local needs and local performance measures. As the Audit Commission developed its role and expertise, there was a shift from an approach based on audit and outcomes to an approach that includes an emphasis on qualitative measures and the process of service delivery.

Social Services Inspectorate

The Social Services Inspectorate (SSI) was created in 1985. Its remit was to disseminate good practice and to undertake the 'systematic investigation of the quality of services received by users and their carers, and the management arrangements for the delivery of these services' (Social Services Inspectorate, 1993, p. 22). Such a systematic framework did not exist. To develop it, the SSI recruited inspectors with a background in management and quantitative analysis. In addition, programmes of research were commissioned to identify key indicators for service planning, delivery and monitoring. The development of the SSI's methodologies was informed by parallel developments in evaluative research, particularly the various special studies of aspects of social services by the Audit Commission.

These methodologies formed the basis of a number of publications aimed at supporting local authorities in developing processes for quality assurance. (See, for example, Social Services Inspectorate, 1990, 1991b, 1993.) The pursuit of quality in social care has continued over the years with a steady stream of publications on the topic from the Department of Health. (These include Department of Health, 1998a and d, 2000b; Social Services Inspectorate/Department of Health, 2001.) The equivalent body in Scotland, the Social Work Services Inspectorate (SWSI), has pursued a programme of themed inspections focusing on strategic issues. (Relevant publications include Scottish Office, 1999, 2000a and b.) The equivalent body in Wales, the Social Services Inspectorate in Wales, is implementing Children First, a programme of national objectives and targets for children's services (National Assembly for Wales, 2000). In Northern Ireland a similar child care strategy is being developed by the Department of Health, Social Services and Public Safety (2002) through its Children First initiative. The aim is to develop good-quality, affordable child care for all children.

As a result of the work of the Audit Commission and the SSI, a range of tools became available to local authorities to support quality assurance before the introduction of the Children Act 1989 – and parallel legislation in Scotland and Northern Ireland – and the NHS and Community Care Act 1990. The Acts required local authorities to establish inspection units for both children's and community care services. National programmes of inspection were conducted by the SSI to support and verify local arrangements. The increased emphasis on inspection within the SSI resulted in the organisation's restructuring in 1992. From then on the policy and inspection functions were separated.

Joint Reviews

A further layer of inspections was added to the separate programmes of inspections carried out by the Audit Commission and SSI with the introduction of Joint Reviews in 1996. Joint Reviews brought together the financial and managerial expertise of the Audit Commission with the professional and technical experience of the SSI 'to look at the overall performance of each local social services authority'. The aim of the Reviews was to 'improve social services by identifying and promoting policies, management and practice which are achieving better outcomes and better value' (Audit Commission/Social Services Inspectorate, 1998, p. 1). Joint Reviews consider the performance of local authority social services against both national standards and those set locally in relation to four key questions:

- Are services focused on meeting individuals' needs?
- Can the authority shape better services for the future?
- Is performance effectively managed?
- Are resources managed to maximise value for money and quality?

(Audit Commission/Social Services Inspectorate, 1998, p. 5)

The Joint Review gathers evidence from a variety of sources including local authority documentation, user questionnaires and interviews, case file analysis and interviews with practitioners and managers. The evidence gathered is evaluated to make a judgement on whether local residents are being well served by their social services. The overall performance of the authority is then plotted on a matrix (Figure 7.1).

The framework used by Joint Review teams allows the performance of individual local authorities to be compared. As well as drawing comparisons, the process also gathers valuable evidence on the effectiveness of particular strategies and approaches. These can then be disseminated.

Quality Protects

As part of the government's drive to improve the quality of health and social care services, the Quality Protects initiative was launched in September 1998. Its overall aim is to improve children's services in England (as stated above, there are also strategies for improving the quality of children's services in Scotland, Wales and Northern Ireland). As part of Quality Protects, all local authorities in England have to submit Management Action Plans (or MAPs) to the Department of Health. In their MAPs, social services departments outline how they have improved children's services in line with government objectives during the previous year, and how they intend to make improvements in the following year.

Funding from the special children's service grant is conditional on local authorities meeting priority areas set by the government. Priority areas for 2001–2, for example, included:

- increasing the choice of adoption, foster and residential placements
- enhancing the development and use of management information systems, and improving quality assurance systems
- improving assessment, planning and record keeping
- improving the life chances of looked-after children.

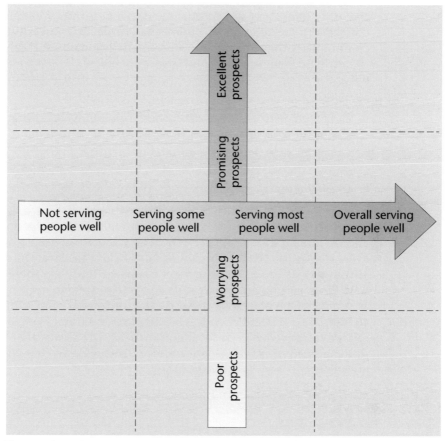

Figure 7.1 **Joint Reviews performance matrix** (Source: Audit Commission *et al.*, 2002, p. 14)

One of the key features of the Quality Protects programme is that it requires the involvement of children and young people, as well as frontline staff, in developing the plans. The detailed and specific information required by Quality Protects – for example, whether a looked-after child or young person has missed more than 25 days of school in the previous year – requires the involvement of frontline staff and managers.

Best Value reviews

The pursuit of quality continued with the introduction of Best Value reviews. Best Value was introduced in April 2000 to replace compulsory competitive tendering. The latter had required local authorities to compare services purely on the basis of cost. Its successor, Best Value, on the other hand, was said to offer 'a relatively permissive regime, allowing councils to develop local approaches, reflecting the diversity of the communities they represent' (Department of Health, 2001e, p. 2).

Best Value requires local authorities to review the services they provide using the 'four Cs':

- *challenging* why and how the service is provided
- *comparing* performance with others (including private and voluntary sector providers)
- *competing* by using open and fair competition in deciding who should deliver the service
- *consulting* with local service users and residents on their expectations of services.

Each local authority must produce an annual Best Value performance plan and undertake a Best Value review of all its services, including social care, every five years. The performance plan sets out the strategic approach the authority will adopt for its services to ensure that they meet the national Best Value performance indicators and to continue to improve the quality of services. The objectives of Best Value reviews are not simply to ensure economic and effective services but to provide a framework for continuous service improvements in local authorities. This means that not only are local authority Best Value performance plans reviewed but also authorities are subject to Best Value inspections.

Key points

- The Audit Commission uses performance indicators to evaluate the performance of public services.

- The Social Services Inspectorate supports – and inspects – quality assurance approaches in local authorities.

- Joint Reviews evaluate how good services are from the point of view of the people who use them.

- The Quality Protects programme aims to improve the quality of children's services.

- Best Value reviews of services are conducted by local authorities using the 'four Cs' (challenging, comparing, competing and consulting).

7.7 Approaches to implementing quality

Quality is more than an empty ideal that managers and practitioners have to live with as a result of various external and internal initiatives. Stripped of the baggage and language that surrounds it, quality is about improving services to users. If it is not about that, it is not about anything. The challenge facing frontline managers is how to develop and maintain a focus on this aspect of quality and how to give it real meaning and application to the work of their teams.

Just as quality is an elusive concept to explain, so it seems to be an elusive idea to promote and put into practice, at least from the top down. Inspections, reviews, special measures and action plans follow one another in pursuit of improving the quality of health and social care services. The question for frontline managers is how best to implement quality. Two approaches seem appropriate to the health and social care field: Total Quality Management and the Excellence Model.

Total Quality Management

Total Quality Management (TQM) focuses on all aspects of quality, both process and outcome. It does so by combining quality assurance and quality control, developing a culture of quality within a team or an organisation. In this approach 'Responsibility for quality rests with each and every member of staff or volunteer and is the first responsibility of every manager' (Warr and Kelly, 1992, p. 5). TQM thus involves the whole organisation. Ideally, all members feel part of, and own, the various levels of the organisation (strategic, operational, customer and development levels).

TQM involves:

- business planning cycles
- performance management systems
- appraisal systems
- quality circles
- codes of practice
- quality manuals
- consumer liaison.

The aim is to develop a culture of quality for the whole organisation. TQM seeks to combine top-down vision and planning with bottom-up involvement and motivation of all staff (Coulshed and Mullender, 2001). The TQM approach was developed in private sector industry. How well does it transfer to the health and social care field? The list in Box 7.1 brings together the common themes and principles of a TQM approach drawn from several sources.

BOX 7.1 Principles of Total Quality Management

Quality is determined by service users

This may appear a difficult concept in social care, which is based on the needs of individuals. However, user groups and research identify a number of common themes that can be used as a starting point for different areas of social care.

Quality is continuous

Quality is not a static issue: it must be the subject of ongoing review and improvement to respond to the changing needs of users.

Quality builds on current strengths

In developing a quality approach, it is important to recognise and build on the strengths that already exist within the organisation and team.

Quality works across boundaries

Developing a quality approach to services provides an opportunity for the team to involve colleagues from within the organisation and external partners. 'Quality has the potential to be part of a shared language, a language able to focus on the common professional concern for the user ... quality can be a channel of dialogue across professional and organisational boundaries which can be potentially neutral' (James, 1994b, p. 211).

Quality is an essential part of good management

Developing and maintaining a quality approach requires not just leadership but an approach that facilitates the involvement of all team members. Managers must create an environment where all can take part and contribute to the quality process.

Quality provides new tools and techniques for practice

A quality approach is not simply concerned with achieving standards and the outcome of services. It is equally concerned with the process by which services are delivered and standards achieved. A quality approach is constantly seeking to improve practice and therefore training is a major feature of such approaches.

(Sources: Dunnachie, 1992; Piggott and Piggott, 1992; Swiss, 1992; James, 1994b; Oppen, 1997)

Although it sounds good, TQM is no panacea. It is essentially a long-term strategy and may be difficult to implement at a unit or team level. There may well be gaps between the rhetoric of 'total quality' and actual day-to-day practice. Box 7.2 sets out a sequence of steps that could be taken to implement a TQM approach within a team or unit. The steps are cyclical, a process illustrated in Figure 7.2.

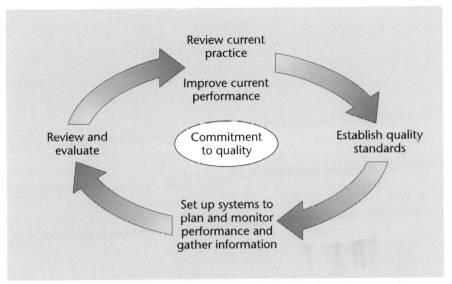

Figure 7.2 **The Total Quality cycle**

BOX 7.2 Implementing TQM

1 Develop a team commitment to quality

At its simplest, this means raising awareness of quality issues in the team. Some team members may approach quality with suspicion, if not hostility, a point made by James:

> The problem is that many of the same mechanisms are used to promote quality as to effect managerial control (information systems, policy and procedural guides, review, inspection, and appraisal). It is all too easy therefore for a manager to talk quality but mean control and for staff to hear quality but understand it as control.
>
> (James, 1992, p. 51)

For this reason, it may help if quality is related directly to improving outcomes for service users. A useful way of developing a culture of quality within the team is to develop a team definition and approach to quality. Quality may also come to be seen as a benefit to workers as well, through job satisfaction for example, or pride in their work.

2 Review current practice

This is best done jointly *as a team*. It means reviewing the areas where the team seems to be performing well. This process could be enhanced by access to information such as the latest performance indicators, recent inspection reports, any user feedback that is available and details of any waiting lists or unallocated work.

As well as identifying where and how the team is performing well, this step also involves the team in discussing how to do things better. Key areas for improvement could be identified through several sources: for example, the organisation's objectives, the requirements of national standards, recommendations from inspections or suggestions from people using the service.

3   Establish quality standards

This is how the team assesses its performance. Although national standards may be set, for example in the Quality Protects programme, these may not be specific enough at a local level. In developing local standards it is important to focus on the practice issues that underpin national indicators. For example, one of the Quality Protects measures is how well looked-after children do in school compared with all the children in the locality. However, the team may feel that this performance indicator is not specific or sensitive enough to get to the heart of the underlying practice issues. Additional quality indicators – such as the number of out-of-school activities and clubs attended – may be needed. Similarly, other national standards may need to be redefined in terms of the practice issues they are trying to address, and could lead to a team developing a number of supporting indicators.

4   Planning better performance

Having identified quality areas, the team can now identify how it will improve its performance. A good way forward is to break down major objectives into smaller tasks and identify a clear timescale. In some cases there may be training or resource implications and, if so, the plan needs to specify how these will be met.

5   Monitoring performance

At some point the team will need to know if it is achieving its planned targets. This requires the gathering of information in a systematic way in order to see how well the team is doing. The most likely sources of information are:

- quantitative data, such as rates of referral, waiting lists, unallocated work, age of service users, ethnicity

- inspection reports

- user questionnaires and surveys of, or consultations with, individuals or groups of service users

- information from partner agencies

- routine audits of specific areas of practice – for example, a review of files to check on the recording of key information. This could be a peer review, so as to make the process less threatening.

6 Review and evaluate

Review and evaluation can take place at a number of levels. At an individual level, supervision and appraisal can be used to review progress against team or individual quality targets, to identify any skills and knowledge gaps that may have arisen and arrange training.

The team could also meet at regular intervals, perhaps having a quarterly team meeting dedicated to quality. This could be used to review progress and to evaluate whether the standards have been met and, if so, whether they have had the anticipated outcomes for service users.

Service users can, and should, play an important role in the evaluation of quality initiatives. These groups may already be established: for example, residents' groups or local support or pressure groups such as Mind. However, it is also possible to establish a local group specifically to consider the issue of quality. The team will also need to consider how best to involve service users in developing quality standards.

7 Improve performance

The objective of TQM is to improve practice at all levels. Having completed its review and evaluation, the final step in the cycle is for the team to identify ways in which it can improve the quality of service it provides.

The Excellence Model

The Excellence Model (previously known as the Business Excellence Model) was launched by the European Foundation for Quality Management in April 1999. It is an approach to quality that enables organisations to assess themselves against a set of criteria for excellence, and to use this self-assessment to do two things: to identify which areas need improving and to consider how best to bring about the changes needed. 'Excellence' in this model is defined as outstanding practice in terms of the core service and how it is managed, delivered and – more to the point – viewed by the people who use it.

The Excellence Model is seen as applicable to the health and social care field. The Quality Standards Task Group, for example, suggests that it has widespread potential:

> The Excellence Model provides a comprehensive framework for continuous improvement and an effective diagnostic tool ... It is potentially suitable for the entire voluntary sector, in all its diversity of scale and function.
>
> (Quality Standards Task Group, 1998, pp. 9–10)

The model provides a broad framework which enables an organisation to incorporate existing or new quality initiatives into its overall pursuit of quality. The Wakefield and Pontefract Community Health NHS Trust, for example, incorporated its existing Investor in People award and status into its model. Similarly, Devon Social Services Department incorporated the requirements of the Quality Protects initiative into its operation of the Excellence Model.

The Excellence Model consists of nine elements (see Figure 7.3). Each element can be used to assess an organisation's progress towards excellence. The first five are *enablers* (concerned with *how* results are being achieved) and the other four are *results* of the process (concerned with *what* is being achieved). The rationale for the model is that leadership drives people management, policy and strategy, and partnerships and resources. Results are seen in terms of people (employees), customers (users) and the impact on society. Good results mean a good service – or excellent performance.

The nine quality criteria are as follows:

1 *Leadership*: how leaders develop and help the organisation towards excellence.
2 *People management*: how the organisation supports its workforce.
3 *Policy and strategy*: how the organisation plans its activities to ensure continuous improvement.
4 *Partnerships and resources*: how the organisation plans and manages its external partnerships and internal resources.
5 *Processes*: how the organisation manages and monitors its activities.
6 *People results*: what the organisation is achieving in relation to its staff.

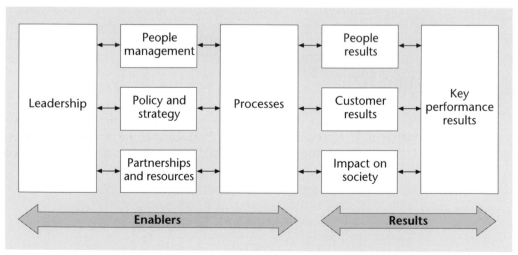

Figure 7.3   **The Excellence Model** (Source: British Quality Foundation, 1998)

7 *Customer results*: what the organisation is achieving in terms of the people who use its services.

8 *Impact on society*: what the organisation is achieving in relation to the expectations of the community.

9 *Key performance results*: what the organisation is achieving in relation to its planned performance.

How well does the Excellence Model work? It has its advocates and indeed it has its merits. It is a whole-systems approach to improvement at team, unit or organisation level, again involving everyone in the process and outcomes. In stressing continuous quality improvement it measures progress over time. Quality models help put systems into place for implementing good practices and, if they work, for delivering good outcomes. But how does the organisation (or team) know it is doing a good job? Is self-assessment, however rigorous, enough to ensure that a good-quality service is delivered? In the final section we look at evaluating quality in practice.

Key points

- Total Quality Management aims to develop a culture of quality for the whole organisation; it combines quality assurance with quality control.

- The Excellence Model enables the organisation to assess itself against a set of criteria for excellence and to use the assessment to achieve excellence.

7.8 Evaluating quality

What does a high-quality service look like – and feel like? How is quality evaluated and by whom? Example 7.2 contains views of some managers we interviewed on how they know whether or not they are delivering a high-quality service.

EXAMPLE 7.2 How is quality evaluated?

'We live as a community, so we are aware of each other, we see each other at home, at work or in our free time. So if someone is not happy, it will show up somewhere – in their work, or in their free time – and because we know the person well, we pick up not only that they are unhappy but also why.

'More formally, we have a review system, an annual review of each resident, where we really go through a person's life, their home life, their work life, their free time, their health, everything. We look at what we said a year ago that we were going to work on, how has that been going, what are we going to work on in the next year, and what people want. The review is really their review of us, the community, and of their life.'

(Manager of a village community for people with learning difficulties)

'We know we're doing a good job from what our service users tell us; that for me is a priority. We have regular reviews in our work: every six weeks or after every six sessions we meet up with the families. We try at the beginning of every piece of work to set a goal – what do they want out of this piece of work – and we then try to measure if we've met that goal, or if we are some way along the line, or haven't met it at all. If we haven't, what do we need to change? So I know if we're doing a good job because of the feedback.

'However, I also know we're doing a good job because we've recently been through a review and an audit. The audit was done by our internal auditors and the review was done by my managers. They sound very similar. The internal audit was by our internal Inspection Unit and they talked a lot with our service users, and with the team, and basically we had a very positive audit report which was really affirming for us as a team, and made us realise how rarely we actually get somebody senior saying, 'Well done, you're doing a really good job'. In fact, we went over the road to the pub and had a drink after it.'

(Manager of a family centre)

'I have a really high expectation of staff and of the project here and of myself, and I feel that I measure quality by my own standard. So I always feel that if I'm a good practitioner it will reflect in the work I do, and it's measured by how young people and how your colleagues receive that. Quality can be measured by the feedback you get from other people. So the quality service is measured by the number of young people that return, and if they didn't return then they didn't value it.

'Quality is measured again by employees: how long they stay, what personal qualities they develop, and what they go on to do. And quality can be measured by the community that you're involved in. So we get a lot of praise from local parents, teachers and other professionals, and the feedback from them is that they value what we are doing.'

(Manager of a project for children and young people)

(Source: manager consultations)

The managers quoted in the example refer to a range of measures of quality:

- feedback from people using the service
- feedback from the wider community
- individual reviews and care plans
- internal audit and review
- staff morale and retention.

This list looks, at first sight, to be unproblematic. However, the first point – feedback from people using the service – is not necessarily straightforward. What happens in situations where people, for whatever reasons, are unable (or unwilling) to say what they think about the service on offer? This could apply to children, especially looked-after and/or disabled children and young people, and also to disabled people, adults with learning difficulties, mental health survivors and people with dementia.

In the learning disability field, for example, several approaches have been used to determine what people think of particular services. In Croydon the Surrey Oaklands NHS Trust worked with 12 people with learning difficulties to develop the skills needed for service reviewing and to identify abuse in homes. The user review group (called Brighter Lives) then visited eight local care homes, talking to residents and finding out what life was like for them. They asked questions, they spent time with residents and they made friends. One of the reviewers explained how it worked: 'They would open up to us and tell us one thing, and the staff another. They could open up because they knew we were like them' (Burrows, 2001, p. 33).

In Kensington and Chelsea the Quality Network (run by the National Development Team and the British Institute for Learning Disabilities) trained 14 people as service assessors, including five people with learning difficulties. Once trained, the assessors visited 18 service users with learning difficulties in their own homes and, with permission, at their work or place of education, or during leisure pursuits. What did this approach mean for the people with learning difficulties involved? The project listed the gains as follows:

- A chance to have a real say and to be listened to
- A model of assessing services that can involve people who do not use language
- A form of assessment that focuses on how it feels to experience a service as a user
- Training to check quality in local services
- Opportunity to develop skills in assessing services ... [becoming a lay assessor]
- Public information about quality in local services.

(Ledger, 2000)

Finally, Example 7.3 illustrates another approach to finding out the views of people who use services, again where it is difficult to do so directly. The approach used here was to conduct a 'care audit' of 12 residential homes for people with learning difficulties, the aim being to explore the quality of residential care from the point of view of the people who experienced it.

EXAMPLE 7.3 Experiencing the residential 'climate'

As a care auditor I was, of course, an outsider to the residential homes I visited. My remit was to listen, and to observe, and to report on what I heard and saw. But supposing some people could or would not speak about their experiences, or their views about their circumstances differed from those of other – more powerful – people? How was I to make sense of silences and omissions, as well as discordant voices? And how was I to be objective in my observations? How could I really know what it was like to live in any of the 12 homes?

[...]

My visits included the finding out, and recording, of basic facts about each home: for example, the number of residents and staff, and the ratio of one to the other; the shift patterns in the home; handover times and procedures; rules, routines and record-keeping. However, the real challenge was to get behind the facts of a home and see, or even feel, what it was like to live there. A care auditor, like an inspector or regulator, has to rely on art as well as science (Clough, 1994). The 'scientific' use of guidelines and checklists is relatively straightforward compared with what the 'artist' has to do: 'to make creative leaps about what it would be like to live in that place and use imagination in searching for clues' (Clough, 1994: 96).

[...]

The following extract from one of my reports focuses on what felt to me to be a free-and-easy atmosphere, or climate, in the home in question:

> During my evening visit there, a small group of people went with two staff to have a drink in the local pub. This is within easy walking distance, so a pub trip can be quite easily, and spontaneously, arranged. There was a very jolly and free-and-easy atmosphere during my visit. Someone put the kettle on to make tea for the TV-watchers; someone else (who normally speaks in a whisper) sang loudly from her bath; someone else demonstrated his gymnastic skills on the lounge floor. Bedtime is usually between 9.30 and midnight, although the resident who enjoys falling asleep on the settee in front of the late night film was already in place when I left at 11 o'clock.

(Source: Atkinson, 1998, pp. 20–1)

This approach to assessing quality is a mix of objective criteria (numbers, ratios, patterns, routines) that can be measured, and more subjective criteria (feelings, experiences) that cannot, but which may be observed. Who checks that the observer is right? Feedback from residents, given directly or indirectly, is needed, but so too is an ability to reflect on the part of the observer. Similarly, who checks that the frontline manager is right about the people who use services, and what constitutes good quality from their point of view? The practice-led manager draws on their own experience of good practice in order to be reflective (and responsive).

Key points

- Managers know they are doing a good job from the feedback they get from a variety of sources, including the people who use their service.

- Sometimes innovative ways have to be found to enable people who use the service to give feedback.

7.9 Conclusion

At one level the concept of quality is uncontentious. The goal of a high-quality service, aspiring to – and reaching – the highest standards of excellence, is one we can readily agree on. This consensus applies from different perspectives, ranging from the people using the service to senior and frontline managers with responsibility for delivering high-quality practice and desired outcomes. The difficulty comes, as this chapter has shown, in knowing how to make this happen. There is no shortage of words on the subject, although much of the advice and guidance is on how to implement quality from the top downwards and, then, on how to monitor and measure it in order to maintain it.

Does this make for a high-quality service? Quality in the end means improving services for the people who use them. This suggests that quality may best be defined and implemented at a unit or team level, where everyone can be involved in the process. Ultimately, it seems to be the quality of the service as it is experienced by the recipient that matters most, and the outcome, or quality of life, that results. In the words of one of the managers quoted in this chapter, quality is 'doing the best we can'; in the words of another, it is doing so in as 'well-informed and respectful' a manner as is humanly possible.

Part 3 People in Social Care

Introduction

The key people in health and social care services are those on the receiving end. The quality of their care, and the quality of their lives, lie at the heart of the whole enterprise. Good outcomes for people who use services depend on the people who deliver and manage those services having the highest standards of practice. Good outcomes – and good practice – come from people who know about and understand the human context in which they work.

This applies particularly to the *practice-led manager*, who is the focus of this book. This person draws on, and is guided by, personal knowledge, experience and awareness of best practice in relation to the children or adults who use their services. The ultimate aim is to deliver high-quality outcomes, which can only be achieved by the manager who supports frontline staff in working in a respectful and responsive way. What works well at the front line of services also works well when it becomes good practice in the hands of the frontline manager. Good practice in this context requires a manager who is self-aware and aware of others, ethically literate and historically reflective.

The human context in which managers and practitioners work is complex and changing. The move to managerialism in health and social care services from the early 1980s has helped sweep away the 'classic professional identity' of doctors and other practitioners. In its place, according to Davies in Chapter 8 'Workers, professions and identity', there is uncertainty and complexity. This may turn out to be 'a good thing', as old certainties relied on devaluing and disparaging other people (the 'incompetent' client and the 'invisible' colleague), whereas the present-day situation allows for new and shifting identities. In a world of partnerships across agencies, multidisciplinary teams and inter-agency collaboration, there is a blurring of professional and occupational boundaries. The manager's role in this is to provide the environment, the 'space' and the support to enable practitioners to value and connect with the people who use services.

To be effective in this role, managers need to know about and understand human behaviour. To understand all of it would be a lifetime's work, according to Skye, Meddings and Dimmock in Chapter 9 'Theories for understanding people'. However, to understand some of it may at least make you a 'good enough' manager – good enough to know how people operate within, and outside, relationships. The authors argue that understanding yourself and others is a prerequisite of providing care and managing staff. Developing and supporting effective working relationships is an essential part of practice-led management. It involves the skills of observing, listening, reflecting and actively engaging with everyone, from team members to service users and senior managers.

Managers in health and social care settings are concerned with human welfare in all its complexity. This means, as suggested in Part 3, understanding yourself and others in order to work flexibly and creatively across professional boundaries. Managers are faced every day with competing and pressing demands, but within restricted resources.

The practice of social care is, according to Dawson and Butler in Chapter 10 'The morally active manager', an essentially moral activity. It requires managers to be *morally active* in exploring situations of need, addressing vulnerability, weighing up consequences and reflecting on the right, and principled, course of action. The morally active manager needs to be ethically sensitive and aware – to act on the basis of internalised values, personal and professional experience and practice wisdom, rather than (or as well as) externally imposed codes of conduct.

Here the authors look at current practice in the light of what has gone before. The morally active manager, and practitioner, can be seen in this wider historical view as a return to the roots of social casework, where good practice depended on the active moral engagement and decision making of the caseworker.

Similarly, Pinnock and Dimmock argue in Chapter 11 'Managing for outcomes' that, although the concept of 'outcomes' is a manifestation of the current context, nevertheless it resonates with the past. A concern with outcomes is a concern with what works best and is most effective. The study of the best and most effective practice is, according to the authors, as old as social work itself. In the present-day context, a focus on outcomes is a focus on results: on what is achieved for (and with) people on the receiving end of services.

The practice-led manager is also the outcome-focused manager – concerned with working with people (staff, service users and their families) to achieve a person-centred service. As the authors argue, the emphasis in this context switches from measuring inputs and outputs to devising and delivering user-defined outcomes. There is a link here with the discussion in Chapter 7 on quality and how to achieve it. One way to achieve a high-quality service is to adopt an outcomes approach. It involves everyone, upstream and downstream, in working together to deliver desired outcomes.

The context in which the present-day manager works owes much to what has gone before. To understand the past is, to some extent, to understand the present. The life-challenging and threatening events of today echo those of the past: loss, separation, the break-up of families, segregation and other transitions. The manager then and now has had to manage staff and other resources to deliver care (and control) in circumstances where people faced difficult, often dire, situations. In Chapter 12 'Taking account of history', Rolph, Adams and Atkinson argue the case, with illustrative examples, for present-day managers to be aware of, and to be informed by, history. After all, as they point out, the history of health and social care institutions and organisations is the history of the people whose lives were touched and shaped by those places.

The manager then and now works within a human context. Some of the solutions of the past are reinvented and come back again; others are overlooked when old problems resurface in a new guise and go unrecognised. The authors argue for historical awareness and historical *reflexivity*. The manager who knows about and reflects on the past can recognise and respond to those universal and recurring human themes, perhaps in a new and creative way.

This, then, in all its richness and diversity, is the human context that is the central concern of Part 3. The frontline manager operates at a certain point in history, drawing on good practice from the past as well as from the present. The practice-led manager works sensitively and flexibly with others to achieve person-centred and desired outcomes.

Chapter 8
Workers, professions and identity

Celia Davies

8.1 Introduction

> BRONWYN'S DIARY
>
> Work sometimes seems like a lonely place – I feel like the meat in the sandwich between our organisation and the workers. I value my manager colleagues and we keep in touch – email, phone and the odd drink after work – but nothing regular. Mostly, I'm getting on with the job on my own, dealing with the day-to-day challenges and routines.

What does it feel like to be a manager in a social care setting today? Do managers have a strong and confident sense of their own contribution? Do they invest a lot of themselves in their work and regard their work roles as part of their personal identity in the same way as those in the front line providing services often do? Why is it, as this extract from Bronwyn's diary suggests, that many managers seem to be caught in the middle and feel, as you have seen in other chapters, that there is tension and conflict both with those above them and with those below them in the hierarchy? Since the early 1980s there has been a relentless process of restructuring public sector services. It has been accompanied by demands that both managers and staff should see themselves differently – whether in the guise of the Conservative government's call to become more entrepreneurial or the more recent Labour government's call to rise to the challenges of performance management. It is the aim of this chapter to look more closely at changing ways of thinking about workers, managers and professionals and at the shifting, and sometimes contradictory, identities that this changing thinking has inspired.

The chapter focuses on a strand of recent theorising about identities which brings to the fore the significance of binary thought. Understanding the ways in which this form of thought locks people into power relations that value some kinds of contribution, while silencing and minimising others, is a key aim of the chapter. I will argue that getting to grips with these ideas can lead to a different way of thinking. This rethinking can help to take forward the vision of practice-led management that is the theme of this book.

The aims of this chapter are to:

- introduce and explore one particular way of theorising identity
- examine professional identities as expressions of this theoretical framework
- show how an overview of changes in policy and practice can be built up using this approach
- begin to demonstrate how some specific daily dilemmas of managing can be cast in a new light.

8.2 Identity: about the self, about the other

Most people, if asked who they are, will have more than one answer. 'I am a mother', one person might say, adding 'a wife and a daughter caring for my parent, and a care assistant working for the local authority'; 'I am a black woman social worker', a second person might say; and perhaps a third might just say, 'I am a doctor'. These different responses give a hint of how people see the world and what culturally available ideas or discourses they draw on to structure and give meaning to their lives. Identity, we can say, is a narrative about the self: a story produced in a social and cultural context.

Identity is a widely used and important concept in the social sciences. Psychology has a long tradition of stressing identity as a developmental process: stages of unfolding of the individual psyche over a lifetime. Sociology, by contrast, has tended for a long time to emphasise roles rather than identities, paying attention to processes of learning what is appropriate behaviour in given social positions and how these positions relate together to form, say, the family or the work organisation. In practice, both the idea of identities as the development of a subjective and individual sense of self and the notion of identities as forged from socially available roles are needed, and these strands have come closer together in recent years. Thinkers who see themselves as part of a post-modern tradition, students in the field of cultural studies and those focusing on the oppressions of race and gender have begun to use identity in a distinctive way. Here, identity retains the same fundamental sense of being a narrative about the self. There is a stress on belonging, and on linking together an internal psychic process with an external social context. But there is a recognition, too, that identities are also complex and shifting and can sometimes sit uneasily together. Identities can be dislodged and overturned. They are never finished products but always subject to revision and change. In a much-quoted comment by Stuart Hall:

> identities are never unified and, in late modern times, increasingly fragmented and fractured; never singular but multiply constructed, across different, often intersecting and antagonistic, discourses, practices and positions.
>
> (Hall, 1996, p. 4)

A crucial point in this theoretical tradition, and the one that forms the basis for this chapter, is that identities also frequently derive their meaning from a logic of pairing: for example mother and child, manager and worker, professional and client. Establishing an identity in this way sets a boundary, stressing the differences between people rather than their similarities and connections. There is always an 'other', symbolically located outside the boundary of a specific identity but in practice helping to give meaning to it. Two things are important here. First, self and other are locked together in this kind of thinking about identity. A narrative about the self comes about in part at least through an understanding of what it is not. Because the other helps give meaning to the self, it has been called a *constitutive other*. Second, this locking together of self and other involves a logic of binary thought – a division that takes the form of 'A' and 'not A' – the valued qualities and the absent qualities. There is a 'them and us' message in identity. The 'other' is a *devalued other*.

This process of creating identity through 'othering' can be seen in myriad ways. It is present, for example, in the framing of the doctor as active and decisive and the patient as passive, compliant and grateful. It is there in the divisions between qualified and unqualified staff. It is also there, of course, in discourses about fundamental social divisions of class, gender and race, where a dominant group defines what is valued and what is normal by reference to itself and hence excludes and oppresses others. The binary thought that underpins it can be masked. Understandings of masculinity that emphasise rationality and detachment can appear to see the insightful and empathetic qualities of femininity as complementary – except that these qualities take on a negative cast (muddled, soft, sentimental, emotional) in a public world of work. Some women decide that the only option is to prove that they can be more masculine than the men. When those who occupy and shape an identity are always white, male and middle class, these factors lend legitimacy and authority to an already powerful and privileged identity.

Focusing on binary thinking in this way suggests a real bleakness at the heart of identity theory. If the very act of establishing my identity devalues and demeans yours, there seems to be little hope that we can relate to each other in a positive way. Yet people do value difference, dialogue does happen, and shifts do occur. How can this be? One explanation lies in the resistance of groups who form to combat their exclusion and the negative portrayal of their qualities. The act of coming together can enable the sharing of an experience of oppression, the naming of it and the identification of strategies to begin to challenge it. In the world of health and social care, the formation of groups of service users and carers, and particularly the emergence of the social model of disability, are cases in point (Shakespeare, 2000). The energy and confidence that comes from naming and supporting that which has been suppressed can have immensely positive results in working to bring new possibilities to fruition. However, there can be negative results too: established ways of thinking are threatened and sometimes the gulf between professionals and service users deepens.

Resistance to binary identities can also come from within. People do not always accept completely the identities they are confronted with: they reflect on them and accept or reject certain aspects. One important consideration here is that identities tend to be destabilised by what is left out. The exclusions which have helped to constitute identities, in the words of one prominent theorist, 'return to haunt the "integrity" and "unity" of the ... "we" ' (Butler, 1992, p. 14). Unease about an identity precipitates action to rethink it by those who find themselves wanting to work against the grain of established understandings. Multiple identities can be a trigger here: where a social worker is black, for example, or where a doctor is female, competing discourses and alternative ways of being can come into play, as will be seen later in this chapter. Psychoanalytical writing also offers the important idea that the construction of the 'other' represents a form of repression and denial, so that the 'return of the repressed' is always a possibility.

Why worry about such highly abstract ideas about identity as these? The struggle to understand theorising is only worthwhile if it sheds new light on practice and helps us to find a deeper understanding of tensions and challenges and to devise new ways of addressing them. The rest of the chapter makes use of the ideas outlined in this section, applying them to the field of social care. Section 8.3 examines how ideas about identity as a boundary-maintaining process that simultaneously constitutes self and others work out when applied to professional identity. You might object that classic professional identity, as set out in the next section, never took full hold in the fields in which you work. That is a valid point, but it does not mean that the idea of professional identity can be discounted. I shall suggest that classic professional identity – while never fully embraced – none the less continues to influence ways of working.

Key points

- Identity is a narrative about the self which involves a sense of belonging.

- Identity constructs a boundary between self and other; it tends to devalue the other so that the devalued other then in part constitutes the identity of the self.

- Identities constructed in this way are not stable and fixed: they can develop and change.

8.3 Self/other boundaries and classic professional identity

The most notable feature of professions today is the extent of criticism levelled against them. Teachers, lawyers and the police are among those being questioned about how they handle their core activities and responsibilities (Foster and Wilding, 2000). Social workers faced an intense bout of hostile media attention in the 1980s (Aldridge, 1994), and this continues, as the media spotlight on child protection cases shows. Most recently, doctors – the group until now held in highest esteem and regarded as the model of professionalism – have found themselves the focus of public criticism. The trust that has been put in the professions, the high hopes that they are somehow apart from the rest of us, able to solve individual and societal problems, now seem misplaced. It is a good moment to explore again the identities that professionals have developed that seemed to work in the past but no longer do so. What are the promises of what I will call 'classic professional identity', and what do these promises say about both the professional and the 'other'?

Expertise lies at the heart of most conventional understandings of professionalism. It derives from a lengthy process of acquiring a body of knowledge which is widely acknowledged to be complex, worthwhile and important. Professionals are accorded respect by virtue of their possession of this knowledge. The process of becoming a professional, the classic model also assumes, has instilled in new members a special sense of *trustworthiness*. The model invites us to see professionals as altruistic and committed to the use of their knowledge for the public good. Trustworthy experts look for *autonomy*, the freedom to apply their skills in ways that they see fit in relation to individual cases. Ideally, they will want to remain unencumbered by resource constraints, by eligibility criteria or by accountability requirements. The demand for autonomy flows from a view that the exercise of expertise is about an *independent* process of thought and *personal responsibility* for decisions. Looked at in this way, the professional becomes a person who is somewhat apart from ordinary people, who commands respect and deference. Professionals are expected to be calm and confident, decisive yet sensitive, and responsible decision makers in key areas of our lives. Instilling that calm and confident demeanour, creating a sense of identity as a professional that overrides other identities, is one part of what the long years of training are designed to achieve.

If professional identity plays up these positive qualities, what does it play down? Doubt and emotional involvement are two key aspects. With so strong a sense of personal and individual responsibility coupled with the high hopes which surround professional activity, professionals need a strong belief in themselves and in the efficacy of their judgements. They are not likely to be humble people! Medicine is the arena where this has been studied most closely. Mackay (1993) provides a sensitive account of the way junior doctors were drawn towards what she called 'the great-I-am' as a lead identity. They adopted a 'persona of decisiveness' and there was a message in their demeanour of 'only I can deal with this'. Scary as it was for the new doctors, this identity served to calm patients and win their trust. Nurses tended to collude in not questioning the doctor in front of the patient. Trying to live up to a goal of infallibility in this kind of identity led the doctor down a path of assuming that others in the team had nothing useful to add. It also made the reality of error particularly hard to acknowledge and deal with in a positive way. Allsop and Mulcahy (1998) tell the story of the GP who had said nothing to anyone about the fact that he was to appear before a complaints tribunal – until his wife questioned him on the day about why he was wearing his best suit. Classic professional identity can thus require almost impossibly high standards, giving no support in achieving them and generating social isolation. However, it can all too easily shade into arrogance and into downgrading the contributions of others.

Identity theory as described in Section 8.2, however, insists that we must not describe identities only in their own terms. We must understand their *relational* character and ask who exactly is seen as 'other' in the process of constituting this identity. I suggest that there are at least three kinds of boundary-maintaining processes at work in classic professional identity as just described. Together they create:

1 the incompetent other
2 the invisible other
3 the unnecessary other.

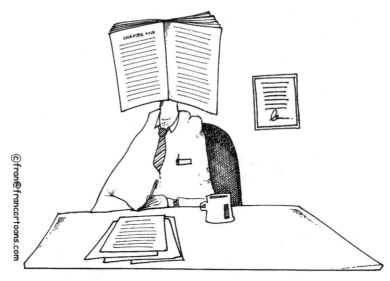

" THE IDEAL PROFESSIONAL- A FACELESS AND
DETACHED EXPERT"

Consider first the question of the client, patient or service user. Classic professional identity calls forth and requires an *incompetent other*, not active but reactive, not knowledgeable but ignorant, vulnerable, needy, grateful perhaps for an expert intervention that can mean the difference in extreme cases between life and death. I have already noted how user groups have challenged this.

Second, there is the matter of those who work with and alongside professionals, without formal qualifications, but often dealing face to face with clients. These co-workers, as I shall call them, often find themselves in the position of the *invisible other*. The work that they do is not given much attention. They are often, for example, grouped together and referred to as 'support' staff. The contact they have with clients and the impact they can have on the wellbeing of clients is not regarded as important or worthy of recognition in the form of significant levels of training or reward. The experience they gain, and the rapport and close contact with the client they often have, are discounted. Nor does their experience readily translate into fast-track routes into professional work.

Third, what of those who seek to manage professionals, or at least manage the contexts in which they work? The classic model of professional identity focuses on the one-to-one relationship with the client as at the heart of professional practice and sees all professionals as of equal competence. Its ideal is independent practice with a system of fees that helps preserve a sense of the professional as apart from the grubby business of commerce and industry, bureaucracy and politics. Doctors, for example, entered the NHS as independent contractors in the case of GPs and with somewhat arms-length contracts as consultants in hospitals. Once again, then, there is a negative 'othering' at work. Several categories of worker are in the position of the *unnecessary* or even *tainted other*: those who do not have the commitment to a profession but are out to make a profit, those who seem nakedly to seek power, and particularly those who are 'mere administrators' or 'bureaucrats'. Managers, according to this model, are a nuisance because doctors have to put pressure on them to ensure that resources and facilities are in place, and because they often seem incapable of providing what doctors need.

The illustration below is from the *Health Service Journal* and makes the point that managers and nurses often buy into the stereotypes depicted. The author of the article (Cole, 2001) urged that it was time to take stock of common ground and work together.

Box 8.1 draws together some of the key ideas of this section, stressing the individualism of professional identity and its strong separation from others. Elsewhere, I have suggested that these features of the classic professional identity drew their coherence historically from a discourse of masculinity. They helped to forge a place for the professions apart from the business and land-owning classes, serving to produce status and prestige in a different way (Davies, 1996). As women take up more positions in professions, and as those from different ethnic minority backgrounds and social classes bring more diversity, it becomes possible to question these features and to see that what has been admired about professions also has its costs.

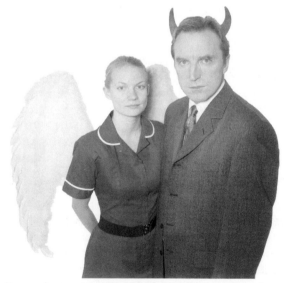

Devils and angels (Source: Cole, 2001, p. 25)

BOX 8.1 The classic professional identity

- A strongly bounded individual: a sense of self apart from others

- Mastery of knowledge: expertise as a hard-won personal acquisition

- Detachment: emotionally controlled and self-referential

- Autonomous practice: a unilateral, personally accountable decision maker

- Interchangeability: a 'company of equals' with presumed equal competence

- A singular identity: professional identity outweighs/transcends all others

(Source: adapted from Davies, 1995, pp. 56–63, 2000)

Just how relevant is this discussion for social work and the field of social care more generally? Is it capable of shedding light on the changes that have been experienced? Does it help to illuminate the contemporary practice dilemmas in any way? These questions are considered in the following sections.

Key points

- Classic professional identity can be identified in terms of the six features outlined in Box 8.1.

- This identity *overvalues* expertise, awarding respect, autonomy and trust.

- It *undervalues* the contribution of clients, colleagues and managers.

8.4 Changing identities in the social care field

Golden age professionals in the post-war years?

The mid-20th century welfare state brought what has been described as the 'golden age' for professionals (Foster and Wilding, 2000), giving them a state-supported mandate to use their discretion in defining and meeting need. The negative aspects of professional identity for others went unnoticed and unchallenged. Respect for the medical profession in particular grew apace, as it made more and more strides in treating disease. The 'support staff' – those who did detailed diagnostic and therapeutic work, those who helped care for and co-ordinate the overall experience for patients – got little attention. The manager at that time, with the lowly title of hospital secretary, was a pale shadow of the doctor, someone who seemed always cautious, deferential and rule-bound. One hospital secretary explained to me in the 1960s how it felt to work with doctors. 'Well,' he ruefully observed, 'sometimes when I go home, I do wonder whether I should consult the worms before I cut the grass!' The NHS has often been called a bureaucratic–professional alliance, but it was an alliance in which the professional was the dominant partner.

Did this golden age extend to the social work field? Yes and no seems to be the answer. Rashid (2000), writing from within social work, sees strong elements of classic professional identity in the rise of psychiatric social work and the development in the post-war period of social casework with its emphasis on therapeutic work with families. On the other hand, he also points out that radical social work turned away from this model, offering instead a community worker identity which stressed client empowerment and political action. Others have identified another significant feature, namely that social workers did not set the terms on which they would work in the way that doctors did. In the main, they were local government employees, working in a hierarchy and with a mix of people, some of whom had professional qualifications and many of whom did not: they have been called 'bureau-professionals' (Parry and Parry, 1979). Yet the top of the hierarchy comprised those with social work training. This to some extent buffered and insulated field social workers, giving them professional support and enabling them to use their professional judgement and discretion. Gender was a factor too. Cochrane, observing the array of professions that developed under the wing of local government in this period, suggests that the presence of so many women was important. It 'helped to confirm the uneasy status of the "new" professions because the dominant image of the old (and by definition legitimate) ones was overwhelmingly male' (Cochrane, 1994, p. 144).

All in all, social work presents a mixed picture in this period. Classic professional identity was not adopted wholesale, but there were enough elements of it to create tensions with clients and colleagues. It can still be useful, as the rest of this section shows, in helping to understand the challenges that today's managers face.

Boundaries between professional and manager

Professions took a hard knock in the 1980s. The election of a Conservative government in 1979 marked the beginning of the end of the golden age for welfare professionals of all kinds. The major changes were discussed in Chapter 3. They included creating the purchaser–provider split, the emphasis on markets and the mixed economy of care, and seeking to instate a new kind of manager as an active entrepreneur, drawing inspiration from successful private business in emphasising how to get results (du Gay, 1996). The criticisms of professional practice and professional competence that were mentioned earlier began to grow in number from this time. This was not only an attack on professions – the start of a 'deprofessionalisation' that many critics in the field have strenuously contested (Dominelli, 1996; Jones, 1999). It was a move that challenged existing forms of management and questioned the role of politicians too.

Clarke and Newman (1997, p. 65) emphasise that the new ideas gained cogency by means of 'vilification of the old and idealisation of the new'. Their summary (Box 8.2) captures well the way in which one identity can set its boundaries by disparaging others. Reading the box from right to left and personalising it – 'we managers are innovative, you bureaucrats are rule bound' – helps to make the point. Recent messages from Labour, less about managerialism and more about modernisation, reflect similar, although not identical, thinking (Department of Health, 1998a).

BOX 8.2 Legitimating managerialism

Bureaucracy is:	**Management** is:
rule bound	innovative
inward looking	externally oriented
compliance centred	performance centred
ossified	dynamic

Professionalism is:	**Management** is:
paternalist	customer centred
mystique ridden	transparent
standard oriented	results oriented
self-regulating	market tested

Politicians are:	**Managers** are:
dogmatic	pragmatic
interfering	enabling
unstable	strategic

(Source: Clarke and Newman, 1997, p. 65)

In the new climate professionals could no longer ignore management and devalue managers. They were being more actively managed, but they also found that they were *becoming managers themselves*. Donna Dustin carried out focus group interviews with eight inner London social work teams in the mid-1990s (see Example 8.1). Respondents reported that they were now operating in a fashion 'dictated by scarcity of resources, demand for tight control of budgets, strict eligibility criteria, high caseloads and maximum output from workers'. Some commented dismally that they had become 'simply council employees' (Dustin, 2000, p. 17). They felt confused and bereft as traditional social work practice and its close personal relationship with the client were overturned.

EXAMPLE 8.1 When social workers become care managers

'You're doing the work and you still feel committed, but sometimes on the worst days, it just feels like a job and it shouldn't just feel like that ... '

'Theory goes out of the window ... '

'We initially came into social work to work with people, not sit behind a computer, write letters and fill forms ... '

'As far as I am concerned, social work is divorced from the community now ... '

'We do more business things, more budgeting ... '

'Whatever you do, wherever you go, you write it down ... '

'The whole system is geared specifically towards (being) less people-centred ... '

(Source: adapted from Dustin, 2000, various pages)

Other studies reported similar findings. Social workers were not just struggling with a new language of resource management and with the business of setting up contracts (Leat and Perkins, 1998), although that was unfamiliar enough. They were also facing a more fundamental challenge to what it meant to be a social worker (La Valle and Lyons, 1996; May and Buck, 2000). Some commentators have viewed this as a moment of profound demoralisation, when managers and workers had become 'alienated from their work environment' and were no longer able to be creative and flexible (Clough, 1998, p. 99). The overall picture is not so bleak, however. Some people, with long experience in social care settings but without formal social work qualifications, were able to move into care management roles and relished their expanded capacity to shape and deliver services. Others, with a variety of backgrounds, seized new opportunities as providers of services in the voluntary and private sectors. Alongside the alienation of social workers, then, there has been active engagement with the new, as different workers in the social care field struggle to create identities that make sense in the new structures (May and Buck, 2000).

Hybrid roles combining managerial and professional skills have now become more significant. Some authors suggest that the trends are towards breaking down the older antagonistic relationships between managerialism and professionalism and creating more integrated roles at different levels in the organisation (Causer and Exworthy, 1999; Gray et al., 1999; Laffin, 1998). Increasingly, the roles that people are asked to adopt are combined ones. The practising professional using therapeutic skills one to one with service users, with no supervisory or budgetary responsibilities, is starting to be in a minority. It seems that managers – classic professionalism's 'unnecessary others' – are becoming not only a necessary but also an *integral* part of an emerging new professionalism. Box 8.3 draws on work by Causer and Exworthy which was discussed in Chapter 1. Perhaps the more hybrid roles like this become a reality, the more the chance of putting into place the practice-led management advocated in that chapter.

BOX 8.3 A growing differentiation of roles and identities?

1 The practising professional

(a) a pure practitioner – no supervisory or budgetary responsibilities

(b) a quasi-managerial practitioner – some supervision and budget work, but main task is practice

2 The managing professional

(a) a practising managing professional – combines practice with management tasks

(b) a non-practising managing professional – professionally qualified but in full-time management

3 The general manager

(a) professionally qualified

(b) not professionally qualified

(Source: adapted from Causer and Exworthy, 1999, p. 84)

Boundaries with colleagues

What, then, has happened to classic professionalism's 'invisible others' – colleagues without professional qualifications? Have they become more visible and more valuable? With care management at the forefront, the boundary between qualified and unqualified has certainly changed. As noted above, opportunities opened up for some people without professional qualifications to build on their experience in the new era that gave more credence to managerial skills. Home carers report a mixed picture of change. Not only are they now giving personal care – washing, dressing, helping with mobility, feeding – they are often also engaged in activities that border on skilled nursing. They remain the least qualified staff, positioned at the bottom of the social care hierarchy, with variable and often minimal training, and working in isolation for an hourly rate of pay that hovers around the statutory minimum (Clough, 1998).

Survey research interestingly indicates that home carers are often more satisfied with their work than social workers, managers or residential care staff (Balloch *et al.*, 1999). In the front line, when services are stretched, however, home carers report going beyond the formal care plan for their clients, getting emotionally and personally involved and blurring the boundaries between worker and friend (Bradley and Sutherland, 1995). Tensions then arise when social workers – in professional-cum-management roles – question the judgements unqualified staff make and refuse to allocate the additional time and resource that home carers say are necessary. Home carers can end up out of sympathy with the 'book learning' of the professional and the resource juggling of the manager that creates the day-to-day dilemmas they face. A study in Norway recorded home carers' concerns about their clients and their requests for more hours. These claims were dismissed by the managers/professionals as stemming from carers' inappropriate forms of thinking derived from their life experience. They were regarded as applying models of 'mother care' to their clients (Rasmussen, 2001). This can be seen as a classic case of 'othering', the professionally qualified staff reinforcing their own identities as experts by devaluing the experience of home carers.

Boundaries with adjacent professions

Classic professional identity, as was seen earlier, involves a vision of making a contribution to care as an autonomous and independent expert. This gives little room for drawing on and valuing the contribution of other professions. Governments have grown ever more critical of what the White Paper *Modernising Social Services* called the 'Berlin Wall' between the different professions in health and social care (Department of Health, 1998a, para. 6.5). There is greater policy determination than ever before to have integrated teams and ensure that shared training takes place. Working effectively across professions and across agencies is a key challenge for today's managers.

Example 8.2 records some comments drawn from three multi-disciplinary mental health care teams when faced with the question of whether they were in favour of what the researchers called 'role blurring' between professions.

EXAMPLE 8.2 Role blurring between professions

For:

'I think we need to overcome some of these, as I see it, ingrained traditional boundary things that are cocking up the way we all work ... we've got to ask who are we working for, are we working for our own traditional boundaries, and maintaining the status quo, or are we trying to move forward and offer the best services to the clients?' (Nurse)

'maybe there is ... a case for mental health workers, rather than being a nurse, being a social worker.' (Nurse)

Against:

'You get a blurring of professional roles, which I think is dangerous ... Because at the end of the day social workers think they know what nurses and doctors do, but they don't. Similarly nurses ... think they know what social workers do, but they don't ... And it's quite common to see where social workers have been meddling in medical matters, and nurses have been meddling in social care matters.' (Social worker)

'I think, when people have got individual caseloads, it's quite easy to fall into the trap, of taking on ... the nursing role for part of a time ... because it's just easier because you know the client and you've always been working with them and perhaps that doesn't get passed back to the relevant professionals.' (Occupational therapist)

Both:

'I think I should concentrate on what I'm good at and allow the other person to do what they're good at. And that way everybody will feel fulfilled in their roles in the team ... There is some blurring, and that's good ... But also we need to be self-aware and know when to stop ... and to clearly identify, well hang on I can't do this any more. I need to hand you over, or I need input from such a one.' (Nurse)

(Source: adapted from Brown *et al.*, 2000, pp. 429–30)

The views of members of these mental health teams clearly varied, but perhaps what comes over most strikingly is hesitancy about connecting with and really valuing others. No one in this context produced a strongly articulated vision that valued the different contributions that members brought or observed that, by working in dialogue, they might both expand their own practice and bring a better resolution for their clients. For all today's rhetoric of teamwork and the restructuring of work, classic professional identity seems alive and well and pulling in the opposite direction.

Finally, what about the way in which the classic professional identity devalues and demeans the service user? The experience of service users was discussed in detail in Chapter 2. It seems that there is a long way to go yet and the position of 'devalued other' is still being strongly felt in a number of spheres. Also, although social work values have long stressed empowerment of clients, policy remains contradictory, particularly in areas such as children's services and criminal justice. The tighter central specification of policies in the wake of high-profile child abuse cases has moved the social worker, some say, 'from therapy and welfare to surveillance and control' (Howe, 1992, p. 497). A probation worker quoted in another study made the bitter comment: 'They're not going to be happy till I'm wearing a uniform and driving around in a car with a flashing light and with a set of handcuffs' (La Valle and Lyons, 1996, p. 7).

All this seems to suggest that professional identity needs a more profound adjustment than merely adding in specific managerial skills at all levels, the trend that Box 8.3 highlighted. What I have done, therefore, is to go back to each of the components of the classic model of professional identity (set out in Box 8.1) and try to respecify them to take account of their weaknesses and make them fit better into the present climate. Box 8.4 suggests that today's practitioner does not need to be someone with a sense of self as possessor of a clearly bounded expertise. Instead, they need to be someone who can value and connect with others, using the multiplicity of experiences of the client and team members to develop adaptive and creative solutions. According to this model, it is not so much what the individual practitioner can do, but what the team, working together, can become. There is an important role for managers here in acknowledging the contradictions of professional identities and in helping to create a climate of respect in which new identities can be negotiated in ways that support the development of services. There is also scope for the roles of professional and manager to come much closer together and for managers perhaps to feel less isolated than this chapter's opening quotation implies.

BOX 8.4 Towards a new professional identity

- A strongly connected individual: a sense of self in connection with others

- Reflective application of knowledge: blending knowledge and experience in a specific context

- Engagement: involvement of self and acknowledgement of emotions

- Team practice: welcoming and valuing the contributions of others

- Specificity: acknowledging unique expertise and experience of all

- Multiple identities: calling on the specificity of team members' experience as a resource for clients

Those who have worked in the field of social care since the 1980s have experienced a deeply unsettling time as contradictions of old identities came into the open and new ones are not clearly apparent. Some of the practical dilemmas of working with and encouraging identity transitions are explored in the final section.

Key points

- In a changing climate, old professional identities have come into question and the ambiguities and uncertainties in them have come to the fore.

- There has been an important process – still under way – of blurring the boundaries between professionals and managers.

- Staff are also struggling with new kinds of role blurring both with co-workers and in multidisciplinary teams, and with the meaning of these for their identities as professionals.

- In a context where social workers and their colleagues in the social care field have never been entirely at ease with the dilemmas of classic professional identity, there is a potential to rethink boundaries between professionals, colleagues and clients.

8.5 Dilemmas of professional identity

In this final section it is argued that using the concepts of old and new professional identity can have practical results in sharpening people's understanding of some of the key dilemmas of contemporary practice and how to manage them better. Two case studies are considered. They are arbitrary choices, designed to begin to illustrate the problems of *not* bothering about the 'other' in professional identity and the possibilities that emerge when people work to bring processes of 'othering' into the open.

The extract in Example 8.3 gives an account by a black woman social worker. She describes the case of her client, a teenage girl of Caribbean descent, previously fostered by a member of her extended family in a mixed-race household and now placed with a white foster carer in a different local authority. As the social worker from the originating authority, she retains a lead role but now has to work with an all-white staff in the second authority.

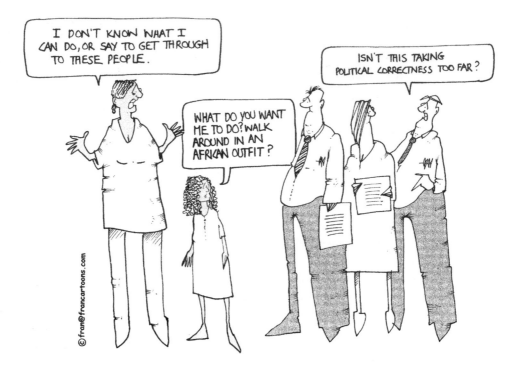

EXAMPLE 8.3 A black social worker speaks

I always have a very hard time, my team manager has accompanied me on a couple of occasions because I had such an awful time. The first time I went there I wanted the case transferred ... I only saw white members of staff up there, there were no black staff in that particular office ... it was very hard work and to have to tell two white male team managers and a white female placements social worker who represented the family that the child was placed with, and another white female social worker, *all* these white professionals, to try and explain cultural needs and identity, because it's a *black child we're talking about*, to try and explain to them was very hard work and at the last meeting the situation, because I am the only one talking about identity and talking about cultural issues at the statutory review, the child turned round to me ... and said: 'What do you want me to do – walk around in an African outfit!' So this is the level, this is what I'm trying to explain to them, that there are concerns, what input is there for her, because she's currently placed with a white family. I'm not pleased about that and... [the lead authority] has a policy that black children are placed with same-race placements where possible. I don't feel that ... [the second authority] had made an effort ... They know that I'm not pleased with her being placed with a white foster parent in an area where there are no black people ... and because she doesn't know anybody, she's not going to seek them out, so issues of her identity which is coming through, different things that she says, and that was a classic for me. Now for me as a

> black worker that's ringing alarm bells, for the white workers it was a case of mockery, that's right you know, erm, you're seen as going overboard on this *black* thing, type of thing. So I felt very angry at that because this child is internalising that all I do is go on about black issues, go on about identity all the time and I'm sort of trying to champion the cause. But it *has* to be prescriptive because she's not going to get it if it's not built into this placement that is *totally* inappropriate, with professionals who she's dealing with who are *all* white ... if it's not put in a prescriptive way it doesn't happen at all and I have, I'm accountable to make sure that her needs are fully met, so because it's put in a prescriptive way it's seen as if that's *all* I do ... I can't convince the white workers, professionals supposedly ... so how am I then going to convince this young person a long, long distance away, if I have to convince her social workers in the first place that she is in great need?
>
> (Source: Lewis, 2000, pp. 144–5)

This excerpt is one of a series of accounts gathered with the aim of exploring how both gender and race are implicated in welfare services and how discourses on these topics can reinforce domination and oppression rather than overcome them (Lewis, 2000). The speaker cannot get her colleagues to acknowledge that there is an issue around black identity for a black young woman in an all-white environment. In the face of this, and with palpable unease, she becomes rigidly prescriptive about the young person's needs. There are several damaging outcomes. The situation:

- accentuates the 'otherness' of black identity and its seeming lack of connection with whiteness
- homogenises and fixes this notion of black/ethnic minority identity
- undermines the authority of the black social worker and marginalises her, so that she is 'reduced to a bundle of ethnically derived (and therefore inherent) capacities' (Lewis, 2000, p. 147)
- prompts the young woman to reject the proffered solution, thus apparently discrediting the solution and further undermining the social worker
- provides no opportunity to acknowledge the multifaceted identity of the client and the complexity of her needs.

Later in the chapter from which this excerpt is drawn, another respondent reflects on the reverse situation, where white workers say, 'I think this case needs a black worker' (Lewis, 2000, p. 150). The results can be equally damaging if black social workers are seen as the only ones able to deal with black clients.

- Black social workers get many of the most complex cases, those least likely to result in positive outcomes.
- Black workers face pressure from black clients to 'befriend' them in contexts where the exercise of professional authority is expected.

- There is no supervision that recognises these distinctive black issues in social work practice for black social workers.
- Black workers remain in basic fieldworker grades, while white workers who do not experience the full range of social work practice, rise up the hierarchy.

Whether 'ethnic matching' should or should not occur, particularly in relation to adoption and fostering, has been a subject of intense debate (see Pinkney, 2000). Lewis argues that neither orthodox social work theory nor the approach adopted by some radical black professionals offers an adequate response. 'Ethnic absolutism', the notion that all an individual's or a group's needs can be derived from and reduced to their ethnicity, should go. It should be replaced with a concern to undo relations of power and domination and with a better understanding of the complexity of the experience of black workers and service users (Lewis, 2000, pp. 133–4).

But if thinking about race needs to change, so too does thinking about professions. Classic professional identity, with its emphasis on possession of a body of expert knowledge, lends credence to the idea that professionals are disembodied experts and interchangeable. It has little vision and no vocabulary concerning differences of class, race and gender among professionals, seeing these as irrelevant and to be transcended in the achievement of knowledge and skills. It also makes little space for a role for a manager in facilitating dialogue and using differences of experience and multiple identities in a positive way. A model such as that set out in Box 8.4, however, offers a better prospect of using the rich individual diversity of a team of professionals in the service of clients' needs. There are some precedents: for example in the arguments about women social workers building on connections with clients to create a woman-centred social work practice (Hanmer and Statham, 1988).

Example 8.4 takes this a step further. In some ways it is much more straightforward and immediately practical in its implications. It deals with a recurring set of dilemmas of how to work across health and social care and with the familiar situation where different groups become exasperated with and blame each other. When faced with people complaining about how 'they' typically act, is it possible to work in more constructive ways?

EXAMPLE 8.4 Tackling existing conflict and misunderstanding

In one of the places we have been working, the 'winter bed crisis' of the previous year had left a legacy of recrimination between general practice, the hospital, the health authority and the social services department as well as a sense of insecurity among local residents, particularly elderly people. Everyone wanted to avoid a repetition the following year but it seemed hard for them to begin co-operating without first dealing with the bad feelings still around.

Before meeting to explore the possibilities for the future, we encouraged them to revisit the past. One hundred and forty people sat at round tables in a large room. They were arranged in 'likeness' groups – general practice together, social services together, elderly residents together and so on.

Each group explored their own perspective of the previous year's 'winter bed crisis' and prepared a three-minute story they could tell everybody in the room. They were asked to tell the story honestly, and to be clear that they were describing not 'the truth' but their own view, using words like 'we believed that ... ' and 'it seemed to us that ... '

People were asked to listen with the intention of understanding the viewpoints of others – not to discover the truth or get the facts right, but to listen for surprises where other people's viewpoint was different from their own. They were asked to listen for how their role was perceived by others, recognising these perceptions might make them angry or upset. They were not asked to respond to what sounded like criticism or to 'set the record straight' but to ask themselves what led to these perceptions. They used this understanding to make posters that showed to the others how we think we are seen/how we would like to be seen/what we would need to do to be seen in this way. Each group who had had 'their say' could tell whether the others had heard by looking at the posters.

> The poster work was an incredible shock to many people. Users were seen as the cause of the problem. The voluntary sector saw the statutory bodies as asleep. The local authority (mainly social services) drew themselves as in the stocks. Everybody was very angry with the council ... Since then people have spent a lot of time talking about it.
>
> (Senior manager)

After lunch the participants were able to work together in a very co-operative atmosphere. The plans they began to formulate have since led to significant improvement in local services.

(Source: Pratt et al., 1999, pp. 38–9)

The authors of this extract favour what they call 'whole systems working', stressing how organisations are living systems that need to find better ways to link the parts to the whole and to adapt and connect (Pratt et al., 1999, p. 3). While this approach does not rest on the theory of identity used in this chapter, its way of working is highly compatible with it. Notice, for example, how the writers do not assume that any one party has the whole of the analysis of the problem or the whole of the answer, and how they actively manage the situation to enable people to contribute and be heard. Notice, too, how connections across self/other boundaries are possible once fears are faced and defences are addressed and dismantled. If strategies like this can be repeated in the way the authors claim, it certainly does seem that they can get results.

Key points

- Viewing co-workers as 'others', for example if they belong to an ethnic minority, can result in damaging outcomes for clients.

- When the processes of 'othering' are exposed, people start to behave more constructively.

8.6 Conclusion

This chapter opened by considering how the creation of an identity often sets a boundary between people and involves binary thinking that simultaneously values the self and devalues the other. Taking the case of doctors, it was argued that a professional identity – even a seemingly benign and positive one – has contradictions. It has potential to devalue others – clients, colleagues and managers – and oppress rather than empower. This 'them and us' feature of identity creation, it was argued, does not work in exactly the same way in the social care field, but it does have some visible counterparts there. Recent policy changes were explored, showing that these can disrupt binary identities but also bring new ones into play.

The message of this chapter, however, is by no means as negative as the idea of binary thinking implies. The theorists stress that identities based on binaries are never simply 'fixed'. They can be explored, challenged and changed. The present climate – with its questioning of professional power, with the rise of hybrid manager/professional roles, and the growing insistence on integrated care teams – is itself creating pressures for change. There is a real opportunity to think afresh about what needs to be preserved from classic professional identity and what tensions in it can now be addressed and changed. Managers, in particular, have a part to play here. If they are aware of the dangers of binary thinking, they can support staff in acknowledging the ambiguities of professional identities, create situations in which tensions can be constructively explored, and develop policies that encourage more inclusive and flexible working across the boundaries that professional identity in the past has set up. 'Bothering about othering', and the rethinking of professional identities that this entails, has a contribution to make in working more positively with client groups and colleagues, and improving the experience of services. Managers can help to make this happen.

Chapter 9
Theories for understanding people

Emily Skye, Sara Meddings and Brian Dimmock

9.1 Introduction

The nature of care services means that managers have to use their understanding of people to enable them to form effective working relationships with service users, staff, their own line managers and people working in other organisations. These relationships are not just a means to an end (delivering a service) but are often an end in themselves (part of a service). For many service users, the quality of their relationship with a care-providing organisation is part of the service. Thus, human relationships and the knowledge that informs people's understanding of themselves and other people are part of the 'stock in trade' of providing care services and managing care staff.

The opportunities for managers to exercise their skills in human understanding will, of course, vary. The intensity of the work being undertaken and the influence of group and team processes are two important factors that have to be considered. Changes of policy or crises that occur in a service also increase the need for a sound understanding of human behaviour, as do differences in terms of power, responsibility and accountability between managers and their staff. However much understanding managers may have, they need to maintain appropriate professional boundaries and acknowledge differences in role. How do people work with and juggle resources, especially their own, in a way that does not lose sight of the humans involved, and how do they respond to human issues within the constraints of a management role? Differences in role become particularly crucial when there are disagreements about how to proceed.

People may occupy multiple roles at different times. The way they present themselves to others depends on the context and their intention to present themselves in a certain way (Goffman, 1969; Perkins and Repper, 1998): for example, as a lover to a partner; as a service user or client to a therapist or doctor; as a manager and supervisor at work but also as someone who is managed and supervised. Some managers are employed in particular because of their expertise and experience of being a service user (Read, 2003). There are ways of thinking and approaching people and situations that can help in understanding different people, including yourself, your managers, the staff you manage, and the users of services. The ways in which you try to understand people has implications, in turn, for how you manage them.

The considerable array of accumulated knowledge about human behaviour and relationships means that we can only touch on the subject in a single chapter. For this reason we have concentrated on discriminating between different approaches and on looking at the wider contexts that affect managers. We address some of the key dilemmas and choices facing managers when looking for knowledge about human behaviour, putting this knowledge into an ethical and culturally sensitive framework. We also examine some key issues for managers requiring a good understanding of human behaviour. Finally, we look at the main skills needed when applying this knowledge.

The aims of this chapter are to:

- locate some of the key sources of knowledge about human behaviour and relationships that managers can use
- argue that knowledge can be used constructively and destructively
- describe the culturally bounded nature of knowledge about human behaviour and the influence of wider processes and systems
- examine the use of knowledge in relation to some key management concerns
- outline the key skills in understanding people.

9.2 Do managers need theories about human behaviour?

Social work theory and managing care

Perhaps the first question to ask before deciding whether theories about human behaviour are of value to managers is 'do they use them at all in practice?' There is evidence that people working in human care services tend not to apply theoretical models, at least not consciously. Taking social work as an example, Stevenson and Parsloe (1978) found that social workers believed their work was informed by 'theory' but that they were not very clear how. One of their research respondents said:

> If you asked me to state a theory here and now, I wouldn't have a clue but my thinking and approach have been informed by them.
>
> (Stevenson and Parsloe, 1978, p. 133)

Another view of the way in which social workers use theory, expressed by Jordan (1989), is that social work is a process of 'violent bodging'. In his view, social workers adapt theories to suit their immediate purposes.

Of course, we are concerned with a much broader canvas than social work and with the management of care services rather than direct practice alone. Nevertheless, current thinking gives greater emphasis to the importance of basing service provision on evidence about what is effective (Sheldon and Chilvers, 2000). One reason why social work provides a useful starting point is that, like other professions involved in care, such as nursing, it does at least use a body of theory for understanding people (see, for example, Payne, 1991 and Davies, 2000), whereas 'care' as such does not. Even social work or nursing theory is often 'second-hand', much of it being adapted from a wide variety of sources in the social sciences and beyond. In so far as care tends to use the body of knowledge drawn from social work or nursing, theories for and about care could be seen as 'third-hand'. Indeed, given that vocational qualifications are probably of more relevance than professional qualifications in the broad field of care, it could be argued that theory of any sort, including that related to human behaviour, is totally absent. Achieving 'competence', certainly up to Level 2 of the Scottish and National Vocational Qualifications in care, is more about ends than means (see, for example, Nolan, 1998), and its knowledge base is implicit rather than explicit.

Arguments about the importance or otherwise of theories of human behaviour tend to be of more interest to educators than to most managers and practitioners. One reason for this is that formal educational and professional qualifications are part of the process whereby an occupation or a profession strives to achieve an identity of its own. Given that professional identity is laid down to a significant extent during training, educators have tended to have an important role in defining what is and is not relevant as far as knowledge is concerned. This is certainly the case in higher education and it partly explains the absence, as yet, of a clearly articulated body of knowledge and theory that applies to care and its management. Given that most care staff receive little or no training and even less 'education' in a college or university, they are often unfamiliar with formal theoretical knowledge and the models of practice built upon it.

Nevertheless, there is a growing culture of 'evidence-based practice' and efforts to build a research base that is directly relevant for managers of care services. If this is to take root, managers will have an important role. Sheldon and Chilvers surveyed social services staff to examine this issue and they conclude:

> A key finding in the questionnaire results is that staff feel that they are given limited support from management for the task of incorporating research findings into their practice.
>
> (Sheldon and Chilvers, 2000, p. 85)

Of course, establishing the habits of evidence-based practice goes back to the early training and education received by social care staff, and the majority of such staff have, to date, received very little formal education of this sort. Sheldon and Chilvers believe that there is a groundswell of enthusiasm at local and national level:

> we now look forward to a point, about ten years away, when the term evidence-based can be dropped, since it will be an automatic and well-founded assumption, that, *of course*, public services are based on current best evidence.
>
> (Sheldon and Chilvers, 2000, p. 86)

Management theory and managing care

There is a massive industry involved in providing training and education for managers working in business and commerce. This has an extensive literature that includes a great deal of theory about human behaviour designed to help managers be better at their jobs. As models of management drawn from business have become more influential in the human services, so has 'management theory'. Like social work theory, management theory tends to draw selectively on the behavioural sciences and adapt them to suit the roles, tasks and contexts of managers. Again, managers of care seem to be getting more 'hand-me-downs', this time from business management, to inform their practice. However, management theory applied to health and social care is beginning to emerge as a distinct area of knowledge (see, for example, Martin and Henderson, 2001). This material tends to be of a practical nature rather than providing explicit knowledge about different approaches to understanding human behaviour as it applies to managing health and social care. Nevertheless, it does encourage managers to reflect on what they are learning rather than argue that management is a purely technical activity.

The systematic application of knowledge to management practice

Is it possible for managers to acquire the kind of knowledge of human behaviour that will enable them to know how to deal with all the possible circumstances they are likely to encounter? We would argue that what managers and experienced staff are aiming for is not the ability to predict and control all possible outcomes but to develop what Schön (1987) terms 'professional artistry'. Using this approach, people can be supervised or coached through practical situations as they arise, although theory or technique cannot prepare them in advance to know how to respond. However, it is important to develop the ability to solve problems through the systematic application of knowledge, skills *and* experience.

We would also argue that most managers and practitioners do apply knowledge about human behaviour that is drawn from a broad range of theory but that they do not always do it in a systematic way. 'Common sense' is very often fragments of knowledge and theory that have become widely applied in everyday discourse. Care staff and managers, whatever their training and qualifications, will have a body of commonsense understandings drawn from attachment theory, learning theory, psycho-dynamic theory, and probably many others. They may not be aware that they know and apply this but they do.

There is a strong case for helping managers to apply theories of human understanding more systematically and to build up their repertoire of knowledge and its application. In the case of some management theory, understanding people can be seen instrumentally as a way of maximising the performance of employees in order to deliver a better service. Understanding people from this perspective is a means to an end. In our view this does not fit well with modern management practice nor with the traditions of human service provision. Services that require staff to go beyond routine tasks, and that involve complex and distressing human circumstances, need to have more than a purely instrumental management strategy. Thus, understanding people in the provision of care is at the heart of the management task and should be apparent in both working relationships and good working conditions. Treating staff well is an integral requirement if an ethos of human concern and respect is to be delivered and if the management of care is to be practice-led. Good and effective relationships between manager and workers are reflected in good and effective relationships between staff and service users.

'Evidence-based practice' is one of the key issues in the current thinking about modernising health and care services and making them more effective. The National Institute for Clinical Excellence (NICE) was established in 1999 in England and Wales to support evidence-based practice in relation to health care. The Social Care Institute for Excellence (SCIE) was set up to perform a similar function for care services. It aims to create for the first time an accessible 'knowledge base' for care services, as outlined in Box 9.1 (overleaf).

BOX 9.1 The Social Care Institute for Excellence

SCIE will create a knowledge base of what works through:

- Rigorous methodology to assess evidence and knowledge from academic research, user and carer expertise and existing practice.

- Assessment of the strength and quality of the evidence.

- A transparent review process.

In translating knowledge of what works into practice guidance, SCIE will:

- Produce good practice guidance, tools and other materials with which individuals and organisations can improve their practice and performance.

- Be clear of the need to treat each case as unique.

- Develop the guidance in partnership.

- Be clear that 'what works' is sometimes hard to define, and different stakeholders may have different opinions about what constitutes a successful outcome.

(Source: SCIE, 2002)

SCIE's position is that there is an important body of knowledge about human behaviour that can be of enormous value to managers, their staff and users of care services. The challenge is to make it relevant and accessible. Theory alone is of little value unless it is made relevant to the contexts in which managers work. SCIE also recognises that this knowledge is contested and that it belongs not just to academics, practitioners and managers but also to service users, carers and the general public.

Key points

- Knowledge about human behaviour for managing care draws on traditions from social work and business management but is beginning to develop its own knowledge base.

- Knowledge of human behaviour alone cannot prepare managers in advance for all the situations they will encounter.

- Knowledge used to 'understand people' is not just a means to an end (greater effectiveness and efficiency) but is valuable in its own right.

- Evidence-based practice for managers is the current approach to improving standards in the provision of care services.

9.3 The pitfalls and possibilities of approaches to understanding people

Do you believe that knowledge about human behaviour is 'a good thing'? This may seem like a strange question in a chapter about understanding people but it is important to be clear about the uses to which this knowledge can be put. Our view is that managers need to use their knowledge, however gained, 'with' people, not 'on' people.

Manipulation or transparency?

If knowledge is power, the abilities that managers have to understand people can be used well or badly. Indeed, such knowledge can be abused just as easily as it can be used positively. Knowledge can be used to manipulate other people to do things, or stop doing things, without them being aware of what is happening. All kinds of euphemisms are applied to the use of knowledge to 'pull the wool over people's eyes'. Apparently innocent words such as 'influence', 'persuasion' and even 'encouragement' might be hiding a degree of covert behaviour and coercion designed to disguise the motivation behind intervention.

Two factors must be uppermost in the minds of ethical managers. First, they have power. Second, many of the people who use their services are vulnerable, for one reason or another, and they have to put their trust in service providers. This combination of power and vulnerability creates all the ingredients for the potential abuse of knowledge of human behaviour, as displayed in a series of scandals in health and care services.

One example of this abuse of the power that knowledge brings was the 'pindown' scandal in children's homes in Staffordshire at the end of the 1980s (Levy and Kahan, 1991). 'Pindown' was the name given to an approach to dealing with children and young people who had what are often referred to as 'emotional and behavioural problems'. It involved confining young people – 'pinning them down' – to a room set aside for this purpose. This serves as a good example because it was an explicit set of interventions loosely based on 'learning theory', but taking its ethos and techniques well beyond acceptable practices to the point where it became abusive. Before looking at how knowledge was abused in the pindown case, Box 9.2 (overleaf) outlines some basic information about learning theory.

BOX 9.2 The basics of learning theory

Learning theory can draw our attention to some readily observable features of human behaviour. In the hands of some learning theorists, there is an emphasis on measurable behaviour and a suspicion of hidden thoughts and motivation because these cannot be known for certain. This theory believes that much of our behaviour is learned (hence the theory's name) and, in the right circumstances, can be 'unlearned'. That is to say, behaviour can be 'conditioned'. Some of our responses happen naturally (for example, our eyes water when we peel onions). However, it is possible to train people to respond in the same way to some other stimulus. The classic example of 'conditioning' is Pavlov's famous experiment on dogs, which he taught to salivate when they heard a bell ring (because they associated this with being fed).

'Instrumental conditioning' focuses on the consequences of behaviour and is the approach most people are familiar with. Certain consequences of behaviour can reinforce it positively, or negatively, i.e. they are 'instrumental'. For example, if a parent responds to a child's temper tantrum by giving them a sweet to keep them quiet, this might inadvertently 'positively reinforce' the behaviour. Thereby, the child learns that temper tantrums get rewarded with sweets ('positive' is used here in the sense of something that is presented and which strengthens behaviour, not in terms of good or bad). Thus, what occurs in reality and is revealed with a focus on observed behaviour might be very different from what was intended. A change in the undesired behaviour might require the positive reinforcement of some behaviour incompatible with having temper tantrums and the omission of rewards for the undesired behaviour.

In 'negative reinforcement' something aversive ceases with the performance of behaviour. For example, a loud sound might be terminated by flicking a switch.

Expressed in a rather simplified form, the technique of 'punishment' involves presenting something aversive after an undesired behaviour. The idea is that the behaviour will thereby weaken. Not only does this raise ethical issues but also it is controversial: is punishment really effective in eliminating undesirable behaviours?

(Source: adapted from Bolles, 1979, pp. 121–2)

There are many complex ethical questions associated with the use of learning theory (as there are with most theories of human behaviour). In the pindown scandal, the improper use of rewards and punishments for children in care formed the crux of the matter. Basic rights for children became rewards and the withdrawal of these rights became punishments. This is what the report of the inquiry into pindown said:

One notes that throughout the Pindown era such matters as communicating with other children and/or staff, going to school, taking
exercise, having reading and writing materials, wearing ordinary
clothing as opposed to night wear, being allowed to have visits, and
going out of the room to go to the toilet without knocking on the door
first and being given permission, are categorised and treated as
'privileges' which have to be earned.

(Levy and Kahan, 1991, p. 117)

Several important lessons can be learned from this case about the uses and
abuses of knowledge. First, knowledge can be used to abuse and
manipulate people (in this case, both children and many of the staff
involved). Second, techniques based on such knowledge should not be
'done to' people but 'used with' them and those who are concerned for
them. Third, there must be checks on the uses of knowledge, and systems
of accountability and questioning at all levels of an organisation. Finally,
staff or others who raise doubts or concerns about such ways of working
should be able to 'blow the whistle' and be listened to.

It is quite possible to use instrumental conditioning in an ethically
acceptable way, and it can be helpful to people experiencing very
distressing behaviour problems. Most parents and others looking after
children use simple systems of rewards for 'desired' behaviour and have
rules about 'undesired' behaviour. The point here is that the uses which
knowledge is put to must be widely acceptable, transparent and open to
questioning.

Neutrality, partiality, objectivity and subjectivity

The use of such words may persuade you that the language in which
theories about human behaviour are written is too difficult to be of use in
the everyday work of a manager. However, if managers are to apply the
amazingly rich and complex body of knowledge about human behaviour
that is available, they must be aware of the 'position' adopted in any
approach to the relationship between the observer and the observed, the
'do-er' and the 'done-to'. Some approaches to understanding human
behaviour – for instance, many medical models, cognitive behavioural
models and approaches based on the work of Freud and the Freudians –
tend to take the view that people providing help have to act as if they are
neutral and objective. Indeed, the whole framework of psychoanalysis that
has been so influential in the development of human services is based on
techniques to ensure distance between helper and helped (Wollheim,
1971). According to this theory, it is only through painstakingly acquired
self-knowledge that people can look at others' lives in a way that enables
them to analyse, observe and help in a neutral way (with no intrusion of
personal grievances or emotions).

Although Freudian ideas have been a strong influence in social work, it is approaches based on learning theory that have been key to much management theory. In short, this tends to use systems of rewards to provide incentives to staff to work in a particular way. Giving positive feedback or even rewards, through additional money or promotion, to staff who have 'done well' is a simple example of the application of learning theory to management practice. Neutrality or objectivity here implies that the system of rewards and incentives is applied fairly and without favour.

Most models of intervention in the human services, whatever the origin of their ideas, tend to take the view that those who are providing services have to strive to be neutral and objective. However, this approach is by no means accepted in all circumstances and by all cultures and traditions of the world.

Is it possible not to let your personal feelings or views affect your judgement? Can you be neutral in your approach to people who abuse children, or men who beat their partners, or white people who put incendiary devices through the letterboxes of their black neighbours? Can you treat staff who do the bare minimum with as much respect as those who 'go the extra mile' on behalf of service users? Alongside traditions about neutrality and objectivity there are those that argue that practitioners should take positions. For instance, Urry (1990) argues that therapists can never be neutral because they are affected by their own age, race and profession. She asserts that, in order to counter public and private gender inequalities between men and women, it is essential to empower women in therapy. Geraghty and Meddings (1999) argue that to remain 'neutral' about lesbian, gay and bisexual issues, in the unequal contexts of Western society, is to take a heterosexist position. Can managers be objective, neutral and professional about cutbacks in their service or changes of policy that lead to discrimination? We would argue that these are situations in which it is not possible or desirable to be neutral.

All approaches to human understanding arise from a historical and cultural context and are developed and adapted over time. There is a 'sociology' of such knowledge that teaches that, along with the possibilities that such knowledge gives, there are limitations and partiality about its use. This suggests that such knowledge should be used with care and some caution, and that you should know its and your limitations. Theories, descriptions and plans are often drawn up by more powerful groups, so you may also need to uncover some of the assumptions behind knowledge bases and training, including the assumptions behind this chapter. For example, ask such questions as 'Who said that?', 'Why?' and 'Did they consider other perspectives?' Some of the answers may be found by reading about the authors at the beginning of a book and reading the editor's introduction, as well as looking at when and where it was published and thinking about the wider context for this (Foucault, 1973, 1980).

> **Key points**
>
> - Knowledge about human behaviour should be used with people (staff and service users), not on people.
>
> - Knowledge gives power, which can be abused.
>
> - The ways in which knowledge about human behaviour and motivation is used should be transparent and open to challenge.
>
> - The need to be 'objective' and to have a commitment to values can create tensions for managers.

9.4 Different contexts for understanding people

Managing care services does not happen in isolation from forces and processes that affect all human endeavour. Most Western theories about human behaviour focus on internal psychological processes or on dynamics and relationships between people. This emphasis is based on the assumption that human behaviour, states of mind and relationships are universal and independent of cultural or historical processes. This is not our view, nor does it fit well with debates about care services, particularly when applying an approach based on anti-discriminatory practice (Dominelli, 1998; Robinson, 1998).

In this section we examine the broader context for understanding people, covering culture and organisations as systems.

Culture

In the field of anthropology it is widely recognised that around the world and throughout history people have grappled with problems that arise from the very nature of being human (Kluckhohn and Strodtbeck, 1961). Broadly speaking, these can be grouped under three headings:

1 relationships with other human beings
2 dealing with the passage of time
3 how we relate to our environment.

In any context, whether large (a country) or small (a care service), culture refers to the familiar and habitual ways in which we engage with these universal challenges. However, it is important to realise that it is the challenges that are universal, not the ways in which we respond. There are great differences both within and between cultures, and culture is a living and dynamic entity. Although all three dimensions are of relevance to understanding people for managers of care services, the first one is of most concern in this chapter.

Trompenaars (1993) is a leading European exponent of a culturally led analysis of diversity in the management of business organisations. In his book *Riding the Waves of Culture*, he draws on sociological, psychological and anthropological theory to outline five orientations covering the ways in which human beings deal with each other (see Box 9.3).

BOX 9.3 Trompenaars' five orientations

1 *Universalism versus particularism.* The universalist approach is roughly: 'What is good and right can be defined and always applies.' In particularist cultures far greater attention is given to the obligations of relationships and unique circumstances, such as friendship and kinship.

2 *Individualism versus collectivism.* Do people regard themselves primarily as individuals or primarily as part of a group? Which comes first in the manager's thinking: the group or the individuals within it?

3 *Neutral or emotional.* Should the nature of our interactions be objective and detached, or is expressing emotion acceptable? Is banging your fist on the table or weeping in frustration in a meeting a sign of commitment or a sign of poor professional control?

4 *Specific versus diffuse.* When the whole person is involved in a working relationship there is a real and personal contact, instead of a specific relationship prescribed by an implicit or explicit contract. In some cultures it is expected that you stay in your specific role (as manager); in others, a more diffuse role is needed before a working relationship can proceed. Do you accept coffee and ask someone about their family before getting down to business? How do you respond if others ask you the same?

5 *Achievement versus ascription.* Achievement means that you are judged on what you have recently accomplished and on your record. Ascription means that status is attributed to you not only by birth, kinship, gender, age, class, race, and so on but also by your connections (who you know) and your educational record (for example, a graduate of Oxbridge with a good degree).

(Source: adapted from Trompenaars, 1993, pp. 8–10)

It is also useful, briefly, to visit the other dimensions of 'time' and 'environment'. In some cultures what a person has done in the past is more important than what they are planning to do next. In others it is what a person is about to do that counts. For some, time goes in a straight line whereas others think of past, present and future circling round together. If you are not sure what difference this might make to a manager, try thinking about planning and it will be clear quite quickly that the way you go about it is fundamentally affected by your view of time.

As for the environment, some cultures focus on the individual as the locus for vice or virtue. Others see the influence of the world on the person as far more powerful. The former see the environment as something to be controlled, the latter as something to be feared and respected. Thus, managers have to understand people (their staff, fellow managers, service users, and so on), who may have very different beliefs about the most fundamental aspects of the business of being a human, and how others should respond. Trompenaars puts this very concisely:

> We cannot strip people of their common sense constructs or routine ways of seeing. They come to us as whole systems of patterned meanings and understandings. We can only try to understand, and to do so means starting with the way they think and building from there.
>
> Hence organisations do not simply react to their environment as a ship might to waves. They actively select, interpret, choose and create their environments.
>
> (Trompenaars, 1993, p. 19)

Organisations and people as systems

General systems theory (von Bertalanffy, 1971) offers one way of thinking about the people in an organisation. The idea is that all organisms are systems, made up of parts (subsystems) that interact with each other. Although originally developed to understand biological organisms, sociologists later used it as a helpful model for human society. A person can simultaneously be a system (an individual human being) and part of a system (for example, a family or care service) and that system can be a subsystem of a super-system (society). When applied to managing care, it helps to see how the groups of people managed (say a team) comprise subsystems (individuals or sub-teams) and are, at the same time, members of larger systems (organisations). This theory gives opportunities to consider matters of human behaviour at different levels and to look at how systems interact.

For a work team to function as an effective system it has to have *boundaries*. More energy must be exchanged within these boundaries than across them in order for it to be seen as a separate system. However, because it is an open system the boundary must be *permeable*. Payne explains this by using an analogy:

> An *open system* is where energy crosses the boundary which is permeable, rather like a tea-bag in a cup of hot water which lets water in and tea out but keeps the tea leaves inside.
>
> (Payne, 1991, p. 135)

For human systems to keep going they have to maintain their integrity and provide some of their own energy, but they also need to exchange energy with other systems. Otherwise they suffer 'entropy' (von Bertalanffy, 1971) and exhaust themselves. To work effectively a system needs *feedback loops* whereby the impact it has on its environment is received back as information to tell it the effect of its outputs. Without this information, systems cannot adapt to their environment. No individual system is ever powerful enough not to have to adapt and respond to exchanges of information and energy with other systems and its own subsystems.

Systems theory attempts to explain how organisations can be both stable and dynamic at the same time. Human systems strive to maintain their equilibrium by ensuring they adapt without losing their integrity. This condition, known as *homeostasis* (dynamic equilibrium), is key to understanding how organisations can adapt to change without falling apart. Human systems also tend to *differentiate* (become more complex over time). The benefits of a system are that when it is in homeostasis, the whole is greater than the sum of its parts. When systems theory is applied to an organisation providing care services, it explains how the organisation taken as a whole will do a better job for service users than if all the individuals within it tried to work without co-operating. This would apply equally well to the need for co-operation between organisations (systems in their own right). However, if the organisation is confronted by too much change too quickly, perhaps through several successive reorganisations, it cannot maintain its integrity, and it becomes less than the sum of its parts and loses its ability to receive feedback and to respond to its environment.

Finally, systems theory is essentially about the interconnected nature of organisms (including human organisations), which is known as *reciprocity*. If one part of a system providing care changes (for example, an agency changes its eligibility criteria for providing intermediate care for older people), this change will interact with other parts of the system (it will affect other organisations that are also involved in providing services, such as day care or home care services). To restore equilibrium to the whole system, changes that require exchanges of information, energy and feedback are needed. This will continue until adjustment is made to the new policy.

One of the advantages of applying systems theory to managing care services is that the notion of reciprocity implies that the same result can be reached in several different ways, and that different results can come out of similar circumstances. This certainly fits with commonsense observations of how the outcome of interaction within a complex network of human organisations is extremely difficult to predict or control. The efforts of the government to reorganise health and care services is a classic example of how difficult it is to predict what impact interventions will have on complex systems. This is particularly so when the building blocks of systems are people – staff, service users, and so on. No matter how well you understand individual human behaviour, or group interaction, wider systems can exert forces on you that can easily make your best efforts come to very little.

It is only by looking at people in a context and at different levels of a system that you can really make sense of behaviour. Sometimes your gaze has to be on a small area of interaction (for example, a team of care workers). At other times you may need to look at the wider organisation or even at a whole service.

Systems theory is helpful to managers as a way of describing what is happening and an aid to modelling complex interactions within and between organisations. Its main weakness is that it does not readily lend itself to making predictions about the outcomes of intervention. It can, however, model possibilities and be an aid in planning and reflecting on complex processes. It is particularly useful when you get 'stuck' with a problem and just cannot understand why people are not responding to your best efforts to help. In these circumstances, systems theory would suggest that you need to look at a different level of system to see whether the issues you are grappling with are better dealt with there.

Managers face several persistent problems in applying their knowledge of human behaviour: some of them are addressed in the next section.

Key points

- Claims that knowledge is universally applicable are challenged by the existence of different cultural traditions and the history of how knowledge about human behaviour has changed over time.

- What is accepted as knowledge about people in any organisation is selected and interpreted.

- Seeing human organisations as complex systems can help in understanding and interpreting human behaviour, although not necessarily in predicting what will happen.

9.5 Persistent concerns for managers of care services

Part of the wider context for understanding people is that care service providers, like all organisations, face new challenges over time. (Some of the old ones even come back again!) These are sometimes called 'the current fashion' in terms of managers' concerns. The language also changes as new influences are brought to bear on service providers. Current 'buzz words' in the care services at the time of writing include 'partnership', 'modernisation', 'joined-up thinking' and 'championing'. Identifying concerns that seem to persist can be difficult, in part because of the distractions caused by too much change happening too quickly but also because jargon can make it look as if changes are happening when in reality they are not. A major continuing concern for managers of care services is the welfare of those using the services, although the language used to describe them changes: for example 'the needy', 'clients' or 'service users'. We have identified three further persistent concerns for managers of care services that are intimately connected with efforts to understand and influence human behaviour:

1 dealing with organisational change
2 motivating staff
3 stress and burn-out in the caring professions.

Organisational change

Martin and Henderson (2001) argue that managing in health and care services has shifted from maintaining the status quo to deliberately stimulating change and encouraging innovation in order to make continuous improvements. In this sense, change is permanent although many people hope that the rate of change will ebb and flow. Thus, understanding how staff and service users react to change is an important part of a manager's job. This requires a certain type of approach to managing people whereby managers:

> establish an open culture in which [they] challenge assumptions, test new ideas and share experience ... This may be especially important if the change involves working with partners in other organisations, and therefore involves understanding different cultures, structures and patterns of working.
>
> (Martin and Henderson, 2001, p. 113)

According to this analysis, understanding people with respect to managing change goes back to looking at behaviour in a context.

The specialist field of organisational change has given rise to a wide-ranging management literature, and there are many possibilities for reflective managers and practitioners to engage with and apply the concepts in this literature to change in social care. Martin and Henderson (2001) apply the work of Lewin (1947) to look at how people respond to change using *force-field analysis*. Put simply, this predicts that in any situation involving change there will be forces (people) driving change, and forces (people) resisting change. This gives rise to an equilibrium between forces: the skilful manager seeks a way to work with and adjust such a balance by reducing the restraining forces. Martin and Henderson suggest that managers can analyse change situations by looking at clusters of forces. Box 9.4 outlines the kinds of forces that might motivate resistance to change.

BOX 9.4 Martin and Henderson's clusters of forces resisting change

- *Personal* (for example, fear of redundancy, loss of competence or loss of pride)

- *Interpersonal* (for example, A does not talk to B)

- *Intergroup* (for example, home care organisers' relationships with care managers)

- *Organisational* (for example, there is an overall shortage of resources or new management structures are being introduced)

- *Technological* (for example, records have been computerised)

- *Environmental* (for example, there are more older people, or the law on mental health has been changed)

(Source: adapted from Martin and Henderson, 2001, p. 128)

They go on to argue that, in any given set of circumstances, people will probably adopt one of the following four positions in relation to change.

1 People who are not, and never will be, committed to the proposed change and will resist it.
2 People who are neither for it nor against it and who will not oppose or support it.
3 People who have some level of commitment and will follow leadership on change but will not lead it themselves.
4 People who are positively for it and will take a leadership position.

Managers do have to make judgements about the extent of resistance to change, and where to focus their efforts in terms of encouraging change or deciding it is not possible.

Box 9.5 (overleaf) shows Martin and Henderson's suggestions for gaining commitment to change.

BOX 9.5 Suggestions for gaining commitment to organisational change

- *Use power.* Reward behaviour that is positive about change.

- *Deal with staff concerns.* If staff whose commitment you need are concerned about proposed changes, listen to them, and engage them in dialogue about possible remedies.

- *Expose the issues.* Explore people's concerns in unthreatening ways. For example, have unstructured, off-the-record discussions that do not require clear outcomes.

- *Use a 'learning' approach.* Explore cross-boundary differences and issues as opportunities for learning and professional debate.

- *Act as a role model.* Behave in ways that give clear messages to staff about where you stand on the issues of change.

- *Use champions.* Make sure that respected colleagues do some of the work of analysis and persuasion.

- *Encourage discussion.* Show that it is legitimate to hold different views about change and give people opportunities to debate and explore different opinions.

- *Be prepared to do deals.* Change often needs compromise and negotiation. Be prepared to bargain.

(Source: adapted from Martin and Henderson, 2001, pp. 133–4)

Motivation and job satisfaction

One reason for understanding people might be to enhance the quality and quantity of their work. There was a view that if managers could understand people better it might be possible to enhance life and job satisfaction and to improve productivity. Taylorism in the early 1900s was one of the first attempts to analyse jobs and to give clear job descriptions to enhance efficiency. The human relations approach of the 1930s and 1940s suggested that what motivates workers is being treated with respect and dignity and that managers should show an interest in them. This may seem very obvious to us now, imbued as we are (or should be) with values arising from a respect for human rights and legislation protecting us from exploitation and unfair dismissal, but at the time it was seen as a radical idea.

Cynics would say that industrial psychology in the mid-20th century was interested in how to increase productivity by increasing motivation instead of improving pay and conditions. Evidence now suggests that understanding people and improved job satisfaction and productivity are not necessarily associated. Babchuk and Goode (1951) comment on this in their study of workers in a men's clothing department in a large store, described in Example 9.1.

EXAMPLE 9.1 Co-operation and job satisfaction

In earlier times, the department was run along individual competitive lines, where much of people's pay was based on sales bonuses, leading to people vying to serve customers. Staff were dissatisfied and wanted a more co-operative system. As a result of changes made by staff to pool work and profit and take equal pay, morale improved, and sales increased. The authors caution that it cannot be concluded from this that self-determining work units have the highest morale – other variables were also important, such as a constant high demand for the product, skilled and knowledgeable workers, with union backing and a liberal management.

(Source: adapted from Babchuk and Goode, 1951, pp. 681–6)

It would be interesting to know whether clients also became more satisfied and whether the shop became a more pleasant place to be. How, if at all, does such a study translate into job satisfaction in the field of health and social care? This is a pertinent question at a time when themes of competition and reward coexist with those of partnership and co-operation. This coexistence can be clearly seen in the voluntary sector in which workers share skills, resources and ideas with colleagues from other independent sector organisations (voluntary and private) with whom they may be competing for the same funding.

Social psychologists have tried to provide frameworks for understanding people in their work contexts. In the 1980s a literature emerged on the value of work, in part spurred by the high levels of unemployment at the time. Jahoda (1982) explains that although pay is one of the important aspects of work, staff also benefit from the 'latent functions of work'. In other words, jobs enforce activity, give employees a structure for day-to-day life and provide shared social goals, social networks and identity or status. Jahoda omits the intrinsic nature of work, which may be particularly important in the fields of health and social care.

In contrast, Fryer (1986, 1987) argues that people are already active and self-organising, and work simply provides the money needed to exercise this agency. In other words, people do not depend on work to provide structure, goals, networks and identity: all that is needed is the means to pursue and develop these aspects for themselves. On a more prosaic level, this debate is often held when considering the impact of a big win on the lottery. Would it change your life? Would you lose your sense of purpose and identity if you decided to give up work? Certainly Jahoda's theory might suggest this. Often winners announce they will continue with their familiar way of life, to avoid the possibility of losing the benefits of familiar structures and routine. On the other hand, would you merely transfer your natural tendencies to create structure and purpose out of life to the new opportunities afforded by your big win, as Fryer's work might predict?

Warr's vitamin model, illustrated in Figure 9.1, describes nine features of the environment that enhance mental health and wellbeing, and may be found at work, increasing life satisfaction as well as job satisfaction.

At low levels, deficiencies in these 'vitamins' lead to both mental and physical ill health. On the whole, increases lead to improved mental wellbeing. For example, within a context of a decent salary, with physical security and safety, people are often more satisfied with their work when they can choose what they are doing. This is particularly true if the organisational environment is easy to understand, and if the goals set in staff appraisal are such that they can predict the impact of what they do. Nevertheless, just as with vitamins A and D, some of these 'vitamins' may be harmful in excess. For example, it is important to have goals and variety but in excess they may lead to work overload, stress and lowered achievement. Warr suggests that all the vitamins have this tendency if used in excess, with the exception of money, physical security and valued social position, for which increases are almost always positive. They might be seen as more akin to vitamins C and E.

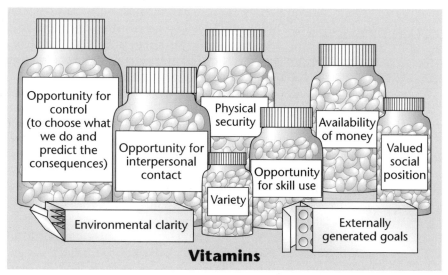

Figure 9.1 **Warr's vitamin model** (Source: adapted from Warr, 1987, Table 15.1)

In summary, people who work in a more co-operative and less competitive environment appear to feel more satisfied, unless they are in a sales context where bonuses are the most effective incentives. Staff working in health and social care organisations are at risk from stress and emotional exhaustion. Evidence suggests that balancing interrelated factors in the work environment protects against this risk. Simply improving work tasks without addressing issues of boundaries and resources is not enough: satisfied staff are equally at risk from burn-out as dissatisfied staff.

Stress and burn-out

Box 9.6 summarises some research on what people find stressful.

BOX 9.6 Stressful events

Atkinson *et al.* (2000) identify five types of stressful event.

1 *Traumatic events* – situations of extreme danger outside the range of usual human experience

2 *Controllability* – the less control we have or perceive ourselves to have, the more stress we will experience

3 *Predictability* – being able to predict a stressful event usually reduces its severity

4 *Challenging our limits* – events that challenge the limits of our capabilities or our view of ourselves are stressful

5 *Internal conflicts* – when our inner needs or motivations conflict with each other

---

McCann and Pearlman (1990) describe burn-out as depression, cynicism, boredom, loss of compassion and discouragement in relation to the psychological strain of working with 'difficult populations'. Managers of care staff doing work that is likely to put them under emotional and psychological strain can reduce the likelihood of burn-out by:

• providing emotional as well as professional support at work
• providing a safe supportive context in which to process issues raised by work
• providing staff with a balance of different types of work (direct work with service users, research, training)
• helping staff to maintain boundaries between different areas of life (sometimes referred to as the personal/professional boundary).

For managers to support staff and reduce burn-out, it is crucial that the difficult emotions that may arise in providing care are seen as a normal response (in most circumstances) and that everyone involved has a responsibility to take this aspect of the work seriously. This is an example of what is often referred to as 'emotional literacy'. Knowledge of common responses to life events and our journeys through the life cycle comprise the components of emotional literacy that are a basic requirement to providing and managing care services.

Human experiences of stress and trauma, and feelings and thoughts about them, can be physically embodied (Kepner, 1987). This is reflected in everyday language such as 'pain in the neck' or 'gets on my nerves'. It is often our sensing, physical selves that we disregard in stressful environments (specifically how our bodies respond to stress). In extreme cases this is referred to as 'post-traumatic stress disorder'.

Onyett et al. (1997) found high emotional exhaustion among mental health workers, especially consultant psychiatrists, social workers, nurses and psychologists, in contrast to their good job satisfaction and motivation. They remind us that job satisfaction and burn-out can coexist (see also Farber, 1983). Worryingly, half of the community psychiatric nurses interviewed for this research fell into the 'high' emotional exhaustion category. Onyett et al. (1997) recommend several environmental factors to address this:

- clearer team goals
- clearer identification with the team
- reduced workload
- appropriate training
- valuing of team members
- adequate resources.

Elsewhere they also recommend that differences between staff in skills and expertise be acknowledged, with clear and different roles for different teams and different professional groups (Onyett et al., 1995). By understanding staff in relation to their work context and how this can be made healthy, it may be possible to support a healthy workforce that can continue to understand and work well with service users.

Key points

- Although the jargon used to discuss how organisations should be managed changes, some concerns seem to persist (dealing with change, motivating staff, stress and burn-out).

- Although change is always with us, the current emphasis is on encouraging change rather than maintaining the status quo.

- The rate of change and the amount of disruption currently being experienced in care services may be counterproductive.

- Managers can have some impact on helping people deal with the process of change.

- There are arguments that work is intrinsically important to people and this may be especially so for those involved in providing care services.

- A range of factors affect the wellbeing of people doing a job, and finding a balance will increase job satisfaction and performance.

- High levels of stress and burn-out can exist alongside job satisfaction and motivation.

- Managers can make a difference in reducing stress and burn-out, although they are subject to it as well.

9.6 The key skills in understanding people

To develop the necessary levels of emotional literacy requires an ability to *observe*, *listen* and *reflect*. This is supported by the literature on service users' experiences of care services which suggests that those responsible for managing services need to ask what they want and what works, and to listen and act on the answers they receive (Harding, 1996). Similarly, one of the best ways of understanding staff is to ask and listen. Managers cannot be expected to have all the answers and always to know what to do. They are there to get the best out of their staff by encouraging a culture of learning through listening, responding and adapting to change.

Meddings and Perkins (2002) found that simply asking service users and staff what 'getting better' meant added to and challenged the professional and research literature on which they predominantly based their practice. This led to an increased understanding of staff and service users and changes in attitudes and practice (see Example 9.2).

EXAMPLE 9.2 Asking people

In mental health, the literature produced by clinicians and researchers often focuses on clinical matters relating to mental state, medication and therapeutic interventions. Yet, in an era of evidence-based practice, it is important not only to look at theories derived by researchers and senior professionals but also to ask people on the ground: staff and service users. We asked what 'getting better' meant to staff and users while searching the literature for an outcome tool which would measure different aspects of recovery. We wanted to look at a range of interventions and how they helped people to get better. With some notable exceptions, tools were drawn from the perspective of professionals and academics, relating to theoretical perspectives more than people's actual experience, and were narrowly focused on reducing symptoms rather than on a broader conception of wellbeing.

We found that both staff and users had quite complex, multifaceted ideas about 'getting better', involving the following:

- improved mental state
- improved wellbeing and relationships
- empowerment
- increased confidence and self-worth
- greater engagement in work and activities
- coping better with everyday life
- getting access to help and support
- improved material circumstances
- better physical health.

Staff rated activities of daily living and access to help and support as more important than did users. Users rated improved material and physical wellbeing as more important than did staff.

Thus, by asking local staff and service users, we were able to understand the meaning of getting better in complex ways, in line with the literature on recovery and psychiatric rehabilitation (Anthony, 1993; Perkins and Repper, 1996). The differences of view between service users and staff also provide important data that could lead to a better understanding of staff and service user interaction.

(Source: adapted from Meddings and Perkins, 2002)

Of course, asking and listening are not sufficient on their own. Service users and staff are not homogeneous groups who all think and act in the same way. Their views change over time, and the quality of the responses is always going to be more or less thoughtful and informed by greater or lesser amounts of experience and expertise. Managers are not passive responders to demands but bring their knowledge, skill and judgement into the process of deciding how to act. Their judgements have to be informed by careful observation and based on a growing body of evidence about what works and why (Sheldon and Chilvers, 2000). They are always constrained by resources and have to make judgements about priorities within a legal and policy framework.

Managers must form their own judgements because they are accountable for their actions to more than one group. This includes service users and staff but managers will also have formal lines of accountability

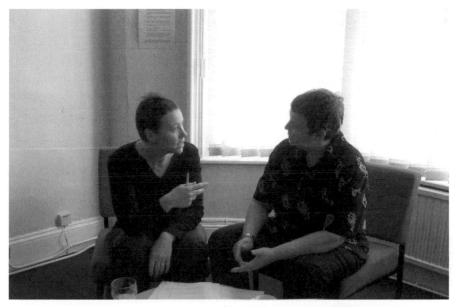

Observing, listening and reflecting are key skills in understanding people

based on the system of governance that applies to their service. They could be accountable to a professional body and have their own set of ethical principles that they have to reconcile with the actions they can, or cannot, take.

Despite the complexities and limitations cited above, we believe that there is much greater scope now than in the past for managers to listen to service users and staff and to act on what they hear.

Key points

- The key skills in the practice of 'understanding people' are listening, observing and reflecting.

- Asking people for their views will not provide all the answers, but there is more scope now to ask service users and frontline staff for their views and to act on what they say.

- Staff and service users are diverse groups of people who do not all think and act in the same way.

- Managers must engage actively and critically when consulting others and bring their own knowledge and experience to bear on what they hear.

9.7 Conclusion

The history of humans' attempts to understand themselves is so complex that it is tempting to resort to 'common sense' and 'muddling through' as the only approach to managing care that is not going to involve a lifetime of study and reflection. Our view in this chapter is that managers of care services are in the 'people business' and that learning about human behaviour is a lifetime's work. We hear a great deal in the human services about the need for 'lifelong learning'. If this is to mean anything then surely it means constantly refining your understanding of yourself and others. This chapter has concentrated on a few aspects of knowledge and its acquisition.

It is often said that 'a little knowledge is a dangerous thing'. This may well be true but it is better than the wilful ignorance and neglect of the struggles of researchers, practitioners and service users to make their labours available for others to use. We leave the last words to a manager. Can you see just how much knowledge and understanding of human beings is implicit in what she says?

BRONWYN'S DIARY

Monday

Fairly gentle start to the week. Met with an ex-client who is due to move to another part of the country for a 'goodbye' session. She is an incredible person who has survived against all the odds. I felt a real mixture of emotions as we had gone through some powerful times together. She was very shaky about the move. I made all the right noises about the positives etc. but I also felt shaky and realised I'll miss her – never get over-involved with your clients, keep the boundaries – and on the whole I do but we're only human and some people touch you – she was one of those.

... Supervision session with a worker from another agency. He's had a bad time with his organisation and we spent a long time looking at the processes. He had sick leave because of it due to panic attacks. Over the months we've been meeting, changes have happened and he's feeling in a stronger place to continue, but at what cost?

Took supervision notes home and ploughed through them fortified by white wine!

Chapter 10
The morally active manager

Angus Dawson and Ian Butler

10.1   Introduction

In the 21st century health and social care managers are required to hold values, to respect the values of others, and to value the people who work in and use services. Services are planned and delivered on 'Best Value' principles, the recent White Paper (for England) in the learning disability field being entitled *Valuing People* (Department of Health, 2001b). As Pattison observes, 'the language of values is everywhere in contemporary society' (1998, p. 352).

Values are not free-floating: they belong to a person, a team, an organisation, a profession and/or to the wider society. Often they are framed in vision and mission statements, in lists of principles and in ethical guidelines. To think and act ethically requires a set of values – and a mindset that values other people. This escalation of values is matched, it seems, by what Davis (1999) calls 'an ethics boom'. The world of health and social care is complex and inevitably throws up ethical issues. Faced with competing demands that require sorting into some order of priority, and confronted daily with vital human needs that somehow have to be met from within restricted resources, health and social care managers need an ethical framework.

This means developing an ethical perspective that is good enough to help cope with the role and tasks that go with the job. In this chapter we pursue the idea of 'the morally active manager' as one way of developing an ethical approach robust enough to cover the dilemmas and difficulties of health and social care at the front line. The terms 'ethical' and 'moral' are used interchangeably in this chapter. Thus, to be morally active is also to act ethically. There is a distinction throughout, however, between the values or principles that guide people's judgement from *within* and external frameworks or guidelines that are imposed from *without*. This idea of the morally active manager builds on Husband's notion of 'the morally active practitioner' (Husband, 1995). In the sense that a manager presides over, and a practitioner works towards, the provision of welfare and other services, both are engaged in an essentially moral activity.

In this chapter we explore what it means to be 'morally active', as a practitioner and as a manager. To be morally active is to act on the basis of internal values, or standards, rather than (or as well as) to act on the basis of externally imposed codes of conduct. 'The morally active manager' makes judgements about, and takes responsibility for, acting in a moral – or a principled – way towards other people. The morally active manager, in drawing on personal and professional experience and wisdom, is also concerned with practice-led management.

We also consider the idea of 'moral management' and look at some of the ethical issues health and social care managers have to deal with. Two key ethical issues are looked at in depth. First, we develop and explore 'an ethics of social care'. This helps underline the point that the practice of social care is intrinsically and fundamentally a moral enterprise. Such an enterprise demands decisions about who is, or becomes, a service user, and when to intervene in people's lives. Second, we develop a more detailed analysis of some of the routine dilemmas that arise in practice, in relation to the ethical distribution of resources. In particular, we explore the concept of need and the role that such a concept may play in determining where resources are directed. Finally, there is a review of the role and place (and potential) of the morally active manager within the health and social care context.

The aims of this chapter are to:

- explore some of the ethical issues in health and social care practice
- trace the origins of care as a moral activity
- develop the concept of the morally active manager
- unpack what an ethics of social care would look like
- address key ethical dilemmas in everyday practice
- consider the concept of need in relation to the distribution of resources
- view ethical issues in a wider social and political context.

10.2   An ethics of social care?

Introducing the morally active manager

Where does the idea of the morally active manager come from? Its origins can be traced back to Bauman's notion of a person's 'moral impulse' or capacity to act morally from within – as opposed to acting in response to externally imposed ethical frameworks (Bauman, 1993, p. 19). This idea was taken up by Husband (1995) who applied it to social work and argued the case for the morally active practitioner. In Husband's terms, such a practitioner acts as an autonomous moral agent rather than purely as an agent of the state, taking responsibility for their professional practice and its implications. The potential of this position to be viewed as anarchic and dangerous was not lost on Husband – but it was countered by the requirement for morally active practitioners to also be reflective in their everyday practice.

This chapter extends Husband's concept into health and social care management by introducing the idea of the morally active manager. In our terms, morally active managers in social care can respond in a flexible but coherent way to the diverse ethical problems encountered in their day-to-day work. The argument here is, following Husband, that ethical management does not come from merely applying an ethical mantra, such as a shortlist of moral principles or a professional code of practice. Although guidelines may be helpful in providing a very loose framework for decision making, they do not help resolve specific issues. In fact, the soundest approach is that managers take responsibility for their own decisions and the consequences that flow from them.

The idea of the morally active practitioner – or caseworker – can be traced back to the origins of social casework in the late Victorian period (Vincent and Plant, 1984). Caseworkers sought then to intervene in the community with the intention of promoting the active citizenship of everyone. This provides a challenging and useful framework for our discussion about contemporary social care management.

One of the complications of current health and social care management is that different professions are working together, often for the first time. Each profession, or occupational group, is likely to have its own values, its particular ways of working and its own ethical traditions. In addition, each professional or occupational group, in turn, is likely to continue to draw on these as their primary guide to action, at least to begin with, which creates one possible area of conflict and confusion. Moreover, it could be argued that all professions in the four countries of the UK have been under a great deal of pressure since the 1980s. There have been significant changes in the nature and identity of the professions and the way in which professionals are viewed. The commodification of welfare and the rise of a market in social and health services; the emergence of the knowledgeable consumer; the promotion of evidence-based practice; and the idea of quality management within these services have all had an impact. These major changes have meant that no profession can automatically rely on gaining the respect or status, or carrying the same moral authority, that it might have had in the past. The members of the professions and occupations related to health and social care are no exception; they are equally likely to be prone to anxiety and insecurity.

A further complication, of course, is that large numbers of people involved in the type of work that is increasingly designated 'social care' do not belong to a traditional profession at all. Indeed, this is evidently a government concern, as steps are being taken to encourage the social care workforce to have further training and attain relevant qualifications. There is clearly not only the potential for conflict between the different professions involved in social care but also the danger that problems will emerge between the professional and non-professional groups working in the field. These 'professional' aspects are relevant to a consideration of ethical issues. It is quite possible, in fact, that one area of potential tension in the future will be deciding what is the most appropriate ethical stance to adopt in health and social care practice against the backdrop of these differing traditions and perspectives.

Health and social care workers and professionals, including social workers, have more or less established sets of ethical principles that might be suitable for application in the developing sphere of social care. One possibility in pursuing the idea of ethical practice is to take one of these 'off the peg' sets of ethical principles and adapt it to the roles and tasks of managers in health and social care. Indeed, this may be what already occurs in practice. Many such codes are in fact derived from the established tradition of ethical scrutiny in the medical profession. It could be argued that medicine has made substantial progress in formulating a general, and more or less consensual, 'basic moral analytical framework and a basic moral language' (Gillon, 1994, p. 184).

A 'principles' approach to ethical issues

The ethical framework that emerges, based on the seminal work of Beauchamp and Childress (2001), is frequently referred to as the 'four principles plus scope' approach.

The four principles are:

1   respect for autonomy
2   beneficence
3   non-maleficence
4   justice.

The 'scope' is the process of deciding how these very different, and potentially conflicting, obligations apply in particular circumstances.

In the simplest of terms, 'respect for autonomy' means the moral obligation to respect the autonomy of each individual in so far as that is compatible with respecting the autonomy of others. It implies treating other people as moral agents in their own right, as ends in themselves and not simply as means to ends. In medical terms, 'beneficence' means doing good and 'non-maleficence' means not doing harm. 'Justice' is the moral obligation to deal fairly in the face of competing claims, especially in relation to equalising claims deriving from people's rights and respecting morally acceptable laws. It prohibits the pursuit of one's own interests at the expense of others' legitimate interests: for example, using scarce resources in unacceptable ways; favouring one's own particular community of interest or association; and disapproving of the moral choices of other people.

These principles can also be seen in combination. When that happens, certain other moral obligations can be discerned, such as the empowerment of other people. Gillon sees this as 'essentially an action that combines the two moral obligations of beneficence and respect for autonomy to help patients in ways that not only respect but also their autonomy' (1994, p. 186). The decision about which prin take precedence, should they compete, or which people any ......, should apply to, and to what degree and in what circumstances, remains the responsibility of the moral agent using the four principles. The model thus leaves 'scope' for how the principles are to be applied – perhaps leaving it open to managers, and practitioners, to act according to their own moral consciences.

There are at least two problems with the principles approach to ethical issues. The first problem is knowing which principles are appropriate in any given situation. The second problem relates to how the approach is used in practice. This problem arises because people who advocate the four principles approach tend to concentrate most on autonomy, at the expense of the other principles. This suggests, at the very least, that there are some background assumptions operating in the use of the four principles approach. These assumptions require some justification, which is often lacking in the literature.

It is interesting to compare the literature on the four principles in health care (Beauchamp and Childress, 2001; Gillon, 1986) with the different sets of principles in social work. The latter include, for example, Biestek's principles of social casework: individualisation; purposeful expression of feelings; controlled emotional involvement; acceptance; a non-judgemental attitude; client self-determination; and confidentiality (Biestek, 1961). These in turn are different from Wilmot's four principles – care and community, justice, autonomy and responsibility (1997) – and Clark's more recent proposal of 'four stocks of ethical practice' – respect, justice, citizenship and discipline (2000).

It is important to note that there are differences in principles even within the broad area of social welfare, not just between the arenas of health and social care. It could be argued that the same principles are just reclassified in a slightly different form. There may be an element of truth in this. However, it is significant that one of the above core ethical principles in social work includes an important element that is not present in the four principles approach in health care: the idea of 'community'.

This observation raises the question 'how can one list of principles be justified over another?' It could be argued that the idea of community is equally as important in health as in social care. Why then does it not feature in the health care list? Perhaps all we can safely say about competing lists is that they give a clearer insight into the priorities of the people who construct them, rather than a true glimpse of what might constitute any fundamental ethical guidelines for life.

The social and political context of the four principles approach

The four principles approach became influential within a particular social and political context – liberal democracy. In this context the central ethical and political issue is to maximise an individual's freedom from the encroachment of any external agencies, such as the state, which might be seen as a potential threat to this liberty. Taking the four principles approach as our example, this means that, although the various principles are supposed to have equal weight, in reality autonomy is nearly always given priority. This can be seen, for example, in Beauchamp and Childress's discussion of paternalistic intervention, when they argue that the action chosen should be that which is the 'least autonomy-restrictive alternative' (2001, p. 186). It could be argued instead that, in at least some situations, a justification for such so-called 'paternalistic' actions could be given by appealing to beneficence.

A similar liberal political philosophy to that underpinning the four principles is at work in some of the recent discussions by members of the disabled people's movement. For example, Shakespeare suggests that 'Disabled people want social independence, which is about autonomy and control over their lives' (2000, p. 59). The focus here is on the 'rights' of disabled people. Full citizenship becomes possible, in this view, not through state or other sorts of social intervention, however caring, but through political action to enable disabled people to achieve their goals. This approach, like any view that appeals to autonomy as the supreme guiding principle for social action, has the potential to distort social relationships.

The problem with concentrating on the principle of autonomy is that those people who, for whatever reason, are thought to be 'dependent' on others, including statutory and voluntary organisations, are in danger of being seen as second-class or marginal members of society. As Campbell (1991, 1994) points out, humans are essentially social beings and we can all be seen as dependent on others to varying degrees. He argues that we should not see dependency as a negative state and freedom from it (autonomy) as the goal. Building on this point, there is no reason to think that when aid comes from other parties, whether family, friends, voluntary organisations or the state, this should necessarily be seen as a threat to an individual's freedom. Of course, such actions *can* threaten people's freedom but such interventions, at best, can enable a 'vulnerable' individual to become, and be seen as, a full and equal citizen in the future: something that might otherwise be difficult to achieve. The language of 'rights' and 'autonomy' might well result in more damage to our humanity and community rather than providing a quick and easy political fix.

role was to 'equalise' the position of disadvantaged people. Green favoured the state doing this by acting as a regulator and an enforcer of minimum standards of wellbeing. This is why his views are of more than historical interest and are relevant to the issues discussed in this chapter.

As well as arguing for what amounts to 'positive freedom' (Berlin, 1969), Green argued for the 'positive power or capacity' of people to develop and 'make the most and best of themselves' within a social context (1986, p. 199). Real freedom, in Green's terms, can only be found by an individual in a social situation. However, even that freedom is not valuable *in itself* but only as a means to an end, namely the common good. Thus, Green's concept of 'positive freedom' was the freedom to realise one's best self and, in community with everyone else, to realise the common good (Himmelfarb, 1995).

Social care as a moral activity

How do these thoughts relate to the case of Maureen in particular and social care in general? They do so because anyone working in the field of social care is explicitly involved in a moral activity. Social care is about human welfare in all its complexity, involving people who, for whatever reason(s), are thought to be vulnerable. Intervention can be seen, therefore, as one way of attempting to equalise the bargaining position of the most vulnerable and disadvantaged people in society. Taking this view, such intervention could be seen as the *morally required* action.

Social care may involve 'interfering' in individuals' lives but, it is argued, this may be justified where it is aimed at restoring the conditions of those people who are otherwise disadvantaged and unable to protect their own interests. Here, social care is, at least partly, directed at producing equality between all. The idea is that true equality involves more than the possession of a set of political rights. It is more like having the capacity to be an active citizen. Supporters of such a view might question Maureen's capacity to act on her own behalf, as a truly active citizen, and may argue instead that residential care would best promote her overall health and general wellbeing and be justified as being in her best interests.

'Care' in such circumstances is rarely straightforward. Practitioners, and managers, face real ethical dilemmas about supporting people 'at risk' in the community. There are questions about if and when to intervene in people's lives and the nature of that intervention. Is it support? Or is it social control? The practice of social care, trespassing as it does on the boundaries of the individual and the state and working day to day with matters of freedom and compulsion, is in itself a moral activity. As such, it cannot be undertaken by merely relying on the 'taken for granted' principles of other people. It requires practitioners – and managers – to be ethically sensitive and aware. Managers make moral judgements about the situations of other people – often where needs are complex and conflicting. In the next section we explore some of those conflicts.

Key points

- To be morally active is to be guided by an internal 'moral impulse'.

- The idea of 'the morally active manager' builds on an earlier idea of the morally active practitioner and originates from social casework.

- Moral or ethical practice transcends the different and competing sets of ethical principles used in the health and social care fields.

- Ethical practice in medicine is based on autonomy, beneficence, non-maleficence and justice. Most people are guided by respect for autonomy.

- The approach leaves 'scope' for how the four principles are applied.

- The 'four principles' approach developed within the context of liberal democracy (which favoured individual freedom).

- In the present-day context, intervention can be seen as empowering (the social inclusion view) or as undermining (the disability rights perspective).

- The British Idealists saw freedom in terms of social relationships with, and social obligations to, other people. They were part of T. H. Green's 'new' liberalism, which favoured social reform.

- Social care is a 'moral activity', based on notions of equality, supporting, advocating for and equalising people who are disadvantaged.

- There are ethical dilemmas about whether and when to intervene in people's lives, and when support becomes control.

10.3   Managing conflicting moral demands

There is a wide range of contexts in which social care managers have to manage competing, as well as absolute, moral demands. Moral dilemmas can arise when obligations to employers conflict with obligations to service users. Whistleblowing in an organisation is an example of such a conflict. Other moral dilemmas involve managers having to weigh up the risk of harm to the individual, set alongside harm to the general public, within a context of possible risk to other people. However, one of the most pressing of the potential moral dilemmas facing managers in social care is the issue of how resources are to be distributed. This moral issue is explored further in this section.

Exploring the concept of 'need'

The emphasis here is on how – and when – to respond to people who are, for whatever reason, 'in need'. The issue of needs is important for two reasons. The first is that the idea of meeting someone's needs provides a possible justification for intervening in their lives, perhaps even in some circumstances against their wishes. The second reason is that recent legal cases have discussed how the idea of needs arises in the context of the statutory duties of social services.

The starting point, however, is to address a more fundamental question. What do we mean when we say that we *need* something? It could be argued that needs have no substance as moral entities. They may be seen as having merely rhetorical force, as though the use of the term 'need' were a way of just clinching an argument, rather than making a real moral claim. This can be seen in such statements as 'I need a swimming pool in my back garden' or 'I need a holiday in the Caribbean'. It may well be true that the word 'need' is used in this type of context only as a way of seeking to add force to a wish or demand. However, this does not mean that needs cannot be given a more substantive basis, in at least some cases. The difficulty comes in trying to separate 'genuine' needs claims from attempts to bolster other types of claim. Various attempts have been made to analyse what needs claims involve but most focus on the idea of needs being instrumental in nature (see Brock, 1998). Many commentators suggest the following as a framework for thinking about needs:

A needs *X* in order to *G*, where *A* is an agent, *X* is the thing needed, and *G* is a goal or a purpose.

This analysis is true of non-moral types of need as well as moral ones. For example, we can substitute 'Pat needs a nutcracker in order to crack nuts' for the far more basic 'Pat needs food in order to survive'. This point leads to two contrasting accounts of 'needs'. An *objective* account argues that we can distinguish 'morally interesting' needs (or needs linked to the idea of universal goals) from relatively trivial means–end activities. According to this view, people (generally) have survival as a goal but they do not all want to crack nuts. In addition, needs are often linked to the idea of avoiding harm. The idea here is that if needs are not satisfied, serious harm of some objective kind will result: that is, harm to some important human interest (Feinberg, 1973, 1984, 1986).

In contrast, the *constructivist* view of needs is that they are created or constructed at a point in time and in particular circumstances. They are recognised as legitimate by the relevant society within which the claim is made. According to the constructivist view, there are no objective needs linked to such a thing as harm unless, of course, the relevant society has chosen to sanction this correlation. The two contrasting approaches to needs are now explored further.

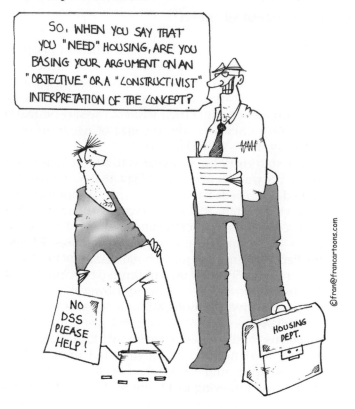

The objective view of needs

This view argues that we can separate the morally interesting uses of the concept 'need' from the trivial by appealing to a distinction between needs and desires. The idea is that 'I may *desire* a swimming pool or holiday but I don't really *need* one'. The argument here is that where needs and desires conflict, or where only one or the other can be satisfied, the need takes priority. Desires and needs are distinguishable and have different types of moral claim on us. A relevant difference between the two types of claim might be the degree of authority the claimant has in such cases. For example, it could be argued that, when judging desires, the person having the desire is the best judge of that state but this is not necessarily so in the case of needs. Needs can be judged just as well, if not better, by someone other than the person directly affected. This contrast is nicely illustrated by Scanlon's example (written before equality was an issue), illustrating the different moral claims that might be made on us in responding to a need and a desire:

> The fact that someone would be willing to forgo a decent diet in order to build a monument to his god does not mean that his claim on others for aid in his project has the same strength as a claim for aid in obtaining enough to eat (even assuming that the sacrifices required of others would be the same).
>
> (Scanlon, 1975, pp. 659–60)

The idea here is that needs can be given some substance independently of whether they are in fact desired as a priority by the person concerned.

Different advocates of the objective conception of needs produce different lists of the needs required to avoid certain types of harm. However, they usually include items such as food, shelter, clothing and health: for example, Maslow's 'hierarchy of needs' (Maslow, 1970). These are precisely the types of issue that will be of direct concern to people working in the area of social care. An appeal is most often made to the idea of a set of 'real' or 'basic' needs, which are universal requirements or necessary conditions for being an agent: that is, having the capacity to pursue any ends. The idea is that such needs are of the type that is *necessary* to people, whatever they actually *want* to do. It is evident how this account of needs might be related to a rich and substantive account of human nature that argues there are certain biological, psychological and socially necessary components to human agency, health and wellbeing.

Again, it is possible to contrast needs and desires. If a desire is not satisfied, no serious harm results, apart from the frustration of having that desire. Desires depend on the way in which individuals perceive the world and there is a sense in which they are incorrigible. However, needs are dependent on facts about the world, including the nature of human beings; they are not dependent on the way in which the world is perceived. In fact, people can be mistaken about what their needs actually are. For instance, to quote a much-used example, a diabetic person might *desire* sugary foods but *needs* insulin. According to this view, needs are independent of people's knowledge of them: even before the action of insulin was understood, and artificial forms were available, it was still true that people with diabetes needed insulin (Doyal and Gough, 1991).

The constructivist view of needs

In opposition to the objective account of needs, some writers have argued that needs are 'socially constructed'. The central claim of this view is that needs are dependent on the prevailing social conditions. This applies in several respects. For example, it is argued that needs come into existence

only where there are resources to meet them. It is also argued that needs
are recognised as such only if they are considered to be basic in the
relevant sense by a particular society. An advocate of such a view is Langan
(1998), who argues that an 'individual can only identify a need for
something when the provision exists' (p. 5). For example, an individual
can claim 'I need a hip replacement' but this is only a genuine need when
the hip can be replaced. Langan goes on to argue that:

> Furthermore, an individual's expression of need is likely to be qualified
> by their judgement of whether or not their demand to have this need
> met would be considered legitimate by the appropriate welfare profes-
> sionals or authorities.
>
> (Langan, 1998, p. 6)

Taking this view, the claim 'I need a car', for example, will only have force
if the person making such a statement expects to have the demand met.
Thus, it can be argued, no morally relevant contrast can be drawn between
needs and desires, and claims based on 'needs' are just the ones that
people choose to respond to. The view taken on this quite theoretical issue
makes a practical difference when considering a real situation – in the next
case, a legal judgment.

The leading legal case about resource allocation for social services went
all the way to the House of Lords. This case was *R. v. Gloucestershire County
Council and Another, ex. P. Barry* [1997] 2 All ER 1. It is important because it
laid down the law about the obligations that social services departments
have in response to the assessed needs of individuals requiring care.
Therefore, it is directly applicable to such decisions in the field of social
care. The case is particularly interesting because the House of Lords'
majority judgment was the exact opposite of the Court of Appeal's prior
judgment on the case. The House of Lords was broadly in favour of a
constructivist view of needs, while the Court of Appeal favoured an
objective account.

The House of Lords held, in the Barry case, that needs under the
relevant legislation are to be determined in relation to the resources
available and suggested that the relevant social services department
should do this. This means where a social services department does not
have the resources to fund a particular service, it is not obliged to provide
it. This applies even in a situation where a person has been assessed as
needing the service, and where the relevant statute places an absolute
obligation on the local authority to provide it.

If the House of Lords had taken an objective view of needs, rather than
seeing them as being socially constructed (as the Court of Appeal did in
the same case), the relevant social services department could not have
pleaded poverty. Instead, it would have been required to meet Barry's
assessed needs. It can be argued that the House of Lords was just making a
practical judgment to reflect the fact that resources are limited. However,
it is interesting that this judgment is based on taking a particular view

within the context of a theoretical disagreement about the nature of needs. Defending an objective account of needs would be one way of protecting service users' interests within the social care context.

Working as a morally active manager

The objective view associates needs with the idea of harm. This can be linked back to the earlier discussion of Green's idea of the state's obligation to ensure that each individual is provided with the minimum necessary to guarantee that they can function as a full citizen. According to this view, where needs exist, there is a moral duty to try to meet them. In the context of social care, this suggests an obligation on frontline managers to be morally active in working towards this end.

Typically, however, social care managers have to contend with the pressure of limited resources. Still, it is important to consider people's needs independently of the legal and financial context as far as possible. Although a manager has responsibility for resources and spending, nevertheless an ethical – or a morally active – approach is to defend core or basic needs. Such a position is morally right as a response to people in need. What does this mean in practice? Example 10.2 illustrates the real-life complexity of assessing and responding to needs.

> ### EXAMPLE 10.2 Harriet
>
> My mum, Harriet, is 84. She lives by herself in a ground-floor flat which, over the last 14 years, has been just right. It isn't too big, it has a small garden, and it has pull alarms in the living-room, sitting-room and bathroom which connect to a service called 'Reallycare'.
>
> Since a serious illness two years ago, Harriet has had a lot of support services as her health has deteriorated. For instance, she has a morning call to help with breakfast, and an evening one to help her prepare for the night. Someone calls once a week to do her shopping and a nurse calls one evening to assist with bathing and dressing. There is also the gardener, the cleaner (privately arranged, who also does the washing), the library lady, the chiropodist and the hairdresser! A social worker calls about every three months to talk about levels of care and billing. This level of support has become more or less permanent. Occasionally, a teatime call is added when things are bad and stopped when things seem better.
>
> The local authority agreed to fund these services. However, last year the funding from central government was cut and the authority is looking to make savings in all departments. They even suggested the withdrawal of Harriet's services altogether. This is not likely to happen this year. However, it all worries Harriet, and with good reason. The billing system is complex and is done quarterly. She still expects a monthly bill and when there isn't

one she frets about being overdrawn. Even though my brother, Tom, and I reassure her, Harriet finds the system confusing and is often on the point of cancelling her services. She says it costs too much, especially on the day the bill arrives – it looks alarming.

This is all very well, except that I live 70 miles away, Tom is 20 miles away, and every so often the co-ordination goes awry. All the individual carers are on the whole kind and caring people, who are doing their best. The GP is very careful and considerate, and he listens. The home care services manager is very skilled and visits Harriet when I am there. She is unhurried, careful about checking things and treats my mum really respectfully. But it is a very fragile system and easily wrecked. There is a high staff turnover, few are qualified and often they are late or off sick. The social worker's role seems entirely administrative. It is rarely the same person twice, and they come to talk packages, benefits and bills. Occasionally there is a good spell when a more proactive social worker suggests day care or physiotherapy, or brings useful things such as a kettle-holder or a height-adjusted stick to enable Harriet to walk in the garden.

The senior manager seems very distant, concerned with budgets and the allocation of resources. The frontline managers are responsible for their various workers but nobody has an overview. No one actually manages the whole set-up. It is called 'inter-agency work' and it has a life of its own. It never seems to connect unless I do the networking!

What are the needs in Harriet's situation? What is the role of the morally active manager? According to the objective account of needs, the primary issue is ensuring that Harriet is given the health and social care that will provide the basis for her to function as an independent and truly free individual. Many of the interventions that are likely to be appropriate are of the type that will support her in managing her everyday life at home – with as much respect for her dignity and autonomy as possible. However, the main practical issue for the manager in such a case will probably be how to establish coherence in Harriet's overall care 'package', given the fragmented nature of services offered by the various agencies involved in her care, especially as they cover the private, voluntary and statutory spectrum.

The other area to consider is the *morally right* way to respond to these needs. There are at least two levels of response. At one level, the worker or practitioner is in a good position to listen to Harriet and her daughter, and to engage with them to meet her needs. However, there are many health and social care workers involved, so a *morally active manager* in this instance is one who is prepared to work across agencies, networking, brokering and co-ordinating services. Above all, a morally active manager would aim to find out the objective and real needs of Harriet and her family, and to work with staff to respond in the most effective way possible in this situation.

> **Key points**
>
> - Needs are different from wishes or desires.
>
> - An objective view of needs sees them as universal human requirements.
>
> - A constructivist view of needs relates them to a particular society at a point in time.
>
> - A morally active manager considers and responds to people's needs.
>
> - The consideration of needs occurs within a social, legal and financial context.
>
> - A moral response takes into account the views of the people most centrally involved.

10.4 Frameworks for moral management

Clearly, it is impossible to ignore the real-life context in which social care managers make their operational decisions. However, there is more to this context than the tensions and dilemmas already discussed. There has been an extraordinary increase in the degree of formal regulation of welfare practices in recent years (see, for example, Parton, 1998, 2000). This can be attributed to the increasing risk-averse nature of modern social life and the demystification (often through well-publicised failures) of professional knowledge. This form of managerialism has produced an increasingly complex web of 'best practice' guidance and formal regulations.

The UK now has four social care councils, each with codes of conduct and practice for social care workers. In England, for example, the General Social Care Council's Code of Practice states that social care workers must:

- Safeguard and promote the interests of service users and carers.
- Strive to maintain the trust and confidence of service users.
- Respect the independence of service users and protect them as far as possible from danger or harm.
- Balance the rights of service users and carers with the interests of society.
- Take responsibility for their practice and learning.
- Justify public trust and confidence in social care services.

(GSCC, 2002b)

In some ways, these regulations could be regarded in similar terms to professional codes of conduct of the sort already mentioned, in so far as they might lessen the actual or perceived scope for moral action by the practitioner and, in turn, the manager. As well as the more fundamental objections already raised specifically about codes of conduct, there are several practical problems that both codes of conduct and other forms of external regulation raise.

The first is a practical objection, in the sense that members of many professions with codes and/or complex forms of external regulation clearly do not know that they have them, or are ill-informed about them, or choose to ignore them in practice. The second problem is that it is not clear whether external professional regulation is the best way of generating ethical conduct (see Dawson, 1994). Such an approach seems to work with a model that assumes a set of principles or a practice guide can meaningfully capture the complexity of ethical decision making. This can be contested on the grounds that most codes and forms of regulation are sketchy and are an attempt to offer a broad outline of only some of the relevant issues. Practitioners and managers will always have to 'fill in' the relevant details and context. The alternative is to have highly detailed codes or regulations that attempt to cover all the features of real life, which is clearly impossible.

The third problem is that regulation and bureaucracy can lead to defensive practice. This means an over-reliance on rules, fulfilling duties defined by the agency and sticking to responsibilities laid down by law (Banks, 2001). This approach is one of meeting obligations – and 'covering one's back' – rather than enabling managers to take actions that are *morally right* (Banks, 2001, p. 157). An alternative model is that of the morally active manager. Such an individual, while perhaps knowing the code for their relevant profession or being familiar with received wisdom on what constitutes best practice, is not necessarily bound by it. They make an ethical judgement informed by all the relevant factors and are willing to accept responsibility for that assessment because it is *their* decision.

What guides ethical decision making? The morally active manager is likely to be guided by the following factors.

- *Ethical awareness*: knowing about ethical dilemmas and conflicts, and how they arise.
- *Values*: being aware of their values and how to stay true to them.
- *Reflexivity*: having the capacity to reflect on their practice and to learn from it.
- *Appreciation of risks*: daring to take risks and being prepared to accept blame.
- *Practice wisdom*: knowledge and experience of good practice in health and social care and how to support it in others.

How does this translate into good practice? A manager of a children's service describes how she works in an ethically sound way, drawing on best practice as she sees it (as a practice-led manager):

I want to go to bed at night with my hand on my heart, saying and feeling that I've done absolutely everything I can to make sure children can stay with their families, if that's in the child's best interests. But equally if it's not in the child's best interests, it's important to make a sound judgement, based on good evidence, and be able to justify the decision. The decision has to be right both now and in the future when the 18-year-old comes back to ask why you did what you did.

(Manager consultations)

Key points

- There is a proliferation of guidance, guidelines, regulatory standards and codes of conduct in health and social care, which is not conducive to developing sound ethical practice in an already complex field.

- Increasing regulation and bureaucracy can lead to risk avoidance and defensive practice.

- The morally active manager is aware of regulations and guidance but can draw on principles and values in order to act in an ethically principled way.

10.5   Conclusion

The relevant ethical issues relating to social care management are manifold and complex. In this chapter we touched on some relevant background issues and gave a few examples of the types of moral issue that might arise for social care managers. We argued that, while lists of moral claims such as the 'four principles' can make some sort of contribution to ethical decision making, they are not without their own problems. Unlike the 'four principles' approach, therefore, we argued for an approach to ethical issues in social care that takes account of the reality of people's lives and the degree of their social exclusion, as well as the wider social and community context.

In contrast to the increasing reliance on external forms of regulation in the social care context (such as guidelines, the sponsorship of best practice, and codes of professional conduct), we argued in favour of the morally active manager. Such an individual has the personal resources to make ethically literate decisions and to take responsibility for their own actions within the social context that surrounds them. In the framework of management this might mean that, where appropriate, managers may well come into conflict with their staff and their employers. Being a morally active manager is not necessarily going to be the route to popularity but it should be a means of ensuring that individual managers can defend their own actions, which will come from critical reflection on the decision to be made.

The idea of the morally active manager, as outlined in this chapter, is a return to the roots of social casework with an emphasis on promoting the conditions for true equality. The aim of such a manager is to be an active citizen in a community of citizens, protecting and promoting the active citizenship of other people.

Chapter 11
Managing for outcomes

Mike Pinnock and Brian Dimmock

11.1   Introduction

How can managers know whether their efforts have made any difference to anyone? When frontline managers first step back from doing a service delivery job they no longer have the immediate feedback from service users that they were used to. An outcome-focused approach can help managers to direct and shape action with greater confidence and certainty. At their simplest, outcomes relate to the impact, effect or consequence of a particular service or intervention over a specific period of time (Utting *et al.*, 2001). A focus on outcomes is not simply about trying to establish whether or not a service has helped service users (outcomes downstream). They are also important in developing a dialogue with existing and potential service users in order to understand what sort of outcomes people want in the first place and how they can be achieved (outcomes upstream).

Managers learn quickly that no service is an island. Good outcomes can only be consistently produced when frontline staff are supported by good organisational arrangements. High levels of interdependence exist both within and between agencies. Good outcomes are rarely achieved by a single team or service, or a single department. Managers should see themselves as 'co-producers of outcomes' (Pinnock and Garnett, 2002), each making a contribution to the achievement of an overall result. In the field of care services this is likely to involve statutory, voluntary and private sector organisations working together with service users.

It can of course be argued that individual examples of good service delivery survive despite management weaknesses and unsupportive organisational arrangements. However, 'islands' of excellence cannot be sustained in the long run and users of services need consistently high standards wherever they live. In an effort to raise standards across the whole of the UK, care services are coming under increasing regulation through the use of care standards (Department of Health, 2002b; Scottish Executive, 2001b). This includes requirements that services in care homes, children's homes, domiciliary agencies, family centres, voluntary and independent adoption and fostering agencies, and day centres meet the standards laid down by the National Care Standards Commission (NCSC). These standards include statements about outcomes.

The aims of this chapter are to:

- explain what outcomes are
- show the use of outcomes at different 'service levels'
- put outcomes into a context of performance management
- examine the pros and cons of their use in planning and shaping services
- explore how to define and evaluate outcomes.

11.2 Outcome-focused management

What are outcomes?

For Nocon and Qureshi (1996) an outcome is defined simply as 'the impact, effect or consequence of a service or policy' (p. 7). However, outcomes involve more than simply assessing the effect of what has already taken place. They are also used to define what people want to see happen in the future. The word 'outcome' is now regularly used as a shorthand for objectives that set out 'desired' or 'hoped for' results: in other words, the 'desired end states' (Martin and Kettner, 1996) that someone hopes to achieve through a care plan, a service plan, an inter-agency strategy or even a national policy.

Chapter 1 introduced the idea of practice-led management based on promoting social inclusion and choice, improving the quality of life and safeguarding people. Management based on outcomes builds on this to show what practice should be aiming to achieve in specific services, and how outcomes can be defined and their achievement evaluated. This is how Bronwyn, a manager of a voluntary organisation providing specialist services for abused children and their families, describes what outcomes mean to her:

> Most of how we measure and decide what our outcomes are going to be is based on the work that we do with our service users, and finding out from them what they want from the work. The agency itself obviously has its own value base, and its own objectives and aims, and they will expect every project to meet these. In deciding on the outcomes for our work we have to make sure they are in line with what the agency is looking for. And then we have to listen to our service users when they say what helped and what wasn't helpful. Then you come, at the end of the day, to a set of outcomes that try to encompass both.

> If you have a service level agreement with another agency, they will say, 'well with this amount of money we're giving you, we expect you to achieve this amount of work'. So that's a different sort of outcome. So, it's a mixture of what service users tell us they want, what we as a project feel we'd like to achieve, what the agency are telling us, and what other agencies also require.

> (Manager consultations)

This manager sees her role as bringing organisational aims and objectives into line with the expressed wishes of service users and agreement with other agencies to come up with outcomes that encompass all three. However, it is not just service-providing organisations and service users that are in the business of defining outcomes. Box 11.1 lists the outcomes defined by the NCSC for the management and administration of care homes for older people. This is just one set of outcomes required for this type of care home (the others include choice of home, health and personal care, daily life and social activities, complaints and protection, environment and staffing).

BOX 11.1 Outcomes for the management and administration of care homes

1 Day-to-day operations

Outcome: Service users live in a home which is run and managed by a person who is fit to be in charge, of good character and able to discharge his or her responsibilities fully.

2 Ethos

Outcome: Service users benefit from the ethos, leadership and management approach of the home.

3 Quality assurance

Outcome: The home is run in the best interests of service users.

4 Financial procedures

Outcome: service users are safeguarded by the accounting and financial procedures of the home.

5 Service users' money

Outcome: Service users' financial interests are safeguarded.

6 Staff supervision

Outcome: Staff are properly supervised.

7 Record keeping

Outcome: Service users' rights and best interests are safeguarded by the home's record-keeping policies and procedures.

8 Safe working practices

Outcome: The health, safety and welfare of service users and staff are promoted and protected.

(Source: adapted from Department of Health, 2002b, pp. 35–42)

This example of an outcome-driven approach to setting standards may seem like stating the obvious at first sight, but these statements can have a powerful impact. Take for example the third one in the list, 'The home is run in the best interests of service users'. Demonstrating that this outcome is being achieved may be far from easy. If the home is privately owned, the managers have to demonstrate that it is not being run in the best interests of the owner or shareholders to the detriment of the best interests of the residents. If it is run by a charity, are the charitable objectives compatible with the best interests of the residents? For example, the charitable objectives might include ideas about religious observance that might not be a priority if residents were consulted. Finally, if the home is run by a local authority, can managers demonstrate that changes of policy resulting from cost cuts are implemented in a way that is driven by residents' best interests?

It is useful to think about outcomes working at three interactive levels:

1   an individual level
2   a service level
3   a strategic level.

The outcomes at each of these three levels should be recursive – that is, we should expect to see them represented at each level of planning, nestling inside each other rather like Russian dolls. How do these levels apply to an example from Box 11.1? The fifth outcome in the list, 'Service users' financial interests are safeguarded', is fairly clear at the level of the individual resident, but less immediately obvious at the other levels. At a service level, is there a policy which ensures that residents' financial interests are reviewed, or is it assumed that they will remain unchanged? In the case of a privately run home that charges above average rates, residents' income from savings and pensions often becomes less than they need. Does the home have a policy to plan ahead with residents? At a strategic level, do all the services that may impact on the financial interests of residents work together? For example, when plans are being made to use local residential homes as part of a policy to reduce 'bed blocking' in hospitals by older people awaiting discharge (intermediate care), is the impact on the financial interests of potential residents a factor? Or is the policy just focused on emptying beds whatever the impact may be on the financial interests of each individual?

Interestingly, the standard that applies to the outcomes in Box 11.1 above (Standard 35, Department of Health, 2002c) requires registered managers of care homes to ensure that service users control their own money. To what extent do strategic plans for services for older people take account of this? Clearly, this will depend on how narrowly the term 'financial interests' is defined. Does it simply mean personal allowances when a person is already resident, or does strategic planning consider 'safeguarding' financial interests when struggling to deal with blocked hospital beds and inadequate community-based care services?

The national context – improving the quality of services

Since the 1980s the approach to measuring public sector performance has started to shift away from examining inputs and outputs (the amount of money spent on a given activity and the number of units of services it produces) towards effectiveness and results. Previously, measuring what outputs were achieved by spending a certain amount of public or charitable funds used criteria defined 'from above', such as the number of meals on wheels delivered, hours of home care input, or the number of chiropody appointments. In the care sector this shift is illustrated by the changes in emphasis in the Department of Health's annual statistical returns to support initiatives such as Quality Protects (Box 11.2).

BOX 11.2 Quality Protects

Quality Protects was launched in September 1998 to deliver effective protection, better quality care and improved life chances for disadvantaged children and young people. The key elements of the Quality Protects programme are:

- new national Government objectives for children's services which set out clear outcomes for children, and in some instances give precise targets to be achieved

- an important role for local councillors in delivering the programme and ensuring, as the corporate parents of children looked after by local authorities, that they receive services of the highest quality

- an annual evaluation of councils' Quality Protects Management Action Plans, which set out how they intend to improve their services

- partnership between and within central and local government and with the health service and the voluntary sector

- government funding of £885m over five years towards a new children's service grant.

(Source: adapted from Department of Health, 2002d)

As a result of the Quality Protects initiative, the Department of Health is now able to collect and report data on, for example, the educational attainments of looked-after children. As a result of this shift, it is becoming possible to see a better balance between data that relate to cost and activity and data that say something about outcomes.

Some commentators see this increasing emphasis on outcome measurement as evidence of the unwelcome intrusion of managerialism and performance measurement into the provision of care services (see, for example, Wilson, 1998). It is certainly the case that the purpose of initiatives such as Best Value are recognisable within the global movement towards what Hood (1991) has defined as 'new public management'. However, in our view it would be wrong to dismiss the growing concern with outcomes as just a 'management thing'. As Sheldon and Chilvers (2000) observe, the study of effectiveness and 'what works' is as 'old as social work itself' (p. 1). In this sense, initiatives such as Best Value can be seen as both a threat and an opportunity. If these reviews provide a real opportunity for staff to work with service users and their advocates to develop better services, they can be a force for good.

However, if you are beginning to feel unclear about how the concepts of 'quality' and 'outcomes' fit together, you are not alone. This is how Bronwyn struggles with this potential confusion:

> Quality means to me delivering a service that is meaningful. It isn't about looking at bits of paper and thinking, that's the goal of this project, we have to achieve it come hell or high water. Not if it's not what our service users actually want. I find at times that there are tensions for us as a project because it's government led; they're looking all the time at output, output, output. What are your outcomes, how are you measuring them, how are you doing this and how are you doing that? At the end of the day, if we've got a parent and a child sitting in front of us who are feeling very stuck, and I'm thinking about how we are measuring outcomes, that for me just goes out of the window. I have to make sure my workers are there, alongside, doing what they can to help that family move on, and the goals might change, and the outcomes might change. I can translate all that on to a piece of paper, but work sometimes takes an awful lot longer than people first envisage and that for me is quality. Sadly, with the funding the way it is at the moment, you sometimes only get one shot at it. You are recognising that this family could do with a year of work and all you get is two months. And where's the quality in that? I find it very frustrating, incredibly so.
>
> (Manager consultations)

The benefits

It is not uncommon for people to get excited by the idea of outcomes. This excitement arises not just from a desire to see where they have been so much as from the relief of knowing where they are supposed to be going: in other words, the sense of purpose and direction that clear outcomes give. As Osborne and Gaebler (1993) have pointed out, if we cannot define success, how do we know that we are not rewarding failure?

Perhaps the most important benefit of focusing on outcomes is that this draws on the knowledge and skill of everyone involved within an organisation and across organisations, including service users, frontline staff, support staff and community representatives. From the perspective of service users, outcomes move on from the passive language of needs and services defined by professionals towards the positive language of results defined by everyone involved. Of course, achieving consensus about outcomes requires great skill and compromise, and a willingness to confront constraints as well as possibilities. Inevitably, the issue of resources will have to be considered as part of the process of defining outcomes. As Schorr observes:

> Attention to results forces the question of whether outcome expectations must be scaled down, or interventions and investments scaled up to achieve their intended purpose.
>
> (Schorr quoted in Annie E. Casey Foundation, 1995)

If realistic outcomes can be defined and agreed, planning can focus on giving each member of an organisation an opportunity to exercise their judgement in finding ways of achieving success. The tendency for managers to try to control complex processes from above removes the opportunities that staff and service users have to feel truly engaged in their part of the attempt to improve services. It is demotivating and deskilling for staff and service users alike. This tendency increases where outcomes are not clear and managers focus more on 'means' than 'ends'. Friedman (2001) points out that disputes between different stakeholders are often about means rather than ends. He comments, 'let's at least get the ends agreed and then we can have a sensible discussion about how best to achieve them'.

It is accepted that the language of performance measurement and the values implicit in 'business models' do not necessarily motivate or attract many people involved in care provision. However, defining purpose in terms of benefits to service users allows staff to make the link between their own personal and professional values and the outcomes that agencies are seeking to achieve. Staff other than those directly involved in service delivery, for example in finance teams, reception areas, information management and human resources, can be clearer about how they can innovate to contribute to achieving outcomes.

Once outcomes are clear, each activity that is undertaken by an organisation can be reviewed in terms of the contribution it makes (or fails to make) to success. When results are the focus, the interdependences that exist between and within organisations are swiftly exposed. For example, in order for a young person with a disability to make a successful transition into adulthood, a number of agencies need to 'get their bit right'. Failure by one agency can jeopardise the whole plan. The process of developing and agreeing these outcomes can in itself have a powerfully integrating effect on newly established services.

Finally, 'what works' is not just about defining outcomes, it is also a matter of the design of research and evaluation and using this to examine the extent to which outcomes have been achieved and what has contributed to success or failure.

Outcomes at work

In the past staff have been encouraged to value uniformity in service provision. Not only is uniformity cheaper to produce, it can also be justified on the grounds that it suggests people are treated fairly. However, services can be, at one and the same time, fair and poor quality. Example 11.1, from an imaginary residential home, illustrates this.

> ### EXAMPLE 11.1 Laundering socks
>
> Under the previous management regime, there was a simple policy on socks – each resident was required to wear black ones. Socks were washed each Monday. End of problem. Costs were reduced by bulk-buying black, stretch-fit socks (the economy criterion). One wash each week in an industrial washing machine was sufficient. Valuable staff time was saved by not having to sort socks into colour washes, or sew name tags, or make 'sock bunnies' and all the rest of those complex sock-drawer management tasks (the efficiency criterion). Everyone got the same quality of clean socks delivered to their room regardless of class, religion, ethnicity, age, disability or gender (the equity criterion).
>
> But of course not everyone wants to wear stretch-fit black socks – particularly if those socks have a history!
>
> The new management recognises that residents wish to adorn their feet (or not) in ways that please them. They buy their own socks with their own money and when they want them washed they, or their carers, can use a normal domestic-scale washer in the laundry room/kitchen that they share with four other people. Socks are placed in mesh bags before they go in the washer so that they never need become estranged. People feel in control of their footwear, which in turn leads to a feeling of greater wellbeing (effectiveness).

What this imaginary example shows is that it is possible to fail with great efficiency and equality. Outcome-focused managers are no longer concerned with 'doing things right' (conforming to procedures); rather, they are concerned with 'doing the right thing' in order to achieve desired outcomes.

Key points

- Outcomes are used to look at what has been achieved in the past and what is desired for the future.

- The process of defining outcomes should be practice-led with meaningful involvement of all stakeholders.

- External standard-setting bodies are increasingly involved in defining broad outcomes for care services.

- Outcomes work at three interactive levels: the individual level, the service level and the strategic level.

- Achieving consensus about outcomes requires considerable skill on the part of managers.

- Outcomes must be related to the resources required to achieve them.

- Outcomes transcend simple measures of efficiency and incorporate values.

11.3   Why measure outcomes?

Evidence suggests that many organisations focus on data about controlling inputs (budgets, staffing, and so on) and recording outputs (units of service produced) (Ward *et al.*, 1998). To move to a focus on measuring outcomes requires the involvement of service users, their advocates and carers. The routine monitoring and evaluation of outcomes has a number of recognised advantages over systems that measure inputs and outputs.

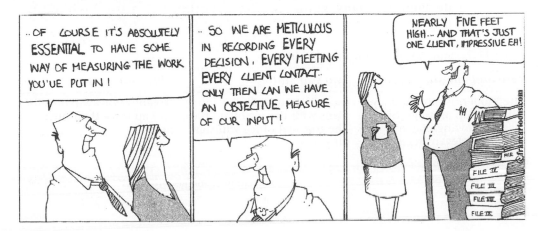

The first and perhaps most important benefit from asking service users and other stakeholders about what outcomes they want, or the extent to which agreed outcomes have been achieved, is that people value 'having a say' (Qureshi *et al.*, 1998, p. 11). Less than perfect progress towards achieving outcomes is more likely to be tolerated if the service is at least trying to go in an agreed direction. Similarly, being told that the service you depend on is achieving its goals is really upsetting if they are not goals that actually provide you with what you want.

Achieving outcomes is unlikely to be a one-off event, and will require good monitoring and evaluation if adjustments are to be made over time. For example, a care service might have an outcome that declares that 'people are involved in decisions that affect their lives'. One of the agreed measures of progress towards this outcome might be attendance at user group meetings and reviews. If attendance was poor, managers would want to find out why and see how the meetings could be improved. Commissioning an external organisation to undertake a user-led review of these meetings could do this. Such a review might show that users see attending personal reviews and having an effective voice there as more important than group meetings. This might help managers to prioritise preparing for reviews rather than changing the way group meetings function. They may decide to have fewer group meetings and look for other ways of getting feedback (perhaps through a survey).

One of the promises constantly being held out to public care services is that effectively managed services based on agreed outcomes will lead to a 'lighter touch' in terms of public inspection and audit, and additional funding. This approach is included in the NHS Plan (Department of Health, 2001f) and the Personal Social Services Performance Fund. This is a controversial area of government policy but one that appears to be here to stay for the foreseeable future. The aim is to encourage joint working between local authorities, health authorities, primary care groups and primary care trusts through incentive payments. A 'star rating' system is used by the Modernisation Agency for the NHS, with greater freedoms for developing plans going to those authorities with high ratings (see Table 11.1).

Table 11.1   **Star ratings for joint working**

Zero and one star status	*Two star status*	*Three star status*
The Modernisation Agency will develop and sign off plans following dialogue with the relevant regional office	Organisations will develop plans with the regional office. The regional office will sign off plans	Organisations will develop and approve their own plans

(Source: adapted from NHS, 2001, para. 6.1)

In this example the degree of autonomy of any agency coming within the jurisdiction of the Performance Fund depends on the assessment of its performance against an agreed set of outcomes. If the organisation has two star status or above it effectively assesses its own performance and sets its own milestones using a set of guidelines. Its performance is published and this is monitored by the body in charge (in this case the Modernisation Agency for the NHS). The scheme is then subject to overall audit by an external organisation.

This approach is coupled with a move towards 'evidence-based practice/management/services' through organisations such as the Social Care Institute for Excellence (SCIE). SCIE will bring information about 'what works' and good practice to the attention of care providers. However, it will also depend on collating information from organisations through routine monitoring and evaluation. Thus, local work on outcomes can also contribute to shaping and directing the future research agenda both locally and nationally.

The routine publication of progress towards outcomes can strengthen public and professional accountability. Reports need to be tailored to suit the needs of different audiences, and some services now routinely report outcomes to service users, their carers and the general public. At the same time government is gathering and publishing reports on progress towards outcomes defined through such frameworks as the NHS Plan and is also moving towards 'league tables' and 'naming and shaming' policies. Again, this is a controversial approach to the measurement of outcomes. It could be argued that there is a tendency for the media to focus too much on the bad news and not enough on the good, and that this is reinforced by the use of league tables and similar forms of reporting on standards.

Key points

- Involving service users in defining outcomes is valuable in its own right.

- Achieving outcomes is a process, not a one-off event.

- The successful use of outcomes involves continuous review and adjustment.

- Government is making increasing use of targets as a measure of the achievement of outcomes.

- The achievement of outcomes is being linked to degrees of autonomy for services.

- Evidence-based practice and outcome-focused or practice-led management are linked through a focus on 'what works'.

- Defining clear outcomes and providing clear results can lead to greater public support for services.

11.4   Outcome-focused planning

Bringing purpose and meaning to the routine work of their staff is one of the key roles of managers. However, providing effective care services can be a complex activity. Often people respond to complexity by either denying its existence ('I don't see what the problem is ...') or retreating from it ('Can we keep it simple please ?' or 'Right, can we get back to reality ?'). Providing care services is often about travelling hopefully rather than arriving.

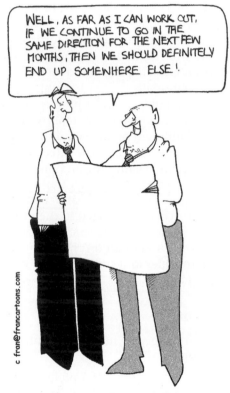

TRAVELLING HOPEFULLY

Even in language, the words people choose to try to share ideas about outcomes seem to get in the way of their understanding:

> It is said that the Inuit of Alaska have as many words to describe types of snow as the Bedouin of the Middle East have words to describe types of camels. Sadly, the English language has been less generous to those involved in the planning and study of social care. Words like assessment, need and outcome have become overloaded and overused to the point where their lack of precision has itself become an obstacle to advancing our understanding.
>
> (Pinnock and Garnett, 2002, p. 96)

We will now look at how the idea of outcomes can be applied to the three levels outlined in Section 11.2:

- the individual level
- the service level
- the strategic level.

Outcomes for individual service users

Where an agency anticipates a continuing involvement with a service user and/or their family, normally some sort of plan is formulated. For example, in learning disability services this may be part of a person-centred planning approach; in child care it may be a 'child in need' plan, a child protection plan or a care plan. In a service for people with mental health problems it might be a part of the care programme approach. Where necessary, separate plans would probably be agreed with carers.

In the past the objectives in these plans have tended to be defined in terms of service needs: for example, to continue to receive meals on wheels four times a week, or to remain in foster care, or to be visited by the outreach service twice a week. This concentration on services rather than outcomes creates a number of problems:

- Plans lack any sense of direction and purpose.
- Since the plan lacks any clear outcome, it is difficult to establish whether progress has been made.
- Service-led plans tend to encourage dependence on services because they do not recognise the resources and strengths of the recipients.
- Service providers have little incentive to bring about progress. In some cases, they may even have vested interests in maintaining evidence of a lack of change in order to justify the continuation of services.
- Service-led plans are often self-perpetuating and fail to consider other ways in which outcomes might be achieved.

In services for children and families the shift towards outcome-focused child care planning began in the mid-1980s through the early work of Roy Parker and his colleagues (Parker *et al.*, 1991). By the early 1990s this work had resulted in the Looking After Children (LAC) materials which included a predetermined framework requiring age-specific objectives across a range of dimensions such as health, education and family and social relationships. This framework provides a context for setting outcome-focused objectives with individual children and young people (Ward *et al.*, 1998).

In social care services for adults Nocon and Qureshi (1996) have developed outcome-focused frameworks for working with a range of adults, including older people and their carers, and people with disabilities and their carers. These frameworks have been developed through extensive consultation and testing with existing and prospective service users. Each framework defines the various outcome domains for different groups. An important feature of Nocon and Qureshi's work for the Social Policy Research Unit (SPRU) is the attention it gives to developing ways of using outcomes at a practice level. The frameworks are accompanied by a range of materials that are intended to help care management staff and service providers engage with the idea of outcome-focused care management practices.

Outcomes in shaping services

Good managers are constantly challenging their services to look for better ways of delivering outcomes. In order to realise the benefits of outcome-focused management they have to connect the conversations about outcomes that are being held at an individual level with the opportunities that exist for the development and improvements of services and practice as a whole. One way of doing this is by working with service users, their carers and staff to develop a clear 'statement of purpose'. An example of this approach is shown in Box 11.3.

BOX 11.3 Service outcomes for North Lincolnshire Children and Families Division

- Children develop and maintain secure and appropriate attachments.

- Children are safe.

- Children achieve their full potential.

- We respond to the needs of children quickly and fairly.

- Children and their carers are involved in making decisions that affect their lives.

- People working with children are given the resources they need to help bring better outcomes.

- The people of North Lincolnshire get value for money from children and family services.

(Source: adapted from North Lincolnshire Council, 2002)

Managing to create and sustain a culture that is constantly looking for ways of delivering better outcomes involves making changes, both big and small. This can be considered at two levels. First, small incremental changes can be made to matters that are within a manager's control and that can often be implemented at little or no cost. Service users and their carers will often be the source of ideas for these improvements. When a service has a mature and deeply held understanding of the outcomes it is trying to produce for service users, change becomes the natural disposition of the team. In teams where the outcomes are clear, change makes sense. Where outcomes are ill-defined or non-existent, change is meaningless and demotivating.

Second, there are bigger, more fundamental changes to the design and pattern of services. These changes are sometimes referred to as 'step changes'. Frontline managers are critical to the successful implementation of changes that lead to transformation of the service through new ways of bringing better results. Managers may find that incremental change only takes them so far before they hit the limitations or 'glass walls' of a particular service model of working. Transformational changes are the opportunity for them to break out of the limitations of certain ways of working.

Strategic planning

At this level, effectiveness can be defined as 'the degree to which the final outcomes of a service or policy match the original objectives for that service/policy' (The Open University, 1992, p. 24). This approach is a useful pointer to the development of broad-based plans across whole communities, often as part of, or to support, government initiatives.

So how would outcome-focused strategic objectives be distinguished from 'run-of-the-mill' objectives? There are no absolute 'rules' as to what does and what does not constitute an outcome. However, for the idea of outcomes to be of any value, they must be about the intended or actual effect that an activity has on the people who are meant to benefit from it. In general, they are better defined in positive terms, focusing on desired futures for individuals, groups and communities. They should also be specific in terms of the results to be achieved. Finally, they should encompass everyone who may benefit from the outcomes, not just those who might appear to be the immediate beneficiaries. For example, good outcomes for a particular community might also benefit those who provide services (because they are more likely to be clear about what they are trying to achieve). Society as a whole might benefit from a reduction in negative effects, such as a decrease in crime or unemployment.

> **Key points**
>
> - Greater precision in the use of language is needed if clear outcomes are to be defined.
>
> - Outcomes designed around existing services are of limited value.
>
> - There has been a move towards an outcome-focused approach to managing care services in both the adult and child care sectors.
>
> - Outcomes for individual service users need to relate to outcomes for the service as a whole (and vice versa).
>
> - Steps towards achieving outcomes can be through small, incremental changes as well as step changes.
>
> - Outcomes for individual services need to fit within broad strategic frameworks. In turn, evaluation of the progress in individual services needs to inform strategic frameworks.

11.5   Defining and evaluating outcomes

When monitoring progress towards outcomes at an operational/service level, Cheetham *et al.* (1992) distinguish between service-based outcomes and client-based outcomes. Client-based outcomes are the 'effects of a provision on its recipients', while service-based outcomes focus on the 'nature, extent and quality of what is provided' (p. 63). Knapp (1984) makes a similar distinction between what he calls 'intermediate' and 'final' outcomes. Intermediate outcomes are 'indicators of performance, service or activity' (p. 32) while final outcomes relate to 'changes in individual well-being compared with the levels of well-being in the absence of a caring intervention' (p. 31).

Cheetham *et al.* propose that service-based outcomes can be further subdivided into different types.

Service-based outcomes

Basic 'health check' measures can help managers understand whether or not the services for which they are responsible are getting the basics right. For example, an outcome sought for children who are being looked after by a local authority might be 'to maximise their life chances by making sure that they achieve their full educational potential'. The very least a manager would need to know in order to measure progress towards this outcome is whether or not children and young people were on a school or college roll or registered for a training scheme. If they were, it would be useful to know if they were actually attending. Similarly, one of the outcomes sought for people with a learning disability might be 'for people to live in valued communities'. One way of measuring this would be to look at how many friends or relationships they had with people outside the service, and how often they were involved in activities in the local community.

This level of detail moves managers into the realm of defining performance measures based on these broader outcomes. Nocon and Qureshi refer to measures of this type as 'destinational outcomes' (1996, p. 21). Although they are fairly limited and need to be supported by other measures, they can begin to reveal whether or not the right people are finding their way into the right services at the right time. In some cases these measures might specify compliance with regulatory or procedural rules (Moore *et al.*, 2000). For example, are children on the Child Protection Register visited regularly and do the reviews take place on time? Clearly, there is a danger that managers may satisfy themselves with measures of this type and look no further for evidence of effectiveness. Simply being in the right place at the right time does not mean that an outcome is being achieved. People with a learning disability may be living in the community, but they may also be living in run-down flats, on poor diets, and afraid to go out the front door. For this reason this class of outcome measure should be used as a starting point – as 'travelling hopefully rather than arriving'.

The achievement of expressed service/programme objectives

Not all progress towards achieving better outcomes can be charted through quantitative and qualitative data. For example, an agency could have an outcome 'to give service users control over decisions that affect their lives'. In order to advance this outcome, the agency might plan to extend a direct payments scheme, introduce a system to involve service users in the appointment of staff or set up a user-led review of arrangements for involving service users in planning. The successful introduction of these developments in themselves can be important measures of progress towards desired results. In these cases it may be useful for the agency to chart the accomplishment of milestones alongside other outcome measures. This style of outcome reporting can be used to track progress towards big, transformational or 'step' changes as well as small, incremental changes. As with the basic measures described above, only limited conclusions can be drawn from this sort of feedback. However, reporting progress in this way can usefully maintain the link between 'work in progress' and desired outcomes.

Quality of service measures

Since the late 1980s considerable attention has been given to developing ways of defining and measuring quality in care services. For the purposes of this chapter it is important that managers recognise the role that quality assurance indicators can play in helping them to understand effectiveness. Their intention should be to measure the extent to which those attributes that they know are valued by service users are actually present within the service. For example, they might have an outcome for an older person that says, 'older people will be helped to live independently in settings of their choice'. Good home care is going to be central to delivering this outcome. So how would they know what constitutes 'good home care'? Home care users consistently talk about how they value aspects such as flexibility around tasks, keeping the same home care assistant, reliability, and so on. If these are the things people say make the service work for them, clearly they are the aspects a service manager would want to monitor.

Service user-based outcomes

Service user-based outcomes are concerned with assessing the extent to which service users have benefited from a given intervention. The definition of final outcomes by Knapp (1984) raises the question of whether it is possible to establish with any certainty if the service had any effect without comparing the results of people receiving the service with a similar group of people who did not. This, of course, raises a number of ethical dilemmas associated with the use of randomised control trials in care settings (that is, trials of a service or an intervention where the effects on service users are compared with a control group of similar people who do not receive the service or intervention). These issues are currently the subject of much debate – a debate that will inevitably intensify as the focus on evidence-based interventions sharpens (Sheldon and Chilvers, 2000).

The idea of defining and assessing outcomes in the provision of care services is fraught with practical and conceptual difficulties. For the frontline manager, however, these are problems of research and, clearly, managers would not want to compromise the pursuit of a given outcome simply because no one has yet developed a satisfactory way of measuring it.

Similarly, there is a small but growing body of knowledge about what sort of outcomes service users want from services and what sort of services are likely to deliver them. In this sense, managers do not have to start from scratch every time they want to engage with the users of a service in producing a statement of purpose. However, there is a danger in relying on 'off the shelf' outcomes that can simply be installed in a service. In order to get a deeper understanding, agreement and ownership of the declared outcomes of a service, staff and users must be involved throughout. Nor is this a one-off exercise for a team 'away day'.

Next we consider some of the main issues that managers need to be aware of in defining and evaluating outcomes.

Defining outcomes

One of the key roles of managers is to develop and maintain clarity and consistency of purpose. Whether in the public, private or voluntary sector, this is a prerequisite of effectiveness. For example, Senge (1990) identifies 'shared vision' as one of his five key competences. Care-providing organisations have been criticised for failing to express their purpose in a way that can be readily understood by service users, their workforce and the general public. This is what is said in *Modernising Social Services*:

> Up to now, neither users, carers, the public, nor social services staff and managers have a clear idea which services are or should be provided, or what standards can reasonably be expected. There is no definition of what users can expect, nor any yardstick for judging how effective or successful social services are.
>
> (Department of Health, 1998a, p. 6)

As discussed in Chapter 3, since the 1980s there has been a move away from administrative approaches to the provision of care services to business management styles of work. One of the more visible manifestations of this shift has been the proliferation of organisational mission statements, vision statements and strap-lines that compete for space in agency publications, annual reports and letterheads. The clumsy style of many of these statements bears witness to the problem of defining the provision of care services in simple terms. Each caveat and conditional clause is a reminder of the complexity of a sector that combines public, private and voluntary organisations together in a bewildering number of permutations.

While the value of mission statements and the like might be questionable, managers should be able to define the purpose of the services they are responsible for in terms of the outcomes these services exist to produce. This should be a set of simple statements – perhaps no more than ten – written in plain language, such as:

'People will be involved in decisions that affect their lives'

'Carers should have lives of their own'

'People will live independently in settings of their choice'.

These statements are deceptively simple. In practice, working with staff and service users to produce such statements can be a difficult and sometimes frustrating process. In order to engage people who do not communicate in conventional ways, staff will need to develop new knowledge and skills. There is a danger that the temptation to 'speak for' others takes over. However, there are ways of avoiding this through the use of *advocacy programmes* (Department of Health, 1996). There is also a growing body of knowledge to help managers to develop effective ways of engaging service users and the wider community in defining outcomes (see, for example, Craig, 2001; Franklin and Madge, 2000; Fajerman *et al.*, 2000).

People's experiences of services in the past may have led them to hold very low expectations of what they can hope for from a service and this may limit their expectations. Similarly, they may not have positive examples to compare with their own services. People with learning disabilities and their carers will often spend their entire lives in contact with health, education and social care services of one form or another and they may be reluctant to make demands or express their dissatisfaction. Comparisons between public and commercial sector services are often misleading in this respect in that they overlook the fact that many users of public sector services do not have the 'power of exit' – in other words, they may be unable to take their business elsewhere. Nor do they necessarily have prior experience of other services which may have been better organised. Numerous examples of this can be found in the stories of people with learning difficulties, as Example 11.2 illustrates.

EXAMPLE 11.2 Anita's story

Well, the Manager turned the meeting round, it was supposed to be about me attending, but when it came down to it what he was on about was that I been offered a place in the sheltered housing and workshop at Cramlington.

And I said I didn't want to go because I was not told that me name had been put down by the social worker, and I didn't want to give up this security so as to share with three other people who I didn't really know. And I might not get on with.

I lost all control of the meeting and I broke down, and like me social worker took me out and told me to pull meself together, and I went back in and the Manager turned round and said: 'You don't want to go.' I said: 'No, I don't, and I don't see why I should give me security up', and he was really nasty after that. And then the Deputy Manager said: 'Oh, I think we'll suspend her for three months', and the Manager said: 'Well, what do you think about that decision?' I said the decision was taken before this meeting.

And like I stayed away for four months, and I went out and told them that I wasn't going back and it's the best decision I've ever made. I've been talking to some of the people who go there now and they hate it, I mean it's just the management's attitude.

(Source: Binns, 1993, p. 169)

Evaluating outcomes

Managers will always have a limited capacity to monitor the effectiveness of their services. They may already be collecting data that contribute to national performance indicators and Quality Protects targets, and it can be frustrating when this proves to be of limited value from an operational point of view. Given the limited value of national indicators, managers may choose to develop their own indicators, tailored to meet the needs and circumstances of the service for which they are responsible. Indeed, the Best Value frameworks require local authorities to develop local indicators to reflect local priorities and to fill the gaps left by national performance indicators.

In designing measures to monitor the outcomes of a service, managers will inevitably be drawn into some of the difficulties that researchers face in evaluating effectiveness. A fundamental difficulty in measuring outcomes for service users is determining when to measure. Some writers take the view that outcomes can only be measured at the point of completion (for example, see Rossi and Freeman, 1993). In the case of the treatment of onset disorders such as depression, it may well be practical to use 'before and after' measurements to evaluate the effectiveness of intervention. Martin and Kettner propose that:

> As a general rule, outcome performance measures should be assessed only on those clients who complete treatment or receive a full complement of services.
>
> (Martin and Kettner, 1996, p. 39)

Often people's involvement with social care services does not have a tidy beginning, middle and end and, as we have seen, in some cases their contact with the service may extend over a lifetime.

Even where interventions have clear start and end points, there can be difficulties in deciding when the intended benefits of an intervention ought to be realised. For example, in the case of the effectiveness of leaving care services, should managers wait a week, a month, a year or more after a young person has left 'care'? Longitudinal studies would not normally be within the scope of routine performance reviews and are more suited to funded research programmes.

Understanding 'what made the difference' is a major difficulty in the study of outcomes. It can be impossible to establish complex cause and effect relationships in social and health care services. Often it is the subtle interaction between a number of different service inputs that leads to a particular outcome. Where outcomes are delivered through partnership arrangements, it may be difficult to isolate the effect of one service or one agency. In circumstances such as these it is important for agencies to understand the critical processes they manage that help bring the overall result. Good outcomes often rely on long chains of events. In the case of a person with a learning disability trying to secure employment, the careers services, outreach services, local transport and local employees may all need to contribute to achieve a successful outcome.

Some services which invest in community-based prevention of crime and other 'preventive' measures may be 'invisible' to service users. If the public are unaware that they are actually receiving a service it can be difficult to evaluate its effectiveness. When faced with difficulties like these there is a danger that managers become paralysed by the difficulty of the task. They have to be pragmatic and accept that their efforts to evaluate the effectiveness of a service will always be less than perfect; however, service users may be willing to settle for 'best available' rather than waiting for some elusive 'ideal solution'.

Designing outcome measures

The design of indicators to measure outcomes – particularly indicators that attempt to measure changes in the health and wellbeing of service users – can be particularly complex. Practice-led managers will want to develop their own approach to measuring the effectiveness of the service area for which they are responsible. The design, collection and use of outcome-based information can also be a resource-hungry undertaking and will almost certainly require specialist skills. For example, in addition to having an understanding of the subject matter itself, designing an outcome measure may require skills and knowledge in information systems, information technology, process mapping, statistical skills and research methods. These are in addition to specialist skills that might be needed to engage with the particular service user group.

Martin and Kettner (1996) suggest six criteria for judging outcome measures.

BOX 11.4 Martin and Kettner's criteria for judging outcome measures

1 **Utility** – do the people who are supposed to use the information think it is useful and relevant? If they do not, it will be ignored.

2 **Validity** – does the indicator measure what it claims to measure? Can we attribute the results that it is reporting to the activity we are evaluating?

3 **Reliability** – does the indicator consistently produce the same result? If it is erratic, it may suggest problems with the definitions on which the indicator is based and/or their interpretation.

4 **Feasibility** – how practical is it to collect the data in question? Does it impose an administrative burden on the staff involved? Does its collection detract from or interfere with direct work with service users? Are there data protection issues related to data sharing?

5 **Cost** – does the cost of data collection outweigh the 'cost of not knowing'? Is the cost of capturing the data electronically prohibitive?

6 **Unit cost reporting** – does the information allow us to understand the cost of producing the outcome in question? Can this be compared with producing the same level of outcome through different means?

(Source: adapted from Martin and Kettner, 1996, p. 60)

Consideration also needs to be given to how the information that flows from indicators can be put to use. An example of this is described in the next section.

Key points

- Measurement of outcomes is required at both the individual level and the service level.

- Regular measurements of a small-scale nature are useful in day-to-day management of services.

- Both quantitative and qualitative measurements are needed.

- The quality of a service should be measured in terms that make sense to the users of that service.

- Measuring the outcomes of a service can create ethical dilemmas.

- As a better 'evidence base' for care services develops, defining and measuring outcomes should become easier.

- People's experiences of services provided in the past may make it difficult for them to imagine different, better services.

- There is a danger of 'over-measurement' of care services, wasting managers' time and depleting resources.

- Deciding when to measure outcomes is a key skill.

- There are clear criteria that managers can use to judge the usefulness of outcome measures.

11.6   Putting outcome measures to use: a case study

In 1999 North Lincolnshire Social and Housing Services introduced a Quarterly Performance Review (QPR). Known affectionately as the 'Quick Prod Round', the process was one of a number of ideas for developing a sharper focus on user-defined outcomes. At the time the system was introduced, managers felt that they were suffocating in a tidal wave of 'badged' initiatives such as Investors in People, the Business Excellence Model, the Charter Mark, and so on. They were also aware of the growing weight and cost of local and central government reviews and inspection programmes (Best Value, Performance and Assessment Framework, Audit Commission Local Authority Performance Indicators). Taken together, these initiatives were distracting managers from day-to-day management and were dissipating efforts to improve service design and delivery.

A common theme ran through all of these initiatives: namely that of good outcomes. Managers agreed that if they could get things right for service users, the rest would follow. In short, Best Value should mean best practice, implying that managers should be practice-led. In designing the QPR process managers wanted to avoid highly 'rational' planning and performance review systems. Experience had taught them that over-elaborate planning systems consumed a disproportionate amount of resources and usually produced disappointing results. Instead, they tried to see planning as a process of organisational learning, thereby focusing their limited capacity on delivering better results rather than on simply servicing an ever more elaborate planning system.

The process started by asking each division (Adult Services, Children and Families and Housing) to agree a set of desired outcomes. For example, the Children and Families Division devised statements that summarised the outcomes it wanted to achieve for service users, together with one outcome related to staff and one that recognised their accountability to the wider community.

Managers then audited what information they had to support their judgement on progress towards each of the agreed outcomes. This included both qualitative and quantitative data. Thus, in addition to routine administrative data, they included an analysis of complaints and representations, the results of any surveys, feedback from user/carer groups, and quality assurance reports. This audit quickly revealed that for outcomes such as 'involving children and young people in decisions that affect their lives', they actually had very little information. This prompted them to make these priority areas for developing feedback loops.

The process adopted used the distinction between service outcomes, client outcomes and overall results (policy impacts) referred to earlier. Managers accepted that they might have to make do with proxy indicators rather than actual client outcomes. For example, ideally the outcome for 'the life chances of children in need' requires annual data on educational attainment and destinations of children and young people. However, month by month they could at least report information on children on a school roll, children attending school, children reporting that they had someone to help with their homework, or someone to attend parents evenings, and so on.

For the managers involved, the purpose of the QPR meeting was simply to provide a routine opportunity to monitor progress towards desired outcomes. Example 11.3 summarises how this attempt to devise an outcome-based approach to management has brought significant benefits to staff and service users.

EXAMPLE 11.3 Benefits from North Lincolnshire's Quarterly Performance Review

- The normally off-putting language of performance review has been turned into an opportunity to examine good practice.

- Having the most senior manager (the Director) chair the meetings gives him an opportunity to feel more in touch with the impact of services in terms of service user outcomes.

- The meetings provide opportunities for managers from support services to see how they contribute to improving the lives of service users. For example, the finance department's performance with regard to getting foster carer payments right is shown to have an important impact on the morale of this vital group.

- Ensuring that the discussion is led by a different operational manager each time encourages shared ownership of outcomes and provides opportunities for 'cross-fertilisation' of ideas.

- The meetings have to identify a limited number of priority actions each time.

The success of the QPR cannot be separated from the culture of the Directorate of the North Lincolnshire Social and Housing Services or indeed its history. In particular, managers believe that the following factors have contributed to its success:

- The Directorate has a well-developed child care information system. Managers are confident in the quality of the data. This means that they do not get sidetracked into interminable debates about the validity or accuracy of the data.
- The Council has a fairly stable workforce. Because of North Lincolnshire's geographical position there is not a lot of staff movement. This is an advantage in terms of organisational learning in that the Council achieves a good balance between knowledge retention and refreshment.

Key points

- Getting 'best value' should mean being led by good practice.

- Part of reviewing outcomes involves auditing existing sources of information rather than devising new ones.

11.7   Conclusion

In this chapter we have argued that a service that is clear about its purpose is more likely to be effective than a service in which outcomes are unclear. We have attempted to answer three key questions. First, are managers clear about the outcomes they are trying to achieve with their intended service users? Second, are they clear about the range, design and level of service that users and stakeholders agree are likely to achieve these outcomes? Finally, how will they know whether or not they are achieving the outcomes that were intended? These three questions are critical to the effective management of care services. The first is about understanding purpose; the second is about understanding what works; and the third is about knowing whether or not services are making a difference. Seen in this way, outcome-focused management is not so much a model or a technique as a way of thinking about the role of managers in relation to the purpose of a service.

Yet how many people have worked in services where they were clear about what they were trying to achieve? Various explanations are given for this lack of clarity. For example, the following comments come from a group of frontline managers of social work services:

> 'The idea of success in providing social care services rests on value judgements and is therefore meaningless.'

> 'The effects of intervention are impossible to measure and so what is the point of defining them?'

> 'Different professional groups define success in different ways and therefore we can't agree what successful outcomes look like.'

> 'Defining success is a hostage to fortune and is best avoided.'
>
> (Manager consultations)

While the arguments behind each of these statements undoubtedly represent a part of the problem of defining success, there is a danger that managers become paralysed by the complexity of providing care services and avoid making any statements about what they are trying to achieve. This chapter has shown how outcomes can be used to make progress towards higher-quality services, better value for money and increased involvement of service users.

Chapter 12
Taking account of history

Sheena Rolph and John Adams (with Dorothy Atkinson)

12.1   Introduction

> Time does contribute something to what we think, but good people are
> never prisoners of their era.
>
> (Chinua Achebe)

On a day-to-day basis, health and social care managers are concerned with
the present and how to manage it. Yet their service, their organisation and
even their practice are part of a long, unfolding history. The concerns of
today's managers are reflected in the concerns of yesterday's managers
because, in spite of the changing nature of services, the people who use
them now have needs in common with those who were on the receiving
end in the past. The themes that recur in the history of managing health
and social care are the same as, or similar to, the ones that are still
prevalent today. No doubt they will continue to be the issues faced by
managers in the future.

This chapter traces key aspects of the history of managing social care by
using selected examples, vignettes and case studies from a variety of social
care settings. The intention is not to give a full historical overview but to
highlight specific management issues and dilemmas. Managers in the
19th, 20th and 21st centuries have faced, and continue to face, the issue of
how to manage staff and other resources in order to deliver 'care', and
often control, in circumstances where individuals, families and children
are facing separation, segregation and other major transitions.

The history of managing social care is important and relevant to
present-day managers for two main reasons. In the first place, it is
instructive. Although present situations never directly mirror the past,
nevertheless there are parallels and similarities between now and then.
Understanding those links is important. In 'taking account of history' in
this way, it becomes possible to understand 'how things came to be'
(Jordanova, 2000, p. 200). In particular, what today's health and social
care managers can learn and understand about past mistakes and abuses
may make them aware of how they arose. It is also possible to learn from
those who defied bad practice and from successful processes in the past.
Past successes can be returned to without having to reinvent the wheel.
Forgetting the good outcomes as well as the mistakes can be dangerous.
The overall aim of this chapter is to encourage managers in health and

social care settings to acknowledge the continuing influence of the past, thus avoiding the trap of becoming 'prisoners of their era'.

In the second place, it is helpful for a manager in health and social care to be aware of the history of an institution, an organisation or a service in order to have a greater understanding of its various complexities. Without knowledge of the context of change and continuity within the organisation, a manager is working in the dark. Ignorance of history can result in confusion, unanswered questions and puzzles, wasteful repetition of solutions, and unawareness of processes that have not worked in the past. This is not to suggest that managers become historians but that they are informed by history. It is important to study the history of management in institutions and in community services, and its effect on service users. Taking account of the history of an organisation is one factor which makes for its smooth running in the present. In this chapter we attempt to place at least some of the concerns of the 21st-century manager in a historical context.

The aims of this chapter are to:

- examine the relevance of a historical approach
- explore what was involved in managing social care institutions in the past
- examine the values and beliefs of people who administered social care
- make links and connections between the past and the present
- take account of contexts and origins in understanding present-day managers' roles.

12.2 Managing adult care

As already stated, the study of the past can be both instructive and enlightening. Not knowing what has gone before can leave the present-day manager in the dark, as illustrated in Sheena Rolph's personal experience in Example 12.1.

EXAMPLE 12.1 Managing in the dark

I worked as a manager of an Adult Education Centre in a large hospital for people with learning difficulties. I arrived there with little knowledge of the history of such institutions or the development of management styles within them. This had repercussions and implications for the way I developed my role.

I wish now that I had known more about the history of the organisation. It would have helped me as a manager in various ways. For example, if I had known more about the establishment of this institution in 1930, the reasons for its existence, and the managerial style at different stages, then I would have seen my future role as manager more clearly. As it was, I remember being confused about the situation I confronted, puzzled by institutional policies, and bewildered by overall hospital staffing issues. If I had learned then about the history of staff recruitment and management, some of the attitudes and work practices would have become clearer, and I would have responded sooner or in a different way.

It is surprisingly easy to overlook the fact that the history of management of social care institutions and organisations is also the history of people: the service users, students, residents and staff. They had often spent many years – sometimes their whole lives – in or close to the organisation. Listening to their stories is a first step for a new manager. Understanding the context in which those stories occurred is the next step. In my case, a deeper understanding of the history of families, their lack of support and the effects of medical attitudes in the 1930s and 1940s would have helped me understand the people with learning difficulties who attended the Adult Education Centre. A knowledge of the Mental Deficiency Acts (1913 and 1927) and the Education Acts would have explained clearly the 'ineducable' label that shocked us all so much, and yet was a part of official policy in the past, with repercussions for managers of the future.

This example refers to managing in a 20th-century institution. The history of institutions – and indeed of community care – goes back much further. The rest of this section traces some of the historical antecedents of today's settings and current practices.

Managing institutions

Although it is possible to see the unfolding story of managing health and social care as a history largely of failures and disasters, we argue that this is a simplistic view and that the picture is far more complex. In fact, history shows there were managers who, despite poor conditions and the local and national policies of the time, defied the many constraints in order to administer a better-quality social care service. Considering that one aspect of effective present-day management is largely concerned with achieving the best possible situation for and with service users in usually less than ideal conditions, these are useful historical pointers. They show how managers have combated neglectful or oppressive policies and lack of resources in the past, and have refused to become 'prisoners of their era'.

The day-to-day management of a Victorian workhouse, which was the responsibility of the Master and Matron, was spelt out in stern detail for the Bromsgrove Union Workhouse in Worcestershire. The Master had to:

keep a register of all the paupers within the workhouse and to enter the names of those leaving or being admitted to the house. He had to take account of the goods and effects of paupers as they entered the building. He had to provide refreshment and medicines for the sick paupers. He ordered all the food and had to account for all of it and to ensure that there was no waste, and if any product was received of a poor quality he had to report this to the Guardians and the suppliers. He had to inspect all the rooms and wards of the male paupers at least twice a day, and he had to list the faults or misdemeanours of every person in the workhouse and report to the Guardians. He was often asked to punish offenders according to the rule book and enter the name, offence and punishment in the official punishment book. He had to oversee the transit of paupers to the church twice on Sunday. He and the porter had to ensure that all gates and doors were locked at night which was nine o'clock in winter and ten o'clock in summer. On entry to the workhouse the Master had to supervise the collection of clothes and the giving out of the workhouse clothing, and also the bathing of the inmate. He also had to give the order to separate the pauper family and direct the members to separate room within the workhouse.

(Land, 1990, p. 20)

The belief in separation of families for their own good is a theme that runs throughout the history of social care and we return to it in a later section of this chapter. Although the workload of managers was, judging from this excerpt, extremely heavy, it was still open to interpretation by individual managers, who could abuse their position or turn it to the advantage of individuals in the workhouse.

Several historians (for example Digby, 1978; Reid, 1994) suggest that even after the notoriously harsh Poor Law Act of 1834, there were still Poor Law Institutions that made a real attempt to address social ills. This was no doubt because of the humane management of guardians, visitors, masters and matrons who had a view of what constituted good care.

Investigations will also reveal that the union workhouse was not an unchanging feature of Victorian society, but one which evolved and developed as a result of national and local factors. It may also become apparent that the image which many people have of the workhouse (based to some extent on its portrayal by Dickens in *Oliver Twist*), though it contains elements of truth, is an over-simple and in some respects misleading one.

(Reid, 1994, p. 1)

Later still, a childhood memory of the West Beckham Workhouse in 1914–18, collected by the Norfolk Federation of Women's Institutes in 1972, describes a happy and festive occasion:

I remember Christmas Days in the Workhouse, some of the happiest of my life. No, I was not an inmate, although at the time, from six years until ten years I was quite sure that to be one was to be as happy as myself.

My grandfather, grannie and auntie were respectively Master, Matron and Assistant Matron at a small county workhouse at West Beckham, near Holt, about four miles from my home. To me it was Heaven and Fairyland all in one, and I certainly saw it through rose-coloured spectacles ...

At last we were there and up the drive to the House – out of the trap stiff and cold and into the warm Lodge ... Then down the flagged passage to the 'Octagon', the centre of the House, around which my grandparents had their quarters. Great swags of evergreen were everywhere strung across the passages ...

The sitting room door would open, and there was granny in black, with a cap of velvet and lace – granddad behind her, tall, benign, with a beautiful silver beard, and auntie in her pink uniform and white apron and cuffs.

... breakfast over, it was time to go with granny on her Christmas rounds with a present for everyone – sweets for the children, tobacco for the men and tea and a cap and apron for the old ladies. To me everyone seemed happy and in my grandparents' special care.

Then to the big kitchen to watch the preparations for dinner, which was served in the dining hall to all the able-bodied. Families were allowed to sit together, a great treat for them which I was too young to appreciate. The great range which cooked the great rounds of beef, and the great cauldron in which the yellow football-sized Christmas puddings were cooked, fascinated us, especially when they were hauled out of the copper on a pulley. My grandfather, father and the porter put on their aprons, sharpened their knives and carved the beef. Potatoes, greens and gravy were got ready and then we were allowed to run backwards and forwards to the dining hall carrying loaded plates. Men and women were allowed a glass of stout or beer and the children lemonade.

(Norfolk Federation of Women's Institutes, 1972, p. 134)

Russell Reeve's childhood memories of the same workhouse only 20 or so years later paint a very different picture. That the regimes described are so different can perhaps be ascribed largely to the different management styles, and the individual ethics of different managers.

My father was a Relieving Officer. Very often we, my mother, my sister and I, went along with him. I actually remember taking lots of people to the workhouse, and socially we got to know the people who kept the local workhouse ... The Master and Matron lived a very grand life. I am talking about pre-war. And they had domestics which were obviously residents from the workhouse. They had very grand quarters. I, as a child, remember he ran a Jaguar car in the days when to have a car at all was really quite extraordinary!

I remember he had a Great Dane dog, which stood as tall as this table and I remember seeing this dog devour great joints of meat, and, at the same time we were well aware that the people in the workhouse ... well, it was probably eating more meat in a day than they might see in a month, you know.

We used to get invited up at Christmas when the local brass band would play in the hall for the residents and everybody was compelled to attend and clap. But, then we are talking about single brick walls painted brown and yellow in the workhouse, as opposed to the carpets and the long luxury polished mahogany tables of the Master and Matron's accommodation.

(Oral history interview with Sheena Rolph, 1999)

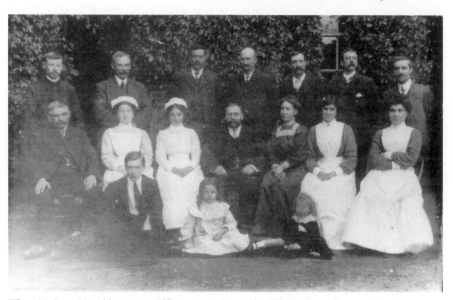

The Union Workhouse: Officers and staff, Mitford and Launditch Union, c. 1910 (Source: Norfolk Museums Service, Gressenhall Museum)

Example 12.2 illustrates the complex history of a social care institution and the people who ran it in its various manifestations. Now called 'managers', these people were variously known as workhouse masters and matrons, wardens, superintendents, organisers and welfare officers. Their stories reveal the long history of issues still being grappled with today by their descendants.

EXAMPLE 12.2 Managing the Heckingham House of Industry

The history of Heckingham Workhouse in Norfolk is a history of social care developments and transformations in microcosm. During the two centuries of its early history it changed from workhouse to hospital for people with learning difficulties, and is now (in new premises but on the same site) a home for older people with learning difficulties. The wheel has turned full circle since Rider Haggard, who had served as a poor law guardian of this workhouse, observed in 1899 that 'it now resembles an infirmary for the aged poor':

It astonished me to-day to see how greatly the conditions of existence at Heckingham have been improved of late years. Now it resembles an infirmary for the aged poor, rather than the last shelter to which the destitute are driven by necessity. In the old days, indeed, it was a dreary place; for instance, I remember the sick ward, a cold and desolate room, where two children to whom I used to carry toys, a twin brother and sister, lay dreadfully ill of some scrofulous disease, with no fire in the grate, and so far as I recollect, no trained nurse to wait upon them. To-day, that ward is bright and cheerful, with a good fire burning in it and a properly certificated attendant to minister to the wants of its occupants ...

In truth, to whatever extent it may be brightened and rendered habitable, one cannot pretend that a workhouse is a cheerful place. The poor girls, with their illegitimate children creeping dirty-faced across the floor of brick; the old, old women lying in bed too feeble to move, or crouching round the fire in their mob-caps, ... all of these are no more cheerful to look on than is the dull appropriate light of this December afternoon.

(Rider Haggard, 1899)

Heckingham changed its function in 1933, becoming an institution for 176 people with learning difficulties. Until 1938 the last workhouse Master and Matron, Mr and Mrs Leslie Hill (shown in the photograph), remained as managers, and vestiges of the workhouse regime were left unchanged, with residents continuing to wear institutional clothing, and the staff, now nurses, wearing dark, high-collared uniforms (Bilyard, 1987). Segregation remained, and the rules concerning care and control, licence and supervision which were passed by the 1913 Mental Deficiency Act, were put in place. In 1953 it became Hales Hospital.

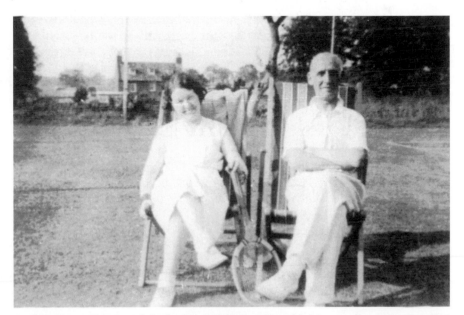

Heckingham House of Industry (1930s): Mr and Mrs Leslie Hill, the last workhouse Master and Matron. The three-storey building in the background is the 'Pesthouse' (Source: Bilyard, 1987, p. 28)

A description of the regime in 1968, given by Frances Kirkpatrick, manager of the hospital, indicates the continuing closeness to the workhouse regime, and the difficulty of making a transition from the Poor Law days:

> It was only slowly that we managed to get domestics to do the grotty jobs, you know, because before that patients did the grotty jobs. It was terribly self-sufficient in those days, and standards were not as good. I mean I was Matron of a boarding school 50 years ago, and the dormitories consisted of a hospital bed and a flock mattress and a chair by the side of the bed! Which is exactly the same, very much the same, as the hospital: there's very little difference. They had a hospital bed, a flock mattress and a chair by the side of the bed. They didn't have individual lockers or individual clothes in those days.
>
> It was terribly regimental. I remember the first day, going to Hales, thinking 'Gosh, I'm never going to live through it' ... the morning parade, and in order to get a comb they had to hand in the old comb and then had to have a clean flannel or clean towel every week. It was part and parcel of looking after a lot of people. There wasn't much difference between schools or the army or anything, it was long lines of people.
>
> (Oral history interview of the manager of Hales Hospital, 1968–95, with Sheena Rolph, 1996)

Hales Hospital was closed in 1995, but a home for older people with learning difficulties was built on the site, a few hundred yards from the hospital. It is therefore an interesting example of a social care organisation with a very long history, which is still in existence. Unlike many other workhouses which have become museums, administrative offices or desirable homes, Hales remains a social care institution. The old workhouse lurks in the background of the new, purpose-built bungalows, as a very immediate symbol of times past, and of the life stories of some of the present-day residents. Some of them have been there since the 1930s, and members of their families have now resumed contact. Recent managers have also been through some of these changes, and an understanding of the past is important in contextualising the present approach, understanding family guilt and grief, and enabling older residents to have choice and independence, reorienting themselves to a new life.

The story of Heckingham is an example of the way one particular workhouse was 'managed' for over a century up to the time the Poor Law was abolished in 1948. It shows that the workhouses did not disappear overnight; many of them simply changed their names.

The old Poor Law workhouse can be seen as the ancestor of most of the institutions which form part of the modern social services. They were used as old people's homes, or occupational training centres, maternity, mental and general hospitals, children's homes and hostels for the homeless. With their workshops, schools and sick wards they constituted the full range of welfare services in microcosm, from which the modern specialised institutions have grown.

(Oxley, 1974, p. 79)

The masters and matrons who ran the workhouses did not disappear either; they became wardens in the post-war institutions. Workhouses were not just the 'ancestors' of present-day institutions: until the 1960s many of them were the institutions, as the buildings were still in use and often run by the same people (Adams, 1999). Similarly, the organisation to which the earliest social care 'managers' belonged also changed its name several times from its inception in 1898 (see Figure 12.1).

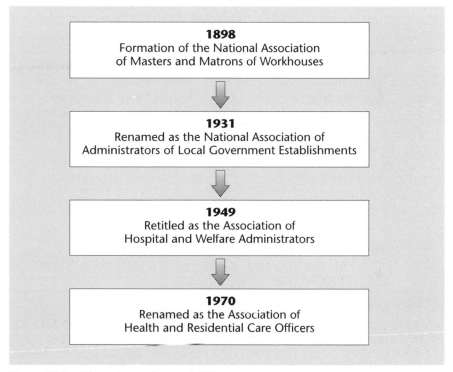

1898
Formation of the National Association
of Masters and Matrons of Workhouses

1931
Renamed as the National Association of
Administrators of Local Government Establishments

1949
Retitled as the Association of
Hospital and Welfare Administrators

1970
Renamed as the Association of
Health and Residential Care Officers

Figure 12.1 **Changing roles and titles**

A short history of Heckingham is readily accessible from two small booklets, written and published locally (Bilyard, 1987; Bilyard, n.d.). Many organisations have now similarly commissioned their own short historical accounts. They are particularly useful for those managers who cannot devote too much time to exploring history. Although, for those who are interested, short periods spent in the Public Record Office or in conducting oral history interviews add to the interest of their job, it is reassuring to realise that local history projects are making history more easily accessible.

Managing community care: the relieving officer

Historians now acknowledge that community care was not an invention of the 1960s and 1970s, but has a much longer history. Many different roles were developed to administer community care in the 18th, 19th and early 20th centuries. In the late 19th century state support for people living in the community was administered by the relieving officer, a key Poor Law official. Relieving officers continued to manage community care until 1948, when their name was changed to 'welfare officer' and 'duly authorised officer', but they retained the same duties.

These duties were onerous and time-consuming. The relieving officer (usually male) was required to visit the houses of all applicants for relief in order to enquire into their state of health, their ability to work, the family background and the means available to them. A report on each case had to be presented at the next meeting of the Board of Guardians. Where relief had already been approved, he was required to administer it weekly by paying the approved sums of money or providing relief in kind, such as bread or meat. If the need for relief was urgent, the relieving officer was required to convey the destitute person to the workhouse or to provide relief in kind if it was more appropriate for the person to stay at home. The relieving officer was also 'duly authorised' to convey 'mental defectives' and psychiatric cases to the local institutions when he or others judged it to be necessary.

A relieving officer was required to maintain six sets of records:

1   Application and Report Book
2   Outdoor Relief List
3   Outdoor Relief List for Vagrants
4   Abstract of the Outdoor Relief List
5   Receipt and Expenditure Book
6   Duly Authorised Officer's lists for detention of persons of unsound mind under the Lunacy Act 1890.

Payment of money, or the provision of medical assistance or relief in kind, could easily make the difference between life and death for destitute people. It could also mean that they were able to stay in their own homes. The regulations concerning the need for a prompt and efficient response from the relieving officer were stark:

> If he neglects his duty and death ensues, he is guilty of manslaughter, and if by reason of such neglect, not death but serious bodily harm or injury or prolonged suffering is occasioned, he is liable to be prosecuted for misdemeanour.
>
> (Little, 1898)

Oral history evidence illustrates the huge caseloads relieving officers were expected to undertake, often to the detriment of people in their care. Present-day managers have similar concerns over their large caseloads and fears that not all service users are being adequately supported or managed in the community. Some oral history accounts also point to the existence of a generic service flourishing well before 1970, and the surprising amount of autonomy granted to community officers in rural districts.

One relieving officer gained his certificate of qualification by correspondence course from the Poor Law Examination Board in 1935. He relished the fact that he was on his own, and had autonomy within his area, and he also enjoyed the variety of his work, the lack of the need to specialise, and the fact that he could usually attend to most of the varied needs in any one family:

> I was on call seven days a week, twenty-four hours a day ... I organised admissions to the local mental hospital, visiting the family first with a GP and a magistrate – we were obliged to visit 'mental defectives' at least once a quarter. I was also responsible for the disabled and the elderly. I had to cover a huge rural district. What I enjoyed about it was the autonomy as an RO. You were your own boss, responsible in your own area ... perhaps even the only person in your area. I didn't see myself as a specialist – I was against specialisms – I liked the joint welfare role and the mental welfare work.
>
> (Oral history interview with Sheena Rolph, 2000)

Two decades later, in 1956, another officer began work in the Welfare Department of Norfolk Social Services Department (known as that even in 1956). His task was to run residential homes for older people and house homeless families, collecting the rent and making sure the children attended school. In 1966 he became assistant local welfare officer, again a generic role that incorporated the mental welfare officer role and included the duty of collecting maintenance from families for children in care:

> I had no administrative or clerical support. I had a huge workload which now included far more administration. I had to manage the Home Care Service for older disabled people in their own homes, assess and allocate houses, recruit support and process time sheets. It took me one whole day a week to collect the charge for home care. Much of it was administrative work rather than professional social work. I covered large areas – the patch was extended to cover a third of Norfolk. I was on duty every evening and every third weekend – on call all the time. But there was little actual support in the community for those with mental handicaps ... two visits a year and little to offer except institutionalisation. There were no care plans, interventions were reactive – the community care was a bit hit and miss.
>
> (Oral history interview with Sheena Rolph, 1999)

These two officers could be seen as generic social work managers well before the Seebohm changes in 1970. They both raised many community care issues which continue to tax social care managers. Although they enjoyed the generic nature of their work, they also admitted to administering a somewhat 'hit and miss' community care service. The history of relieving officers is also notable for the fact that these early administrators of community care were almost always male, a tradition which continued in many counties as the relieving officers metamorphosed into duly authorised officers in 1946 and then mental welfare officers in 1959 (Rolph *et al.*, 2002).

Key points

- Community care has a long history: today's health and social care staff and managers were foreshadowed by relieving officers and their successors.

- History contains evidence of good practice in spite of constraints.

- Key themes in the past – such as the separation of families – still recur today.

- The history of institutions sheds light on management style and practice over time.

- People were maintained in their homes through a combination (or 'package') of care, assistance and cash.

- Generic services flourished in some areas long before the inception of social services departments.

12.3   Managing child care

There are many pressing concerns for those involved in managing child care today. They include how to keep families together rather than separating children from them – even though the practice of separation continues in some cases, albeit for many different reasons. There are also concerns about the moves from one form of care to another and the separation of children from siblings or local areas and friends. These issues are not new, however, and often they echo the concerns of past managers. In this section we discuss some of the issues facing child care and rescue societies in the past, noting the relevance of this history for today's managers.

There is a vital need not only to know and understand the past with its successes and failures but also to pay greater attention to historical suggestions and solutions. This is because of the inability of successive generations of policy makers to solve some of these problems and the frequency with which failed solutions recur. Present-day managers, in being able to reflect on the past, need not be blinkered in their approach, but can afford to be creative and courageous in seeking to break long traditions of failure. Furthermore, historical reflexivity means being able to innovate from a strong position. Knowledge of the history of child care management is thus a key tool in enabling change in the management of transitions of all kinds, and in questioning the need for such transitions in the first place.

Managing separations and migrations

In her study of the Waifs and Strays Society (later the Church of England Children's Society), Harriet Ward emphasises the relevance of her history as a working tool rather than simply an academic exercise:

> In recent years there have been heated debates over issues such as access between separated children and their parents, the relative merits of fostering and residential care, and the extent to which parents physically or sexually abuse their children. It is salutary to note that all these questions were also being debated a hundred years ago ... an analysis of the historical material may increase our awareness of the intractability of some of the problems caused by the need to care for separated children.
>
> (Ward, 1990, p. 420)

The need to separate children from their parents has now been called into question in view of the fact that, very often historically as well as today: 'the only participants who were ultimately obliged to show a permanent commitment towards the most problematic children were their own parents' (Ward, 1990, p. 422). Preventive measures to avoid separation were suggested in the past but not taken up. Yet there have always been managers who have tried to implement change. Ward's history reveals that there were several managers who were able to challenge received wisdom and even the accepted policy of the Society, such as Miss A. Lee, who is described in Example 12.3.

EXAMPLE 12.3 Managing the Marylebone Home for Girls

Miss Lee was involved in management between 1882 and 1895. During this time she was a strong advocate of the admission of pauper children. She was the superintendent of the Society's Marylebone Home for Girls, managing it for 14 years, and ensuring that it received destitute children, thus 'saving' them from the workhouse. She spoke out against the detrimental effects of both large institutions, such as the workhouse, and smaller homes where the children were boarded out. Instead, she advocated the establishment of small, certified homes in villages as the most sympathetic environment for separated children, emulating an ideal family life, ensuring fewer intermediate moves, and offering a supported transition into work and independence when they were older.

Miss Lee was also remarkable in that she was against severance and was convinced that many children were unnecessarily removed from their parents. In 1883, in an article in the Society's magazine, she said that the reason poor children living with their families were 'vastly superior in health, appearance, vivacity, and intelligence' to those in Poor Law or children's homes was 'because, even in the most wretched homes, social and family affects were not dried up. Someone cares for the children, if only to scold them. They have a home, they are relations of someone' (p. 140). She made the point that the best, in fact the only, way to improve the lot of difficult or promiscuous girls, was to work with and co-operate with the whole family. She claimed that 'where the parental tie does exist, no matter how bad we may think the parents to be, it is only through using it, and acting with it, and through it, that success in our work can be expected' (p. 141).

(Source: Ward, 1990)

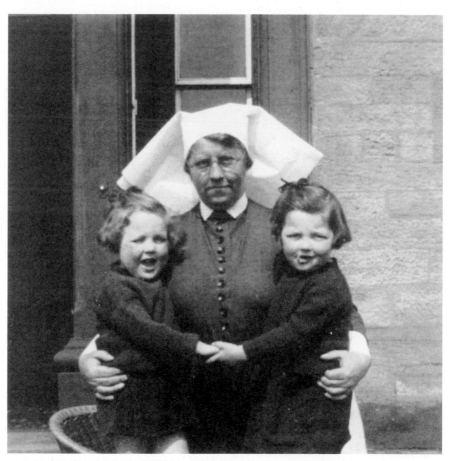

A matron of the Waifs and Strays Society (Source: Bowder, 1980, p. 68)

The dark side of managing child care was the practice of 'emigrating' the children. One of the major transition issues facing managers of the Waifs and Strays Society was that of emigration. Over 100,000 children were moved to Canada between 1870 and 1930, with others being sent to Australia, New Zealand, Southern Rhodesia and South Africa (Bowder, 1980). Speed was important in ensuring that, as far as possible, 'unspoilt' children would arrive to 'fill the empty lands of the Empire' (Bott, 1998, p. 205).

It is clear from the evidence that transitions and separations punctuated the lives of children in care. The philosophy of the time did not allow for compassion or preparation for these separations, managers often only rarely allowing themselves to show signs of affection:

> It seems I was born in London, but my earliest recollections are of the Isle of Wight. When my grandmother died ... in 1905 – I found myself being taken across to the mainland ... There I was placed in the care of an elderly widow for six years.

> I was taken to St Aldelm's Home for boys. There were about forty-eight boys in the Home and I enjoyed being with the others but discipline was strict and food scanty.

> In the spring of 1913, someone asked: 'Who would like to go to Canada?' I grasped the opportunity. Just a few of us were taken to Liverpool by the superintendent who showed us more affection than at any other time. I was fourteen years old and weighed all of eighty pounds. On May 16 about twenty-five of us sailed on the Tunisian.
> (Boy from Children's Society home quoted in Bowder, 1980, p. 51)

The practices of some of the managers of the Waifs and Strays Society were openly criticised even at the time. Maria Rye's emigration society began sending children to Canada in 1869. Although her methods were lampooned by George Cruikshank, Dickens' illustrator, who depicted her snatching heartbroken children from parents 'befuddled by drink' (Ward, 1990, p. 119), her agency was used by the Waifs and Strays Society. A government inspector, sent to Canada to investigate the rumours, found that children were being summarily taken off the street and emigrated so fast that their parents did not know where they were. He also found that, once there, there was no supervision of the emigrants, leaving them open to abuse by Canadian employers.

The Society established two receiving homes in Canada. Its founder, Edward Rudolf, had to be seen to support the policy in order to gain sponsorship, but he was less than enthusiastic about the practice of 'emigrating'. His story is an example of a hands-on but behind-the-scenes manager, who was never in the public eye like Dr Barnardo, but who nevertheless had considerable influence in reducing the more extreme tendencies of some of his staff, as well as the sponsors and supporters (see Example 12.4).

EXAMPLE 12.4 Managing the Waifs and Strays Society

Edward Rudolf established the Society in 1881 and spent the next 38 years running it, setting up 113 homes and ultimately caring for 4531 children. According to Ward (1990), he ran the Society in the manner of the first-class civil servant he had once been. He issued forms and lists of regulations, foster parent agreements, notices of discharge or transfer, service after-care reports and formal parental consents for emigration. Individual homes were continuously updated on policies through circulars, and Homes Committees were told to remain in contact with girls who had left for domestic service 'by treating them to letters and possibly at times to presents' (Ward, 1990, p. 144).

Rudolf was thus aware of the importance of smoothing transitions of all kinds made by the young people in his homes, and the need to maintain affectionate contact with ex-residents. The formal regulations and the Society Constitution are evidence that he was also uneasy about the bad practices surrounding emigration, severance, separation and depriving families, parents and children of their rights. In this he steered the Society away from some of the practices engaged in by other societies, for example Dr Barnardo's, which insisted on parental agreement to the possibility of emigration at some future date before admission of their child to a home was considered. Power was thus transferred from parents to Dr Barnardo's, and the parents, in need perhaps of temporary help at a time of poverty, hardship or bereavement, were entrapped. In contrast, the Waifs and Strays Society's form merely asked: 'Is there any objection to its [the child] being emigrated if this is thought to be desirable by the Society?' This enabled parents to refuse to consent to emigration, but at the same time enabled them to refer their child to the Society.

Ward suggests that, although there is evidence that some bad practice continued in the Waifs and Strays Society, Rudolf's influence as a manager was a deterrent, and 'at least some attempt' was made to respect the rights of parents (Ward, 1990, p. 150). He is presented as a manager who was at odds with the philosophy of other contemporary societies, and whose fair-mindedness meant that 'the considerable pressures from those of his supporters who were in favour of exceeding the legal mandate and denying parents their rights, were relatively ineffective' (Ward, 1990, p. 151).

The migration of children and young people into and around the UK remains a concern for managers, as local authorities use facilities in many different parts of the country. Concerns about how to manage these moves, maintain family contact and enable a relationship with a new and unfamiliar community remain major elements in a manager's brief. Supervision of the young people is notoriously difficult to manage for reasons of cost, the availability of personnel, difficulties of inter-agency co-ordination and general problems of communication and reporting. Management of the staff who liaise with many different agencies to maintain contact with young people sent to institutions in different parts of the country is fraught with problems, and comparisons can be made with accounts of transition in the past. A manager struggling with dogmatic asylum laws may at the very least take heart from those in the past who challenged inhumane 'emigrating' policies.

A new definition of 'separated children' has emerged recently (Refugee Council, 2001). Unaccompanied children represent a small but significant proportion of the immigrants and asylum seekers entering the UK now. Today's managers are confronted with concerns as to how and where to place the children, how to keep siblings together, how to arrange their education, and above all, how to supervise their placements and maintain contact with them when they move through several different counties.

Another established practice in some West African countries relates not to unaccompanied children but to children who are relinquished by their impoverished parents into the hands of relatives living abroad who promise them a better life. The tragic case of Victoria Climbié, murdered by her aunt and partner in London in 2000, renewed grave concerns as to how this type of reverse child migration is to be managed. 'Managerial errors' at all levels were blamed for Victoria's death. It happened despite the involvement of several managers and services, none of whom proved able to prevent it.

It could also be said that the managers lacked awareness of complex ethnic issues. This showed itself in across-the-board assumptions, for example that a Jamaican social worker would be familiar with West African customs and religions. This seemed to show a lack of understanding by the managers of cultural differences between ethnic groups. We have already highlighted some of the same issues of separation from family, isolation and hidden abuse. In a reversal of 19th-century history, immigrant children are now arriving *here*, just as they arrived in Canada and Australia in the first half of the 20th century. Some are being placed in inappropriate adult accommodation, even in prisons, while others, like Victoria, are in danger of being hidden from view, living in abusive situations with relatives or family contacts. In a climate of increasing use of agencies, charities and private organisations, it is useful to reflect on management issues which arose in charities and rescue societies in the past, and in particular to listen to the voices of those who experienced similar difficult transitions.

Managing transitions and change

Transitions and separations were also a major feature of the management of both Dr Barnardo's Homes and the Thomas Coram Foundling Hospital, founded in 1741. Babies received into the hospital were almost immediately sent out to foster parents for five years. At the end of this time they were separated from their foster parents and returned to the hospital, staying until they were 14, when another move meant that they were placed in either military or domestic service. The sudden break with their foster family often caused great pain to the children, although some experienced abusive foster homes which they were pleased to leave. Many remembered their foster parents with great affection:

> That was lovely ... Memories of happiness, yes. Bill [her foster brother] was my sort of guiding light and I went everywhere on his shoulders ... happiness, that's the main thing I remember. And I remember the summer, not the winter.
>
> (May, aged 72, quoted in Oliver and Aggleton, 2000, p. 18)

The shock and trauma of leaving often idyllic, though poor, foster homes in the country for the harsh life of the hospital is clear from people's memories. The move, taken for granted as essential, was managed insensitively, causing heartbreak for the children. They were not told in advance of their admission back into the hospital; they were given no explanation of this sudden separation from foster mothers and siblings; their 'hair was cut severely short, their clothes were removed, they were bathed and given their school uniform' (Oliver and Aggleton, 2000, p. 19):

> And the next memory ... was this very big building and having all our hair shaved off ... I can remember this big stone room that had iron beds and there were two bed-heads put together like that. And there was a little boy in the other bed and he was crying all the time, 'I want my mummy, I want my mummy.' And I remember putting my hand through and holding his hand and thinking I must not cry. I had promised Bill I would not cry.
>
> (May, aged 72, quoted in Oliver and Aggleton, 2000, p. 20)

Ronald, another 'foundling', describes the shock he had in experiencing the kind of care he received on his return to the home, offering insights into the management style:

> It wasn't the care we had at home [i.e. in the foster home]. It was military style. It was 'here is a job I've got to do, get on with it' ... The staff were not unkind, but certainly not loving. They'd got a job to do. You had to obey orders whatever they said and if you didn't, you were in trouble. It was a monastic sort of existence. As long as you kept going you were okay.
>
> (Ronald, aged 75, quoted in Oliver and Aggleton, 2000, p. 21)

Many of the personal memories of social care management endow it with military characteristics, such as regimentation and lack of affection. These characterise care for older people (as in Example 12.2) as well as children and young people. The 'short sharp shock' policies of the 1980s – which aimed to change and improve individuals by means of sudden forceful transitions – are another recent feature indicating that solutions from the past can resurface alarmingly and are never far away.

The voices of those experiencing child care highlight the pain of the separations and transitions. At the same time, though, they often acknowledge the benefits of the schools or societies at a time when there were no alternatives, and when families received no help. Danny Ross, for example, went to the Blue Coat School in Liverpool when his father died and his mother was unable to feed and clothe all her children. He describes the separation from his family:

> And so it was that one day in July 1924, Mary [his sister] and I, accompanied by our mother, presented ourselves for admission. We were parted almost immediately ... I can still hear the Headmaster saying 'Now boys, say goodbye to your mothers', and still see my mother with tears in her eyes holding the small case into which she had put my home clothes which I had just discarded.
>
> (Ross, 1996, p. 8)

Managing such dramatic life changes was a challenge for staff. It appears from the evidence that very often the aim was to make such tasks as easy as possible for the staff, who were not encouraged to make any special effort to help the children to bear the separations. Although philosophy and practice are now very different, there remains the issue of how to train and manage social care staff who are putting painful decisions into practice, managing adoption or fostering, or admitting young people into care homes.

Yet, in a way, the history of the children's homes and orphanages is the story of an attempt at a visionary approach to a management experiment set up to oppose the poverty and hardship of the workhouses. It is a story of dreams that often went wrong, visions that are now discredited. However, it was also sometimes the chance of a new life. Danny Ross from the Blue Coat School paid tribute to the role the school played in preparing him for adult life:

> When we left we were kitted out as indeed all the boys were, with a new suit, a couple of striped flannel shirts, two stiff collars, studs and a tie, two pairs of socks, one pair of boots and a bowler hat. Whether one was going to be an apprenticed plumber, or away to sea, or an office job, all were given a bowler hat.
>
> As I reached the tall iron gates and walked off the School premises, I looked back over my shoulder and the memories crowded in, both happy and sad, and had I realised then what I have realised since, I must surely have said to myself, 'Thank God for the Blue Coat School'.
>
> (Ross, 1996, p 114)

Some transitions, when well-managed and when the children were well-prepared, could offer hope and a future to young people.

Key points

- Key themes in child care today – family life and how to support it – are echoed in historical accounts.

- Some past practices (such as child emigration to other countries) reflect a different and no longer accepted philosophy of child care.

- Migration of children into the UK is an issue for today's managers.

- Past transitions for children in care often meant sudden breaks.

- Sudden breaks were reinvented as 'short sharp shocks' for young offenders in the 1980s.

12.4   Managing social care

Example 12.5 illustrates inter-war community care for people with learning difficulties. It sheds light on an early style of hostel management and the vision and beliefs of a particular manager. It also represents an early example of the management of the transition of people with learning difficulties from long-stay institutions into smaller homes, employment and a degree of independence in the community. In addition, it suggests that sometimes service users' voices were heard and choices given.

EXAMPLE 12.5 Managing a women's hostel

Eaton Grange in Norwich opened in 1930. It was a small 'certified institution' with the role of 'working hostel' for women with learning difficulties. Between 1930 and 1948 it was managed by a Matron-Superintendent who lived in the hostel. Miss Yeadon was a State Registered Nurse and held both the Medico-Psychological Certificate and the Certificate of the Central Midwives Board. However, in keeping with the tradition of female superintendents and matrons, her job also included the role of housekeeper. The word 'management' was given importance in the job description: her duties were to include 'house-keeping and general management as well as supervision of the nursing' (job advertisement for Matron, 24 January 1930).

Another important aspect of her managerial role was her duty under the Mental Deficiency Acts (1913 and 1927). The legislation, with its eugenic overtones, required not only the institutionalisation of 'mental defectives' but also that they were strictly monitored and controlled, whether in hostels, homes or with their families in the community. A sustained campaign in the early years of the 20th century (led by the National Association for the Care of the Feeble-Minded and the Eugenics Society) had culminated in the Mental Deficiency Acts which were to be implemented by a Board of Control. There were moral panics and fears of criminality, violence, a 'rising tide of illegitimacy' and 'racial degeneracy', all of which were largely attributed to 'mental defectives', who therefore had to be controlled and monitored.

Juggling the two management roles of nurse supervisor under the Acts and housekeeper within the 'Cinderella' service of 'mental deficiency' nursing presented many challenges to the new Matron. Nevertheless, despite the constraints of working under the local Mental Deficiency Committee, Miss Yeadon began to develop her own management style. Evidence from elsewhere has shown the significant role women played in managing small private institutions, suggesting that their regimes continued a 19th-century focus on education and training, rather than on custody and control alone (Stevens, 2000). The new Matron aimed to do the same but within a local authority-funded hostel.

The management issues faced by the new Matron related to the day-to-day running of the hostel. Miss Yeadon did not hold the budget – that was the remit of the Town Clerk in the City Treasurer's department – but she was responsible for every other aspect of management. She oversaw the wellbeing, training and employment of residents, as well as the work and welfare of a comparatively large complement of eight staff; and she was responsible for the upkeep of the building and grounds and the laundry. The Matron's role, in many ways, fits with a modern approach. Since the 1980s, for example, the emphasis on the manager's role has resulted in 'welfare professionals ... being required to manage the day-to-day operations of their particular operational units' (Butcher, 2000, p. 25). This has been seen as 'creating managers out of professionals' (Hoggett, 1991, p. 254).

Although based firmly within the eugenicist context of the time, the Matron's management style in the hostel suggested a more liberal approach. Miss Yeadon's early speeches and reports indicate her ambitions for the women and outline the way she envisaged her role. She saw the hostel as providing a homely family atmosphere, combined with a degree of independence, freedom, education and preparation for work.

(Source: oral history interviews with Sheena Rolph, 1998; Norfolk Record Office, 1932)

Historical dilemmas in managing social care

The example is based on documentary and oral accounts which present a vivid picture of the day-to-day management of the hostel. Several important themes emerge from the records and oral history testimonies. They were key issues for the Matron then and they are key issues in the health and social care field today. These issues are: how to manage a 'home'; how to manage transitions; and how to manage time. We will take each theme in turn.

Managing a 'home'

The Matron had a vision of the hostel as 'an Eldorado' for the women, who, until coming to live there, had led deprived lives in colonies, workhouses and institutions for 'mental defectives'. Miss Yeadon's style of management seems to have been very relaxed: she shared social events and outings with the women, and photographs show her out of uniform enjoying days out at the seaside. She wanted the hostel to be as homely as possible, with herself at the centre of a large 'family'.

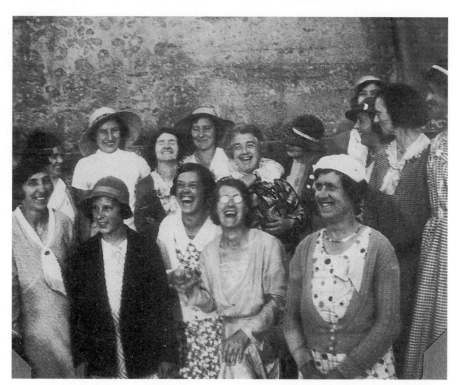

A day at the seaside. Miss Yeadon is fifth from the left, at the back (Source: Brigham *et al.*, 2000)

One of the issues faced by the Matron was that of creating a balance between care and control: a 'homely' as against a 'custodial' style of management. Very real limitations on freedom still existed. The moral panics of the 1930s were clearly reflected in the purpose of the hostel, and therefore the role of the Matron was to ensure segregation: although the women could have experience of work and opportunities for outings and leisure, this was supervised and they were excluded from most aspects of ordinary life. One of the residents was prevented from returning to live with her family, despite pleas from her mother. The woman remembers:

> Every week I go out, and then I didn't want to go back. We used to go out every Wednesday and Saturday. I went to the Market Place. Police ... they brought you back ... My mother wanted me home.
>
> (Oral history interview with Sheena Rolph, 1998)

Her story illustrates the extent of the control over the women in the 1940s, and the limits of the 'freedom' described in official speeches and reports.

Managing transition

By 1942 Eaton Grange was identified as a 'training hostel for domestic service' (Board of Control Inspector, 24 August 1942, Norfolk Record Office). Although she did not define it as such, the Matron was also anxious to provide training and support for *transition* from institution to community for those for whom, as she said in a speech given in March 1932, 'the outside world was an imagination' because:

> Whilst away from home (in the colony or workhouse) no opportunity presented itself for [them] to be given a chance amongst their more fortunate friends in civil life. After only a short stay in the hostel, A.C. has now been able to go out to service for the first time to a freedom which hitherto has been unknown to her.
>
> (Norfolk Record Office, 1932)

The Matron instigated a gradual progression route whereby the women could move from jobs within the hostel to daily outside work and then, if this was successful, to live-in positions. Miss Yeadon had to manage a register of prospective employers, meet them to assess their suitability, not only in terms of conditions of work and living but also in terms of their ability to supervise the women. Once the women had been placed in work, the Matron was on call and also visited the families at intervals to encourage the success of the placement and the fair treatment of the women. Although Miss Yeadon did not refer to it as such, she was in effect setting up and managing an early system of supported employment.

Managing time

Even before the outbreak of the Second World War, time management was an issue for a manager undertaking so many new tasks. By 1938 there were 47 women at Eaton Grange and of these 29 were employed on a daily basis outside the hostel, and two lived in with their employers. In 1945 these figures had grown so that of the 49 women living there, 33 undertook daily work and 12 were in outside positions (Norfolk Record Office 1932, 1948). As numbers grew, so there was a corresponding decline in staff because of wartime conditions. The Matron appeared to continue to run the hostel under these conditions by dint of devotion to duty, never taking a holiday – unless it was with the women – and involving the residents far more than before in running the hostel. One woman was trained as a fire-watcher, another as a cook, while others did the gardening and were in charge of the laundry. Although this style of management could be said to have exploited the women, it could also be seen as giving them status and empowerment in running their own home.

Taking account of the past

What does this reveal about the management style of a Matron in a hostel for women labelled as 'mentally defective' in the period 1930 to 1948? What continuities can be seen between her role and that of social care managers now? Her role was a socialising, training, educating one similar to that of learning disability nurses and managers of care homes today. Wartime conditions called for a special type of single-handed management, resulting in problems of time and supervision that are familiar to hard-pressed managers of care homes now. The documentary and oral accounts reveal the tensions that existed within this early management role. Although training and employment routines were managed so as to enable the women to enjoy a better life, nevertheless their opportunities were still fundamentally limited. This example therefore offers an opportunity to explore the contradictions of care and control in social care management which are still a major concern.

Issues surrounding de-institutionalisation and transitions of all kinds are still high on the agenda of social care managers involved with long-stay hospital closures and the development of community care. The Matron of Eaton Grange was both dealing with incoming residents in transition from long-stay institutions and running a halfway house, where her major role was to ease further outward transitions. Miss Yeadon's ideal of a participative approach which focused on engaging with at least some of the residents as regards their placements; her enthusiasm for education and training; and her determination to enable as many as possible to go out into the world with supervision and support – these aims are comparable with some of those of today's managers.

Although we might argue that the constraint on the Matron to ensure strict social control over the women, even when out in the community, no longer exists, it is salutary to consider present-day constraints which sometimes have a similar effect and which oblige managers to limit choice. Such recurring constraints on managers include: limited finance; lack of, or substandard, daytime activities; rules in some homes regarding the need for all residents to be out of the home all day; and problems with transport or the availability of staff. There are also even more distressing policies for people on the receiving end, such as the change of use of small homes and the seemingly arbitrary dispersal of people with the final closure of the old institutions. Once again, the issue is often one of choice and advocacy.

The story of Eaton Grange has an immediacy and a continuity that is unusual for small facilities in that it is still open and has existed in various forms and guises until the present, its role varying between offering a home in the community and a halfway house. The major job of the current and last manager is to prepare people whose home it has been since they moved into the hostel from the local hospital to move into smaller and more appropriate group homes and flats. The end of Eldorado or the beginning?

> **Key points**
>
> - Managing care, in the past and in the present, often involves balancing the need for control with the wish to create family-style regimes in institutional settings.
>
> - The role of manager, then and now, involves managing a 'home', managing transitions and managing time.
>
> - Managing care always takes place in the context of restricted finances and other resources.

12.5 Conclusion

In this chapter we have highlighted continuity and change in the unfolding, often cyclical, history of social care management. Although progress is apparently made in some areas, in others history reminds of the need for constant vigilance.

We have explored the rules, values and beliefs of some of the people involved in managing institutional and community care in the past. In so doing, we have made links between the concerns then and the concerns of health and social care managers today.

The Victoria Climbié story, although set in the 21st century, includes almost all of the more difficult challenges to management covered in this chapter. From all accounts, her voice was never heard nor sought, let alone listened to. She was separated from her family through a new form of child migration. The trial highlighted ethnic issues that were not addressed and the buck that was passed from one key adult to another.

That case is the worst (known) tragedy of all. How could it have happened in 2000, with society's supposed greater awareness of the needs of children? History shows that there will always be change in health and social care; it suggests that change will continue into the future through globalisation, world events and the migrations of people. There will continue to be new challenges for those at the front line of services, including managers.

Victoria Climbié's story illustrates new and changing circumstances triggered by world events. So how can taking account of history help prepare managers for the future? Such awareness might enable them to recognise patterns or familiar issues even when they present within a new context (as with Victoria Climbié). All the old and much-debated issues were there but seemed to go unrecognised because this was a new situation with new fears. At the very least, today's managers might be better prepared so that they are not prisoners of the past or present, but are ready for the future.

Appendix: The consultation process

As part of the consultation process to inform the development of the course material, course team members met with groups of workers and service users across Scotland, England, Wales and Northern Ireland. This Appendix briefly outlines the consultation process and gives context to some of the quotations from managers, practitioners and service users presented throughout this book and its companion volume, *Managing Care in Practice*.

Adult service user consultations

The user consultation strategy for adult services involved (among other less structured meetings) four workshops with groups of people with experience of using mental health, disability, learning disability and older people's services. A facilitator with direct experience of services was identified for each workshop and participants were contacted by facilitators through informal networks. Some people already knew each other and others met for the first time at the workshops. Everyone had experience of several services, including health, voluntary sector, community-based and residential settings.

Some people had experienced compulsory services, and several people in the mental health group had been 'sectioned' under the Mental Health Act. The names of some participants and all projects, centres, wards and professionals have been changed. Some participants were happy for their names to be used. It was clear that, although services are split along similar lines to those chosen for the consultations, people do not fit into neat service delivery boxes. For example, Lou, a woman in the learning disability group, also had a visual impairment. Judith, from the older people group, had a physical disability and had cared for her elderly mother. Because people have diverse experience of services we have chosen to identify them by name alone alongside quotations in the chapters. For example, to have identified Judith as belonging to a 'physical disability' service user group would deny the range of her experience and contribution. By using names only we hope to highlight the commonalities of experience and emphasise people rather than service categories.

The groups had the following remit:

> To consider a set range of questions from their specialist viewpoint as users of services for a specific group of people. Views on their experiences of involvement (or lack of it) in consultation and planning services will be particularly useful.

For adult groups, Jeanette Henderson (a member of the course team) met with facilitators to talk through the consultation process with the aim of ensuring that participants as well as the course team would find the experience useful and relevant. Group members were sent the course outline and information about the materials likely to be developed for the course. Each member was paid a fee for taking part as well as travel expenses. Following the workshops a representative or facilitator from each of the groups was invited to a meeting at The Open University to discuss the content and process of the consultations. A report was produced for each of the groups outlining the themes discussed and containing a selection of quotations illustrating the views of the group, and an overall report summarising the sessions was circulated.

Young people, children and families consultations

The parent and young people user views are drawn from several consultations co-ordinated by Janet Seden (a member of the course team). In one, a Home-Start staff member interviewed six families with children under five years who were receiving services from Home-Start (a voluntary befriending agency, accessed by referral from commissioning agencies). These families had all experienced a crisis in their family life that had led them to ask for help. The agencies they experienced included social services, health, education, housing and the benefits agency. The families' experiences of the statutory agencies were mixed, ranging from the helpful (sensitive responses) to the incompetent (initial telephone calls not returned). They were unanimous in valuing responsive, respectful encounters with professionals and valued highly the peer support of the befriending agency.

In another consultation, Maya Joshi and Rukshana Owen (with Janice Whyne at the Family Service Unit) interviewed five young women who had attended a group for teenagers who had experienced sexual abuse. The therapeutic group had now ended and been evaluated. It was thought that these young women, who besides attending the group had also experienced a range of other interventions in their lives, would be able to tell the researchers what they thought about the services and professionals they knew about. The researchers prepared questions relating to the areas of:

- benefits received from services
- the positives and negatives of the experience
- the young women's feelings about the services they received and improvements they might like to suggest.

The researchers found they needed to adjust the language of the questionnaire and make space for the respondents' own areas of concern as the research progressed, and that making space for free narrative was a useful way to work. These consultations were undertaken as face-to-face interviews which were then transcribed.

In both adult and children's consultations the respondents had a rich experience of very current meetings with a range of professionals from several agencies. This makes their valuable views and insights both genuinely felt and grounded in direct personal experience. Material from these consultations is referred to in this book as 'service user consultations' and 'children's consultations'.

Regional and individual manager consultations

Regional consultations were held in Leeds, Edinburgh and Belfast. The regional sessions were held with groups of people working in or using care services. Participants were identified and contacted by regional academics in the School of Health and Social Welfare.

Two workshops were held with groups of managers and practitioners in the north-east of England. The first consisted of managers and practitioners from a local authority that had moved to integrated health and social care adult teams. The second workshop was made up of groups of senior managers, frontline managers and practitioners from adult and children's services in one local authority.

Workshops with managers discussed a set of questions that focused on expectations – what senior managers and staff expect of frontline managers, and what managers think is expected of them – and experiences – what senior managers and staff consider they get from frontline managers.

Twenty-six semi-structured interviews were held with individual managers in the Midlands and north east of England. Additional material from managers was gathered with the help of the BBC in preparing audio and video cassettes for use by students of the course. Material from these interviews and workshops is used throughout this book and is referred to as 'manager consultations'.

Finally, three managers were asked to keep written diaries of their work for several weeks, and one manager kept an audio diary over a period of several months. These are all drawn on in both course books.

Some managers and service users continued their involvement with the development of the course by becoming critical readers of course materials.

References

Achebe, C. (2000) quoted in Jaggi, M., 'Storyteller of the savannah', *The Guardian*, 18 November. [Ch. 12]

Adams, J. (1999) 'The last years of the workhouse', in Bornat, J., Perks, R., Thompson, P. and Walmsley, J. (eds) *Oral History, Health and Welfare*, London, Routledge. [Ch. 12]

Aldgate, J. (2001) 'Safeguarding and promoting the welfare of children living with their families', in Cull, L.-A. and Roche, J. (eds) *The Law and Social Work – Contemporary Issues for Practice*, pp. 31–42, Basingstoke, Palgrave/ The Open University (Set Book for K269 *Social Care, Social Work and the Law: England and Wales*). [Ch. 1]

Aldgate, J. and Bradley, M. (1999) *Supporting Families through Short Term Fostering*, London, The Stationery Office. [Ch. 2]

Aldgate, J. and Tunstill, J. (1995) *Making Sense of Section 17*, London, HMSO. [Ch. 1]

Aldridge, M. (1994) *Making Social Work News*, London, Routledge. [Ch. 8]

Allsop, J. and Mulcahy, L. (1998) 'Maintaining professional identity: doctors' responses to complaints', *Sociology of Health and Illness*, Vol. 20, No. 6, pp. 802–24. [Ch. 8]

Altman, I. (1975) *The Environment and Social Behaviour*, Monterey, CA, Brooks/ Cole. [Ch. 6]

Annie E. Casey Foundation (1995) *Getting Smart, Getting Real: Using Research and Evaluation Information to Improve Policies and Programs*, Baltimore, Annie E. Casey Foundation. www.aecf.org/publications [accessed July 2002] [Ch. 11]

Anthony, W. A. (1993) 'Recovery from mental illness: the guiding vision of the mental health system in the 1990s', *Innovations and Research*, Vol. 2, pp. 17–24. [Ch. 9]

Arnold, J., Cooper, C. L. and Robertson, I. T. (1998) *Work Psychology. Understanding Human Behaviour in the Workplace*, London, Financial Times and Pitman. [Ch. 5]

Atkinson, D. (1998) 'Living in residential care', in Brechin, A., Walmsley, J., Katz, J. and Peace, S. (eds) *Care Matters: Concepts, Practice and Research in Health and Social Care*, London, Sage. [Ch. 7]

Atkinson, R. L., Atkinson, R. C., Smith, E. E., Bem, D. J. and Nolen-Hoeksema, S. (2000) *Hilgard's Introduction to Psychology* (13th edn), London, Harcourt College Publishers. [Ch. 9]

Audit Commission (1986) *Making a Reality of Community Care*, London, HMSO. [Ch. 7]

Audit Commission (2000a) *Getting Better All the Time: Making Benchmarking Work*, London, Audit Commission. [Ch. 3]

Audit Commission (2000b) *Charging with Care: How Councils Charge for Home Care*, London, Audit Commission. [Ch. 3]

Audit Commission/NHS (2000–1) 'Joint Reviews of Social Services', www.audit-commission.gov.uk/home [accessed April 2002] [Ch. 2]

Audit Commission/Social Services Inspectorate (1998) *Reviewing Social Services: Guiding You Through*, London, The Stationery Office. **[Ch. 7]**

Audit Commission/SSI/National Assembly for Wales (2002) *Guiding You Through: A Guide to Preparing for a Joint Review of Social Services*, February. www.joint-reviews.gov.uk [accessed July 2002] **[Ch. 7]**

Babchuk, N. and Goode, W. (1951) 'Work incentives in a self-determined work group', *American Sociological Review*, Vol. 16, pp. 679–87. **[Ch. 9]**

Baggini, J. (2000) 'Target trouble', *The Stakeholder*, Vol. 4, pp. 14–15. **[Ch. 3]**

Balloch, S., McLean, J. and Fisher, M. (eds) (1999) *Social Services: Working Under Pressure*, Bristol, Policy Press. **[Ch. 8]**

Bamford, C., Qureshi, H., Nicholas, E. and Vernon, A. (1999) *Outcomes of Social Care for Disabled People and Carers*, Outcomes in Community Care Practice No. 6, York, University of York Social Policy Research Unit. **[Ch. 2]**

Banks, S. (2001) *Ethics and Values in Social Work* (2nd edn), Basingstoke, Palgrave. **[Ch. 10]**

Barnes, M. (1999) 'Users as citizens: collective action and the local governance of welfare', *Social Policy and Administration*, Vol. 33, pp. 73–90. **[Ch. 2]**

Barnes, C. and Mercer, G. (eds) (1997) *Doing Disability Research*, Leeds, The Disability Press. **[Ch. 2]**

Barnes, M. and Bennett-Emslie, G. (1997) *'If They Would Listen ...': An Evaluation of the Fife Service User Panels*, Edinburgh, Age Concern Scotland. **[Ch. 2]**

Barry, M. and Hallett, C. (eds) (1998) *Social Exclusion and Social Work*, Lyme Regis, Russell House Publishing. **[Ch. 1]**

Bauld, L., Chesterman, J. and Judge, K. (2000) 'Measuring satisfaction with social care amongst older service users: issues from the literature', *Health and Social Care in the Community*, Vol. 8, No. 5, pp. 316–24. **[Ch. 2]**

Bauman, Z. (1993) *Postmodern Ethics*, Oxford, Blackwell. **[Ch. 10]**

Beauchamp, T. and Childress, J. (2001) *Principles of Biomedical Ethics* (5th edn), Oxford, Oxford University Press. **[Ch. 10]**

Bebbington, A. and Miles, J. (1989) 'The background of children who enter local authority care', *British Journal of Social Work*, Vol. 19, pp. 349–68. **[Ch. 1]**

Beresford, P. (2000) 'Service users' knowledge and social work theory', *British Journal of Social Work*, Vol. 30, No. 4, pp. 489–504. **[Ch. 2]**

Beresford, P. and Wilson, A. (1998) 'Social exclusion and social work: challenging the contradictions of exclusive debate', in Barry, M. and Hallett, C. (eds), pp. 85–96. **[Ch. 1]**

Beresford, P., Croft, S., Evans, C. and Harding, T. (1997) 'Quality in the personal social services: the developing role of user involvement in the UK', in Evers, A., Haverinen, R., Leichsenring, K. and Wistow, G. (eds) *Developing Quality in Personal Social Services: Concepts, Cases and Comments*, pp. 63–80, Aldershot, Ashgate. **[Ch. 7]**

Berlin, I. (1969) *Four Essays on Liberty*, Oxford, Oxford University Press. **[Ch. 10]**

Berridge, D. and Brodie, I. (1998a) 'Children's homes revisited', in Department of Health (1998b), pp. 68–70. **[Ch. 5]**

Biestek, F. (1961) *The Casework Relationship*, London, Unwin University Books. **[Ch. 10]**

Bilyard, J. (1987) *Hales Hospital, A History: Workhouse to Hospital*, Norwich, Norwich Health Authority. **[Ch. 12]**

Bilyard, J. (n.d.) *Thirty Years of Friendship: The Friends of Hales Hospital 1960–1990*. **[Ch. 12]**

Binns, A. (1993) 'Anita's story', in Walmsley, J., Reynolds, J., Shakespeare, P. and Woolfe, R. (eds) *Health, Welfare and Practice: Reflecting on Roles and Relationships*, London, Sage (K663 Reader). **[Ch. 11]**

Boaz, A., Hayden, C. and Bernard, M. (1999) *Attitudes and Aspirations of Older People: A Review of the Literature* (Department of Social Security Social Research Summary), London, DSS Social Research Branch. **[Ch. 2]**

Bolles, R. C. (1979) *Learning Theory*, New York, Holt, Rinehart and Winston. **[Ch. 9]**

Bott, A. (ed.) (1998) *Flo. Child Migrant from Liverpool*, Warwick, Plowright Press. **[Ch. 12]**

Bowder, B. (1980) *Children First*, London and Oxford, Mowbray. **[Ch. 12]**

Bowes, A. M. and Dar, N. S. (2000) 'Researching social care for minority ethnic older people: implications of some Scottish research', *British Journal of Social Work*, Vol. 30, No. 3, pp. 305–21. **[Ch. 2]**

Bradley, J. and Sutherland, V. (1995) 'Occupational stress in social services: a comparison of social workers and home help staff', *British Journal of Social Work*, Vol. 25, No. 3, pp. 313–31. **[Chs 6, 8]**

Brandon, M., Owers, M. and Black, J. (2001) *Learning How to Make Children Safer: An Analysis for the Welsh Office of Serious Child Abuse Cases in Wales*, Norwich, UEA Monographs. **[Ch. 4]**

Bray, S. and Preston-Shoot, M. (1995) *Empowering Practice in Social Care*, Buckingham, Open University Press. **[Ch. 5]**

Brechin, A. (1998) 'Introduction', in Brechin, A., Walmsley, J., Katz, J. and Peace, S. (eds) *Care Matters*, pp. 1–11, London, Sage. **[Ch. 1]**

Brigham, L., Atkinson, D., Jackson, M., Rolph, S. and Walmsley, J. (eds) (2000) *Crossing Boundaries: Continuity and Change in the History of Learning Disability*, Kidderminster, BILD Publications. **[Ch. 12]**

Bright, L. (1999) 'The abuse of older people in institutional settings: residents' and carers' stories', in Stanley, N., Manthorpe, J. and Penhale, B. (eds) *Institutional Abuse: Perspectives Across the Life Course*, pp. 191–204, London, Routledge. **[Ch. 6]**

British Quality Foundation (1998) *Guide to the Business Excellence Model*, London, BQF. **[Ch. 7]**

Brock, G. (ed.) (1998) *Necessary Goods: Our Responsibilities to Meet Others' Needs*, Lanham, Maryland, Rowman & Littlefield. **[Ch. 10]**

Brody, R. (1993) *Effectively Managing Human Service Organizations*, London, Sage. **[Ch. 5]**

Brooks, I. (1999) 'Managerialist professionalism: the destruction of a non-conforming subculture', *British Journal of Management*, Vol. 10, pp. 41–52. **[Ch. 3]**

Brown, D. (2002) 'New Care Standards body to be axed in favour of merged inspectorate', *Community Care*, 25 April, p. 16. **[Ch. 6]**

Brown, B., Crawford, P. and Darongkamas, J. (2000) 'Blurred roles and permeable boundaries: the experience of multidisciplinary working in community mental health', *Health and Social Care in the Community*, Vol. 8, No. 6, pp. 425–35. [Ch. 8]

Burrows, G. (2001) 'Making a brighter future', *Community Care*, 21–27 June, pp. 32–3. [Ch. 7]

Burton, J. (1998) *Managing Residential Care*, London, Routledge. [Chs 5, 6]

Burton, M. and Kellaway, M. (1998) *Developing and Managing High Quality Services for People with Learning Disabilities*, Aldershot, Ashgate. [Ch. 7]

Butcher, T. (2000) 'The public administration model of welfare delivery', in Davies, C., Finlay, L. and Bullman, A. (eds) *Changing Practice in Health and Social Care*, London, Sage/The Open University (K302 Reader). [Ch. 12]

Butler, J. (1992) 'Contingent foundations: feminism and the question of "post-modernism"', in Butler, J. and Scott, J. W. (eds) *Feminists Theorize the Political*, London, Routledge. [Ch. 8]

Campbell, A. (1991) 'Dependency revisited: the limits of autonomy in medical ethics', in Brazier, M. and Lobjoit, M. (eds) *Protecting the Vulnerable*, London, Routledge. [Ch. 10]

Campbell, A. (1994) 'Dependency: the foundational value in medical ethics', in Fulford, K., Gillett, G. and Soskice, J. (eds) *Medicine and Moral Reasoning*, Cambridge, Cambridge University Press. [Ch. 10]

Campbell, P. (1996) 'Challenging loss of power', in Read, J. and Reynolds, J. (eds) *Speaking Our Minds: An Anthology*, pp. 56–62, Basingstoke, Macmillan. [Ch. 2]

Carpenter, J. and Sbaraini, S. (1997) *Choice, Information and Dignity: Involving Service Users and Carers in Care Management in Mental Health*, Bristol, The Policy Press. [Ch. 2]

Causer, G. and Exworthy, M. (1999) 'Professionals as managers across the public sector', in Exworthy, M. and Halford, S. (eds) *Professionals and the New Managerialism in the Public Sector*, pp. 83–101, Buckingham, Open University Press. [Chs 1, 8]

Cheetham, J., Fuller, R., McIvor, G. and Petch, A. (1992) *Evaluating Social Work Effectiveness*, Buckingham and Philadelphia, Open University Press. [Ch. 11]

Clark, C. (2000) *Social Work Ethics*, Basingstoke, Macmillan. [Ch. 10]

Clarke, J. and Newman, J. (1993) 'Managing to survive: dilemmas of changing organizational forms in the public sector', in Deakin, N. and Page, R. (eds) *The Costs of Welfare*, pp. 46–65, Aldershot, Avebury. [Ch. 1]

Clarke, J. and Newman, J. (1997) *The Managerial State: Power, Politics and Ideology in the Remaking of Social Welfare*, London, Sage. [Chs 3, 5, 8]

Clarke, A., Hollands, J. and Smith, J. (1996) *Windows to a Damaged World: Good Practice in Communicating with People with Dementia in Homes*, London, Counsel and Care. [Ch. 6]

Clough, R. (1994) 'Being an inspector', in Clough, R. (ed.) *Insights into Inspection: The Regulation of Social Care*, London, Whiting and Birch Ltd/SCA Copublication. [Ch. 7]

Clough, R. (1998) 'Social services', in Laffin, M. (ed.) *Beyond Bureaucracy? The Professions in the Contemporary Public Sector*, Aldershot, Ashgate. [Ch. 8]

Clough, R. (1999) 'The abuse of older people in institutional settings: the role of management and regulation', in Stanley, N., Manthorpe, J. and Penhale, B. (eds) *Institutional Abuse: Perspectives Across the Life Course*, pp. 205–22, London, Routledge. **[Ch. 6]**

Cochrane, A. (1994) 'Managing change in local government', in Clarke, J., Cochrane, A. and McLaughlin, E. (eds) *Managing Social Policy*, London, Sage. **[Ch. 8]**

Cole, A. (2001) 'Going to the devil', *Health Service Journal*, 18 January, pp. 24–5. **[Ch. 8]**

Community Care (2001) 'Public concerns', 29 November–5 December, p. 5. **[Ch. 3]**

Coulshed, V. and Mullender, A. (2001) *Management in Social Work* (2nd edn), Buckingham, Palgrave. **[Chs 5, 7]**

Craig, G. (2001) *What Works in Community Development with Children?*, Ilford, Barnardos. **[Ch. 11]**

Crepaz-Keay, D. (1996) 'Who do you represent?', in Read, J. and Reynolds, J. (eds) *Speaking Our Minds: An Anthology*, pp. 184–5, Basingstoke, Macmillan. **[Ch. 2]**

Cutler, T. and Waine, B. (1997) *Managing the Welfare State: Text and Sourcebook*, Oxford, Berg. **[Ch. 3]**

Cutler, T. and Waine, B. (2000) 'Managerialism reformed? New Labour and public sector management', *Social Policy and Administration*, Vol. 34, pp. 318–32. **[Ch. 3]**

Davies, C. (1995) *Gender and the Professional Predicament in Nursing*, Buckingham, Open University Press. **[Ch. 8]**

Davies, C. (1996) 'The gender of professions and the profession of gender', *Sociology*, Vol. 30, No. 4, pp. 661–78. **[Ch. 8]**

Davies, C. (2000) 'Care and the transformation of professionalism', in Davies, C., Finlay, L. and Bullman, A. (eds) *Changing Practice in Health and Social Care*, pp. 343–54, London, Sage/The Open University (K302 Reader). **[Ch. 8]**

Davies, M. (ed.) (2000) *The Blackwell Encyclopaedia of Social Work*, Oxford, Blackwell. **[Ch. 9]**

Davis, M. (1999) *Ethics and the University*, London, Routledge. **[Ch. 10]**

Davis, J., Rendell, P. and Sims, D. (1999) 'The joint practitioner – a new concept in professional training', *Journal of Interprofessional Care*, Vol. 13, No. 4, pp. 395–404. **[Ch. 2]**

Dawson, A. (1994) 'Professional codes of practice and ethical conduct', *Journal of Applied Philosophy*, Vol. 11, No. 2, pp. 145–53. **[Ch. 10]**

de Winter, M. (ed.) (1997) *Children as Fellow Citizens*, London, Radcliffe Medical Press. **[Ch. 2]**

Department of Health (1991a) *The Children Act 1989 Guidance and Regulations, Volume 3, Family Placements*, London, HMSO. **[Ch. 2]**

Department of Health (1991b) *Working Together in Child Protection*, London, HMSO. **[Ch. 4]**

Department of Health (1992) *National Assistance Act 1948 (Choice of Accommodation) Directions 1992*, Local Authority Circular, London, Department of Health. **[Ch. 4]**

Department of Health (1996) *Directions: A Directory of Agencies which Provide Information or Advocacy to Disabled People in England and Wales*, London, Department of Health. **[Ch. 11]**

Department of Health (1998a) *Modernising Social Services: Promoting Independence, Improving Protection, Raising Standards*, Cm. 4169, London, The Stationery Office. **[Chs 1, 3, 7, 8, 11]**

Department of Health (1998b) *Caring for Children Away from Home*: Messages from Research, London, John Wiley. **[Ch. 5]**

Department of Health (1998c) *Quality Protects: Transforming Children's Services*, London, Department of Health.
www.doh.gov.uk/quality.htm [accessed July 2002] **[Ch. 7]**

Department of Health (1998d) *Objectives for Social Services for Children*, London, The Stationery Office. **[Ch. 7]**

Department of Health (1999a) *The Health Act 1999*, London, The Stationery Office. **[Ch. 1]**

Department of Health (1999b) *Fit for the Future? National Required Standards for Residential and Nursing Homes for Older People*, Consultation document, London, The Stationery Office. **[Chs 1, 6]**

Department of Health (1999c) *Caring about Carers: A National Strategy for Carers*, London, The Stationery Office. **[Ch. 2]**

Department of Health (1999d) *Mental Health: Modern Standards and Service Models*, National Service Frameworks series, London, Department of Health. **[Ch. 7]**

Department of Health (2000a) *The National Health Service Plan 2000: A Plan for Investment, A Plan for Reform*, Cm. 4818–1, London, The Stationery Office. **[Chs 1, 3]**

Department of Health (2000b) *A Quality Strategy for Social Care*, London, Department of Health. **[Chs 2, 3, 7]**

Department of Health (2001a) *Transforming Children's Services: An Evaluation of Local Responses to the Quality Protects Programme*, London, The Stationery Office. **[Ch. 1]**

Department of Health (2001b) *Valuing People*, London, The Stationery Office. **[Chs 2, 10]**

Department of Health (2001c) *The Children Act Now: Messages from Research*, London, The Stationery Office. **[Ch. 2]**

Department of Health (2001d) *Care Homes for Older People. National Minimum Standards*, Care Standards Act 2000, Norwich, The Stationery Office. **[Ch. 6]**

Department of Health (2001e) *Quality on the Way: A Report of an Inspection of Service Quality Improvements in Social Care*, London, Department of Health. **[Ch. 7]**

Department of Health (2001f) *The NHS Plan*, London, Department of Health. **[Ch. 11]**

Department of Health (2002a) 'Guidance on the Implementation of Regulations and National Minimum Standards by the NCSC', Letter from Jacqui Smith MP, 29 January 2002, Newcastle, National Care Standards Commission. **[Ch. 6]**

Department of Health (2002b) *National Care Standards Commission Implementation Project*, Norwich, The Stationery Office. **[Ch. 11]**

Department of Health (2002c) 'Service users' money', Standard 35, *National Minimum Standards: Care Homes for Older People*, London, The Stationery Office.
www.doh.gov.uk/ncsc [accessed July 2002] **[Ch. 11]**

Department of Health (2002d) 'Work programme', *Quality Protects*.
www.doh.gov.uk/qualityprotects/index.htm [accessed March 2002] **[Ch 11]**

Department of Health and Social Security (1989) *Caring for People: Community Care in the Next Decade and Beyond*, London, HMSO. **[Ch. 7]**

Department of Health/Social Services Inspectorate (1991) *Care Management and Assessment: Practitioners' Guide, Managers' Guide, Summary of Practice Guidance*, London, HMSO. **[Ch. 4]**

Department of Health, Social Services and Public Safety (Northern Ireland) (2002) *Children First*, Belfast, Health and Social Policy Unit. **[Ch. 7]**

Department of Social Security (1998) *Opportunity for All: Tackling Poverty and Social Exclusion*, London, The Stationery Office. **[Ch. 1]**

DHSSPS (Department of Health, Social Services and Public Safety) (1999) *Fit for the Future – A New Approach*, London, The Stationery Office. **[Ch. 3]**

Digby, A. (1978) *Pauper Palaces*, London, Routledge & Kegan Paul. **[Ch. 12]**

Dimmock, B. (2002) *The Integration of Health and Social Care: Implications for the Provision of Awards and Qualifications in Higher Education*, Unpublished paper, Milton Keynes, School of Health and Social Welfare, The Open University. **[Ch. 1]**

Dominelli, L. (1996) 'Deprofessionalizing social work: anti-oppressive practice, competencies and postmodernism', *British Journal of Social Work*, Vol. 26, pp. 153–75. **[Ch. 8]**

Dominelli, L. (1998) 'Anti-oppressive practice in context', in Adams, R., Dominelli, L. and Payne, M. (eds) *Social Work: Themes, Issues and Critical Debates*, pp. 3–22, London, Macmillan. **[Ch. 9]**

Donabedian, A. (1980) *Explorations in Quality: Assessment and Monitoring, Volume I. The Definition of Quality and Approaches to Its Assessment*, Ann Arbor, University of Michigan. **[Ch. 7]**

Doyal, L. and Gough, I. (1991) *A Theory of Human Need*, Basingstoke, Macmillan. **[Ch. 10]**

du Gay, P. (1996) 'Organising identity, entrepreneurial governance and public management', in Hall, S. and du Gay, P. (eds) *Questions of Cultural Identity*, London, Sage. **[Ch. 8]**

Dunnachie, H. (1992) 'Approaches to quality systems', in Kelly, D. and Warr, B. (eds) *Quality Counts: Achieving Quality in Social Care Services*, London, Whiting and Birch/SCA Copublication. **[Ch. 7]**

Dustin, D. (2000) 'Managers and professionals: another perspective on partnership', *Managing Community Care*, Vol. 8, No. 5, pp. 14–20. **[Ch. 8]**

Edwards, M. (2000) *Partnership Arrangements Under the Health Act 1999 and Care Trusts – Main Features and Implications*, London, King's Fund. **[Ch. 3]**

Ells, P. and Dehn, G. (2001) 'Whistleblowing: public concern at work', in Cull, L.-A. and Roche, J. (eds) *The Law and Social Work: Contemporary Issues for Practice*, Basingstoke, Palgrave/The Open University. **[Ch. 4]**

Evans, C. (1999) 'Gaining our voice: the developing pattern of good practice in service user involvement', *Managing Community Care*, Vol. 7, Issue 2, pp. 7–13. [Ch. 2]

Evans, C. and Fisher, M. (1999) 'Collaborative evaluation with service users', in Shaw, I. and Lishman, J. (eds) *Evaluation and Social Work Practice*, pp. 101–17, London, Sage. [Ch. 2]

Fajerman, L., Jarrett, M. and Sutton, F. (2000) *Children as Planning Partners: A Training Resource to Support Consultation with Children*, London, Save the Children. [Ch. 11]

Farber, B. A. (1983) *Stress and Burnout in the Human Service Professions*, Oxford, Pergamon. [Ch. 9]

Farrell, C. M. and Morris, J. (1999) 'Professional perceptions of bureaucratic change in the public sector: GPs, head teachers and social workers', *Public Money and Management*, Vol. 19, December, pp. 31–6. [Ch. 3]

Faulkner, A. and Layzell, S. (2000) *Strategies for Living: A Report of User-Led Research into People's Strategies for Living with Mental Distress*, London, Mental Health Foundation. [Ch. 2]

Feinberg, J. (1973) *Social Philosophy*, London, Prentice-Hall. [Ch. 10]

Feinberg, J. (1984) *Harm to Others*, Oxford, Oxford University Press. [Ch. 10]

Feinberg, J. (1986) *Harm to Self*, Oxford, Oxford University Press. [Ch. 10]

Flekkoy, M. G. (1991) *A Voice for Children*, London, Jessica Kingsley. [Ch. 2]

Foster, P. and Wilding, P. (2000) 'Whither welfare professionalism?', *Social Policy and Administration*, Vol. 34, No. 2, pp. 143–59. [Chs. 3, 8]

Foucault, M. (1973) *The Order of Things: An Archaeology of the Human Sciences*, London, Tavistock. [Ch. 9]

Foucault, M. (1980) *Power/Knowledge: Selected Interviews and Other Writings*, New York, Harvester Wheatsheaf. [Ch. 9]

Franklin, A. and Madge, N. (2000) *In Our View: Children, Teenagers and Parents Talk about Services for Young People*, London, National Children's Bureau. [Ch. 11]

Friedman, M. (2001) 'Results based accountability meets community strategy', Paper given at Lessons From America conference, Scunthorpe, 29 June. [Ch. 11]

Fryer, D. (1986) 'Employment deprivation and personal agency during employment', *Social Behaviour*, Vol. 1, pp. 3–39. [Ch. 9]

Fryer, D. (1987) 'Editors introduction', in Fryer, D. and Ullah, P. (eds) *Unemployed People: Social and Psychological Perspectives*, pp. ix–xiii, Buckingham, Open University Press. [Ch. 9]

General Social Care Council (GSCC) (2002a) *Standards and Values Expected of Employees and Employers (Draft Standards)*, London, GSCC. [Ch. 1]

General Social Care Council (GSCC) (2002b) *The Draft Code of Conduct for Social Care Workers*.
www.codes-consultation.co.uk [accessed July 2002] [Ch. 10]

Geraghty, W. and Meddings, S. (1999) 'Lesbian, gay and bisexual issues in systemic therapy: reflections on the wider context', *Context*, Vol. 45, pp. 11–14. [Ch. 9]

Giddens, A. (1999) *Runaway World*, Reith Lectures, London, BBC. www.news.bbc.co.uk/hi/english/static/events/reith_99/week4/week4.htm [accessed March 2002]. **[Ch. 1]**

Gillon, R. (1986) *Philosophical Medical Ethics*, Chichester, Wiley. **[Ch. 10]**

Gillon, R. (1994) *Principles of Health Care Ethics*, Chichester, Wiley. **[Ch. 10]**

Glendinning, C., Halliwell, S., Jacobs, S., Rummery, K. and Tyrer, J. (2000) 'Bridging the gap: using direct payments to purchase integrated care', *Health and Social Care in the Community*, Vol. 8, No. 3, pp. 192–200. **[Ch. 3]**

Goffman, E. (1961) *Encounters: Two Studies in the Sociology of Interaction*, Indianapolis, The Bobbs-Merrill Co. Inc. **[Ch. 6]**

Goffman, E. (1969) *The Presentation of Self in Everyday Life*, London, Penguin. **[Chs 6, 9]**

Government Statistical Service (1998) *Community Care Statistics 1997: Day and Domiciliary Personal Social Services for Adults, England*, Statistical Bulletin, London, Department of Health. **[Ch. 3]**

Gray, A., Banks, S., Carpenter, J., Green, E. and May, T. (1999) *Professionalism and the Management of Local Authorities*, Durham, University of Durham, Centre for Public Management Research. **[Ch. 8]**

Green, T. (1986) 'Liberal legislation and freedom of contract' (first published 1882), in Harris, P. and Murrow, J. (eds) *T. H. Green: Lectures on the Principles of Political Obligation and Other Writings*, Cambridge, Cambridge University Press. **[Ch. 10]**

Greig, R. (2000) 'Promoting effective service user engagement for people with learning difficulties', *Managing Community Care*, Vol. 8, Issue 1, pp. 44–7. **[Ch. 2]**

Hales, C. (1993) *Managing through Organisation*, London, Routledge. **[Ch. 5]**

Hall, S. (1996) 'Introduction: who needs "identity?",' in Hall, S. and du Gay, P. (eds) *Questions of Cultural Identity*, London, Sage. **[Ch. 8]**

Handy, C. (1993 and 1999) *Understanding Organizations* (4th edn and 4th edn revised), Harmondsworth, Penguin. **[Ch. 5]**

Handy, C. (1995) *Inside Organisations*, London, BBC Books. **[Ch. 5]**

Hanmer, J. and Statham, D. (1988) *Women and Social Work: Towards a Woman-Centred Practice*, London, Macmillan. **[Ch. 8]**

Harding, T. (1996) *The Standards We Expect: What Service Users Want from Social Services Workers*, London, National Institute for Social Work. www.elsc.org.uk/users_carers_floor/standards/ [accessed August 2002] **[Ch. 9]**

Harding, T. and Oldman, H. (1996) *Involving Service Users and Carers in Local Services: Guidelines for Social Services Departments and Others*, London, National Institute for Social Work/Thames Ditton, Surrey Social Services Department. **[Ch. 2]**

Hardy, B. and Wistow, G. (1997) 'Quality assured or quality compromised? Developing domiciliary care markets in Britain', in Evers, A., Haverinen, R., Leichsenring, K. and Wistow, G. (eds) *Developing Quality in Personal Social Services: Concepts, Cases and Comments*, Aldershot, Ashgate. **[Ch. 7]**

Hardy, B., Turrell, A. and Wistow, G. (1992) *Innovations in Community Care Management*, Aldershot, Avebury. **[Ch. 5]**

Hardy, B., Young, R. and Wistow, G. (1999) 'Dimensions of choice in the assessment and care management process: the views of older people, carers and care managers', *Health and Social Care in the Community*, Vol. 7, pp. 483–91. [Ch. 3]

Hasenfeld, Y. (1983) *Human Services Organisations*, Englewood Cliffs, NJ, Prentice-Hall. [Ch. 5]

Hatton, C., Azmi, S., Caine, A. and Emerson, E. (1998) 'Informal carers of adolescents and adults with learning difficulties from the South Asian communities: family circumstances, service support and carer stress', *British Journal of Social Work*, Vol. 28, No. 6, pp. 821–37. [Ch. 2]

Hemmings, S. and Morris, J. (1997) *Community Care and Disabled People's Rights: Training Project (NISW Briefing 22)*, London, National Institute for Social Work. [Ch. 2]

Henderson, J. and Seden, J. (2000) *What Do We Really Want from Social Care Managers? Aspirations and Realities*, Paper presented to Dilemmas 2000 International Conference, 1–3 September, University of East London. [Ch. 5]

Henderson, J. and Seden, J. (2003) 'What do we want from social care managers? Aspirations and realities', in Reynolds *et al.*, pp. 85–94 (K303 Reader). [Ch. 3]

Henwood, M. and Hudson, B. (2000) *Partnerships and the NHS Plan – Cooperation or Coercion? The Implications for Social Care*, Leeds, Nuffield Institute for Health Community Care Divisions. [Ch. 3]

Himmelfarb, G. (1995) *The De-moralization of Society. From Victorian Virtues to Modern Values*, London, IEA Health and Welfare Unit. [Ch. 10]

Hoggett, P. (1991) 'A new management for the public sector?', *Policy and Politics*, Vol. 19, pp. 243–56. [Ch. 12]

Holman, B. (1998) 'Neighbourhoods and exclusion', in Barry, M. and Hallett, C. (eds), pp. 62–73. [Ch. 1]

Home Office (1998a) *The Human Rights Act*, London, The Stationery Office. [Ch. 1]

Home Office (1998b) *Getting It Right Together: Compact on Relations Between Government and the Voluntary and Community Sector in England*, Cm. 4100, London, The Stationery Office. [Ch. 3]

Home Office (1999) *The Stephen Lawrence Inquiry: Report of an Inquiry by Sir William Macpherson of Cluny*, London, The Stationery Office. [Ch. 1]

Home Office (2000a) *Race Relations (Amendment) Act*, London, The Stationery Office. [Ch. 1]

Home Office (2000b) *Human Rights Act: An Introduction*, London, Home Office Communication Directorate. [Ch. 4]

Hood, C. (1991) 'A public management for all seasons?', *Public Administration*, Vol. 69, Spring, pp. 3–19. [Ch. 11]

Howe, D. (1992) 'Child abuse and the bureaucratisation of social work', *Sociological Review*, Vol. 40, No. 3, pp. 491–508. [Ch. 8]

Hudson, B., Hardy, B., Henwood, M. and Wistow, G. (1999) 'In pursuit of inter-agency collaboration in the public sector: what is the contribution of theory and research?', *Public Management*, Vol. 1, No. 2, pp. 235–60. [Ch. 5]

Humphries, B. (1996) *Critical Perspectives on Empowerment*, Birmingham, Ventura Press. [Ch. 5]

Husband, C. (1995) 'The morally active practitioner and the ethics of anti-racist social work', in Hugman, R. and Smith, D. (eds) *Ethical Issues in Social Work*, London, Routledge. [Ch. 10]

Jahoda, M. (1982) *Employment and Unemployment*, Cambridge, Cambridge University Press. [Ch. 9]

James, A. (1992) 'Quality and its social construction by managers in care service organisations', in Kelly, D. and Warr, B. (eds) *Quality Counts: Achieving Quality in Social Care Services*, London, Whiting and Birch/SCA Copublication. [Ch. 7]

James, A. (1994a) *Managing to Care*, London, Longman. [Ch. 5]

James, A. (1994b) 'Reflections on the politics of quality', in Connor, A. and Black, S. (eds) *Performance Review and Quality in Social Care*, pp. 200–14, London, Jessica Kingsley. [Ch. 7]

Jones, C. (1999) 'Social work, regulation and managerialism', in Exworthy, M. and Haldord, S. (eds) *Professionals and the New Managerialism in the Public Sector*, Buckingham, Open University Press. [Ch. 8]

Jordan, B. (1989) 'Review of David Howe: an introduction to social work theory', *Journal of Social Policy*, Vol. 18, No. 3, pp. 462–3. [Ch. 9]

Jordanova, L. (2000) *History in Practice*, London, Arnold. [Ch. 12]

Joseph Rowntree Foundation (1998a) *Deaf People from Minority Ethnic Groups: Initiatives and Services (Findings 818)*, York, Joseph Rowntree Foundation. [Ch. 2]

Joseph Rowntree Foundation (1998b) *Deaf and Hearing People Working Together in Statutory Organizations (Findings 428)*, York, Joseph Rowntree Foundation. [Ch. 2]

Joseph Rowntree Foundation (1998c) *The Experiences of Mental Health Service Service Users as Mental Health Professionals (Findings 488)*, York, Joseph Rowntree Foundation. [Ch. 2]

Joseph Rowntree Foundation (1999) *Evaluation of the National Service User Involvement Project (Findings 129)*, York, Joseph Rowntree Foundation. [Ch. 2]

Judd, S., Marshall, M. and Phippen, P. (1997) *Design for Dementia*, London, Hawker Publications Limited. [Ch. 6]

Kakabadse, A., Ludlow, R. and Vinnicombe, C. (1988) *Working in Organisations*, Harmondsworth, Penguin. [Ch. 5]

Kellaher, L. A. (2000) *A Choice Well Made: 'Mutuality' as a Governing Principle in Residential Care*, London, Centre for Policy on Ageing/Methodist Homes. [Ch. 6]

Kenny, D., Pettitt, G., Brooker, M., Marshall, G., Kinniburgh, J., Field, S., Chell, M., Barer, R. and Stanton, R. (2000) *Social Care in London 3: Trends in Social Services' Activity 1993–1998*, London, London Research Centre. [Ch. 3]

Kepner, J. I. (1987) *Body Process: Working with the Body in Psychotherapy*, San Francisco, CA, Jossey-Bass. [Ch. 9]

King, M. and Trowell, J. (1992) *Children's Welfare and the Law: The Limits of Legal Intervention*, London, Sage. [Ch. 4]

Kitchener, M., Kirkpatrick, I. and Whipp, R. (2000) 'Supervising professional practice under new public management: evidence from an invisible trade', *British Journal of Management*, Vol. 11, No. 3, pp. 213–26. **[Ch. 5]**

Kluckhohn, F. and Strodtbeck, F. L. (1961) *Variations in Value Orientations*, Connecticut, Greenwood Press. **[Ch. 9]**

Knapp, M. (1984) *The Economics of Social Care*, London, Macmillan. **[Ch. 11]**

Knuttson, K. E. (1997) *Children: Noble Causes or Worthy Citizens?*, Florence, Arena and UNICEF. **[Ch. 2]**

La Valle, I. and Lyons, K. (1996) 'The social worker speaks: the management of change in the personal social services', *Practice*, Vol. 8, No. 3, pp. 5–14. **[Ch. 8]**

Laffin, M. (ed.) (1998) *Beyond Bureaucracy? The Professions in the Contemporary Public Sector*, Aldershot, Ashgate. **[Ch. 8]**

Land, N. (1990) *Victorian Workhouse: A Study of the Bromsgrove Union Workhouse 1836–1901*, Studley, Brewin Books. **[Ch. 12]**

Langan, M. (ed.) (1998) *Welfare: Needs, Rights and Risks*, London, Routledge/ The Open University. **[Ch. 10]**

Le Grand, J. (1990) *Quasi Markets and Social Policy*, School of Advanced Urban Studies, Bristol, University of Bristol. **[Ch. 3]**

Learning Disability Advisory Group (2001) *Fulfilling the Promises: Proposals for a Framework of Services for People with Learning Disabilities*, Cardiff, National Assembly for Wales. **[Ch. 2]**

Leat, D. and Perkins, D. (1998) 'Juggling and dealing: the creative work of care package purchasing', *Social Policy and Administration*, Vol. 32, No. 2, pp. 155–81. **[Ch. 8]**

Ledger, S. (2000) *Quality Network 2000 in Kensington and Chelsea*, Unpublished report, Royal Borough of Kensington and Chelsea. **[Ch. 7]**

Levitas, R. (1997) 'Discourses of social inclusion and integration: from the European Union to New Labour', Paper presented at the European Sociological Conference, University of Essex, August. **[Ch. 1]**

Levy, A. and Kahan, B. (1991) *The Pindown Experience and the Protection of Children: The Report of the Staffordshire Child Care Inquiry 1990*, Staffordshire County Council. **[Chs 1, 9]**

Lewin, K. (1936) *Principles of Topological Psychology*, New York, McGraw-Hill. **[Ch. 6]**

Lewin, K. (1947) 'Frontiers in group dynamics: concept, method and reality in social science; social equilibria and social change', *Human Relations*, Vol. 1, pp. 5–41. **[Ch. 9]**

Lewis, G. (2000) *'Race', Gender, Social Welfare: Encounters in a Postcolonial Society*, Oxford, Polity. **[Ch. 8]**

Lewis, G. and Gunaratnam, Y. (2000) 'Negotiating "race" and space: spatial practices, identity and power in narratives of health and social welfare professionals', Paper presented to the Social Policy Association Conference, 19 July, Roehampton. **[Ch. 6]**

Lindow, V. (1996) *Service User Involvement: Community Service Users as Consultants and Trainers*, Leeds, NHS Executive Community Care Branch. **[Ch. 2]**

Lindow, V. and Morris, J. (1995) *Service User Involvement: Synthesis of Findings and Experience in the Field of Community Care*, York, Joseph Rowntree Foundation. [Ch. 2]

Ling, T. (2000) 'Unpacking partnership health care', in Clarke, J., Gerwitz, S. and McLaughlin, E. W. (eds) *New Managerialism, New Welfare?*, Milton Keynes, The Open University/Sage Publications. [Ch. 3]

Lipsky, M. (1980) *Street-Level Bureaucracy*, New York, Russell Sage Foundation. [Ch. 5]

Lister, R. (1998) 'In from the margins: citizenship, inclusion and exclusion', in Barry, M. and Hallett, C. (eds), pp. 26 38. [Ch. 1]

Little, J. (1898) *The Poor Law: Comprising the Law Relating to the Poor Law Authorities: The Relief of the Poor, Including Pauper Lunatics, the Settlement and Removal of the Poor by John Frederick Archbold*, London, Shaw and Sons. [Ch. 12]

Loney, M., Bocock, R., Clarke, J., Cochrane, A., Graham, P. and Wilson, M. (1991) *The State or the Market: Politics and Welfare in Contemporary Britain. A Reader* (2nd edn), London, Sage/The Open University (Set Book for D211 *Social Problems and Social Welfare*). [Ch. 1]

Mackay, L. (1993) *Conflicts in Care: Medicine and Nursing*, London, Chapman & Hall. [Ch. 8]

Marshall, M. (2001) 'Dementia and technology', in Peace, S. M. and Holland, C. (eds) *Inclusive Housing in an Ageing Society*, pp. 125–44, Bristol, The Policy Press. [Ch. 6]

Martin, L. and Kettner, P. (1996) *Measuring the Performance of Human Service Programs*, Thousand Oaks, CA, Sage Publications. [Ch. 11]

Martin, V. and Henderson, E. (2001) *Managing in Health and Social Care*, London, Routledge/The Open University (B630 Set Book). [Chs 5, 7, 9]

Maslow, A. (1970) *Motivation and Personality*, New York, Harper & Row. [Ch. 10]

May, T. and Buck, M. (2000) 'Social work, professionalism and the rationality of organisational change', in Malin, N. (ed.) *Professionalism, Boundaries and the Workplace*, London, Routledge. [Ch. 8]

Mayo, E. (1933) *The Human Problems of an Industrialised Civilisation*, New York, Macmillan. [Ch. 5]

McCann, I. L. and Pearlman, L. A. (1990) 'Vicarious traumatisation: a framework for understanding the psychological effects of working with victims', *Journal of Traumatic Stress*, Vol. 3, pp. 131–49. [Ch. 9]

McCurry, P. (2001) 'Room for manoeuvre?', *Community Care*, 18–24 January, pp. 26–7. [Ch. 6]

McDonald, A. (2001) 'Care in the community', in Cull, L.-A. and Roche, J. (eds) *The Law and Social Work – Contemporary Issues for Practice*, pp. 146–54, Basingstoke, Palgrave/The Open University (Set Book for K269 *Social Care, Social Work and the Law: England and Wales*). [Ch. 1]

McHarron, A. and Nettles, M. (1999) *Payments to Service Users*, Birmingham, Partnerships in Mental Health. [Ch. 2]

McIntosh, B. and Whittaker, A. (2000) *Unlocking the Future: Developing New Lifestyles with People Who Have Complex Disabilities*, London, King's Fund. [Ch. 2]

Meddings, S. and Perkins, R. (2002) 'What "getting better" means to staff and users of a rehabilitation service: an exploratory study', *Journal of Mental Health*, Vol. 11, No. 4, pp. 319–25. **[Ch. 9]**

Mintzberg, H. (1981) 'Organisation design: fashion or fit?', *Harvard Business Review*, January/February, pp. 103–16. **[Ch. 5]**

Mintzberg, H. (1992) 'Structuring of organisations', in Mintzberg, H. and Quinn, J. B. (eds) *The Strategy Process*, London, Prentice Hall. **[Ch. 5]**

Mintzberg, H. (1994) *The Rise and Fall of Strategic Planning*, London, Prentice Hall. **[Ch. 5]**

Moore, T., Rapp, C. and Roberts, B. (2000) 'Improving child welfare performance through supervisory use of client outcome data', *Child Welfare*, Vol. 79, No. 5, pp. 475–98. **[Ch. 11]**

Morgan, G. (1997) *Images of Organisation*, London, Sage. **[Ch. 5]**

Morris, J. (1991) *Pride Against Prejudice*, London, The Women's Press. **[Ch. 1]**

Morris, J. (1994) 'The shape of things to come? Service user-led social services', *Social Services Policy Forum Paper No. 3*, London, National Institute for Social Work. **[Ch. 2]**

Morris, J. (1995) 'Creating a space for absent voices: disabled women's experiences of receiving assistance with daily living activities', *Feminist Review*, Vol. 51, pp. 68–93. **[Ch. 1]**

Morris, J. (1997) *Encouraging Service User Involvement in Commissioning: A Resource for Commissioners* (produced for NHS Executive on behalf of the National Service User Involvement Project), London, Department of Health. **[Ch. 2]**

National Assembly for Wales (2000) *Working Together to Safeguard Children. A Guide to Interagency Working to Safeguard and Promote the Welfare of Children*, Cardiff, National Assembly for Wales. **[Ch. 7]**

NHS (2001) '6.1 Plans and evaluations', *NHS Performance Fund: Guidance for 2001/2001*.
www.doh.gov.uk/nhsperformance/perffund [accessed March 2002] **[Ch. 11]**

Nocon, A. and Qureshi, H. (1996) *Outcomes of Community Care for Users and Carers*, Buckingham and Philadelphia, Open University Press. **[Ch. 11]**

Nolan, Y. (1998) *Care: NVQ Level 2*, Oxford, Heinemann. **[Ch. 9]**

Norfolk Federation of Women's Institutes (1972) *Within Living Memory: A Collection of Norfolk Reminiscences*, Northgate, Blackburn Times Press. **[Ch. 12]**

Norfolk Record Office (1932) Ref. no. N/TC 52/41, Eaton Grange files 1, 2 and 3. **[Ch. 12]**

Norfolk Record Office (1948) c/ss 2/5 East Anglian Regional Hospital Board Committee Minutes, 30 September. **[Ch. 12]**

North Lincolnshire Council (2002) 'Principles and objectives', *Children and Families Services*.
www.northlincs.gov.uk [accessed August 2002] **[Ch. 11]**

O'Halloran, K. (1999) *The Welfare of the Child: The Principle and the Law*, Aldershot, Ashgate/Arena. **[Ch. 4]**

Oliver, C. and Aggleton, P. (2000) *Coram's Children. Growing up in the Care of the Foundling Hospital, 1900–1955*, London, Thomas Coram Research Unit. **[Ch. 12]**

Onyett, S., Pillinger, T. and Muijen, M. (1995) *Making Community Mental Health Teams Work*, London, Sainsbury Centre for Mental Health. **[Ch. 9]**

Onyett, S., Pillinger, T. and Muijen, M. (1997) 'Job satisfaction and burnout among members of community mental health teams', *Journal of Mental Health*, Vol. 6, pp. 55–66. **[Ch. 9]**

The Open University (1992) D212 *Running the Country*, Unit 16, *Running Hospitals: The Rise and Fall of Planning*, Milton Keynes, The Open University. **[Ch. 11]**

Oppen, M. (1997) 'Towards a new client orientation through continuous improvement', in Evers, A., Haverinen, R., Leichsenring, K. and Wistow, G. (eds) *Developing Quality in Personal Social Services: Concepts, Cases and Comments*, Aldershot, Ashgate. **[Ch. 7]**

Osburne, D. and Gaebler, T. (1993) *Reinventing Government: How the Entrepreneurial Spirit Is Transforming the Public Sector*, New York, Plume. **[Ch. 11]**

Oxley, G. W. (1974) *Poor Relief in England and Wales, 1601–1834*, Newton Abbot, David and Charles. **[Ch. 12]**

Parker, R., Ward, H., Jackson, S., Aldgate, J. and Wedge, P. (1991) *Looking After Children. Assessing Outcomes in Child Care: The Report of an Independent Working Party Established by the Department of Health*, London, HMSO. **[Ch. 11]**

Parry, N. and Parry, J. (1979) 'Social work, professionalism and the state', in Parry, N., Rustin, M. and Satyamurti, C. (eds) *Social Work, Welfare and the State*, London, Edward Arnold. **[Ch. 8]**

Parton, N. (1994) '"Problematics of government", (post) modernity and social work', *British Journal of Social Work*, Vol. 24, No. 1, pp. 9–32. **[Ch. 7]**

Parton, N. (1998) 'Risk, advanced liberalism and child welfare: the need to rediscover uncertainty and ambiguity', *British Journal of Social Work*, Vol. 28, No. 1, pp. 5–27. **[Ch. 10]**

Parton, N. (2000) 'Some thoughts on the relationship between theory and practice in and for social work', *British Journal of Social Work*, Vol. 30, No. 4, pp. 449–64. **[Ch. 10]**

Pattison, S. (1997) *The Faith of the Managers: When Management Becomes Religion*, London, Cassell. **[Ch. 7]**

Pattison, S. (1998) 'Questioning values', *Health Care Analysis*, Vol. 6, No. 4, pp. 352–9. **[Ch. 10]**

Payne, M. (1991) *Modern Social Work Theory*, Basingstoke, Macmillan. **[Ch. 9]**

Peace, S. (1998) 'Caring in place', in Brechin, A., Walmsley, J., Katz, J. and Peace, S. (eds) *Care Matters*, London, Sage Publications. **[Ch. 6]**

Peace, S. M. (2000) 'Residential care for adults', *Research Matters*, October 2000–April 2001, pp. 30–2. **[Ch. 5]**

Peace, S., Kellaher, L. and Willcocks, D. (1997) *Re-evaluating Residential Care*, Buckingham, Open University Press. **[Ch. 6]**

Pearn, M., Roderick, C. and Mulrooney, C. (1997) *Learning Organizations in Practice*, Maidenhead, McGraw-Hill Europe. **[Ch. 1]**

Perkins, R. E. and Repper, J. M. (1996) *Working Alongside People with Long Term Mental Health Problems*, Cheltenham, Stanley Thornes. **[Ch. 9]**

Perkins, R. and Repper, J. (1998) *Dilemmas in Community Mental Health Practice: Choice or Control*, Abingdon, Radcliffe Medical Press. [Ch. 9]

Peters, T. and Waterman, R. H. (1988) *In Search of Excellence: Lessons from America's Best Run Companies*, New York, Harper & Row. [Ch. 7]

Pfeffer, J. and Salancik, G. R. (1978) *The External Control of Organisations: A Resource Dependence Perspective*, London, Harper & Row. [Ch. 5]

Piggott, J. and Piggott, G. (1992) 'Total Quality Management (TQM): the way ahead', in Kelly, D. and Warr, B. (eds) *Quality Counts: Achieving Quality in Social Care Services*, London, Whiting and Birch/SCA Copublication. [Ch. 7]

Pinkney, S. (2000) 'Anti-oppressive theory and practice in social work', in Davies, C., Finlay, L. and Bullman, A. (eds) *Changing Practice in Health and Social Care*, London, Sage/The Open University (K302 Reader). [Ch. 8]

Pinnock, M. and Garnett, L. (2002) 'Needs led or needs must: the use of needs-based information in planning children's services', in Ward, H. and Rose, W. (eds) *Approaches to Needs Assessment in Children's Services*, London, Jessica Kingsley. [Ch. 11]

Pollitt, C. (1986) *Beyond the Managerial Model: The Case for Broadening Performance Assessment in Government and the Public Services*, London, Centre for the Evaluation of Public Policy and Practice, Brunel University. [Ch. 7]

Pollitt, C. (1990) *Managerialism and the Public Services: The Anglo-American Experience*, Oxford, Basil Blackwell. [Ch. 3]

Pollitt, C. (1997) 'Business and professional approaches to quality improvement: a comparison of their suitability for the personal social services', in Evers, A., Haverinen, R., Leichsenring, K. and Wistow, G. (eds) *Developing Quality in Personal Social Services: Concepts, Cases and Comments*, Aldershot, Ashgate. [Ch. 7]

Pratt, J., Gordon, P. and Plamping, D. (1999) *Working Whole Systems: Putting Theory into Practice in Organisations*, London, King's Fund. [Ch. 8]

Priestley, M. (1998) 'Discourse and resistance in care assessment: integrated living and community care', *British Journal of Social Work*, Vol. 28, No. 5, pp. 659–74. [Ch. 2]

Quality Standards Task Group (1998) *A 'White Paper' on Quality Standards in the Voluntary Sector*, London, QSTG. [Ch. 7]

Qureshi, H. and Henwood, M. (2000) *Older People's Definitions of Quality Services*, York, Joseph Rowntree Foundation. [Ch. 2]

Qureshi, H., Patmore, C., Nicholas, E. and Bamford, C. (1998) *Overview: Outcomes of Social Care for Older People and Carers*, Outcomes in Community Care Practice Series, York, Social Policy Research Unit. [Ch. 11]

Rashid, S. (2000) 'Social work and professionalisation: a legacy of ambivalence', in Davies, C., Finlay, L. and Bullman, A. (eds) *Changing Practice in Health and Social Care*, London, Sage/The Open University (K302 Reader). [Ch. 8]

Rasmussen, B. (2001) 'Corporate strategy and gendered professional identities', *Gender, Work and Organisation*, Vol. 8, No. 3, pp. 291–310. [Ch. 8]

Raynes, N. V. (1998) 'Involving residents in quality specification', *Ageing and Society*, Vol. 18, Part 1, pp. 65–78. [Ch. 2]

Read, J. (2003) 'Mental health service users as managers', in Reynolds *et al.*, pp. 12–20 (K303 Reader). [Ch. 9]

Refugee Council (2001) *Separated Children*, London, Refugee Council and Save the Children. **[Ch. 12]**

Reid, A. (1994) *The Union Workhouse: A Study Guide for Teachers and Local Historians*, British Association for Local History, Chichester, Phillimore Press. **[Ch. 12]**

Reith, M. (1998) *Community Care Tragedies: A Practical Guide to Mental Health Inquiries*, Birmingham, Venture. **[Ch. 4]**

Reynolds, J. and Walmsley, J. (1998) 'Care, support or something else', in Brechin, A., Walmsley, J., Katz, J. and Peace, S. (eds) *Care Matters*, pp. 66–80, London, Sage. **[Ch. 1]**

Reynolds, J., Henderson, J., Seden, J., Charlesworth, J. and Bullman, A. (eds) (2003) *The Managing Care Reader*, London, Routledge (K303 Reader).

Rider Haggard, H. (1899) 'A description of Heckingham Workhouse, Suffolk', in *A Farmer's Year* (1933), London, Longmans Green and Co. **[Ch. 12]**

Riley, C. and Riley, J. (1998) 'Outcome indicators: friends or enemies?', *Managing Community Care*, Vol. 6, No. 6, December, pp. 246–53. **[Ch. 3]**

Robinson, L. (1998) 'Social work through the life course', in Adams, R., Dominelli, L. and Payne, M. (eds) *Social Work: Themes, Issues and Critical Debates*, London, Macmillan. **[Ch. 9]**

Rogers, A., Pilgrim, D. and Lacey, R. (1993) *Experiencing Psychiatry: Users' Views of Services*, London, Macmillan/Mind. **[Ch. 2]**

Rolph, S., Atkinson, D. and Walmsley, J. (2002) '"A man's job?" Gender issues and the role of Mental Welfare Officers, 1948–1970', *Oral History*, Vol. 30, No. 1, pp. 28–41. **[Ch. 12]**

Rose, D. (2001) *The Perspectives of Mental Health Service Users on Community and Hospital Care*, London, Sainsbury Centre for Mental Health. **[Ch. 2]**

Ross, D. (1996) *A Blue Coat Boy in the 1920s*, Roby, Pharaoh Press. **[Ch. 12]**

Rossi, P. and Freeman, H. (1993) *Evaluation: A Systematic Approach*, Newbury Park, CA, Sage. **[Ch. 11]**

Rouse, J. (1999) 'Performance management, quality management and contracts', in Horton, S. and Farnham, D. (eds) *Public Management in Britain*, pp. 76–93, Basingstoke, Palgrave. **[Ch. 6]**

Scanlon, T. M. (1975) 'Preference and urgency', *The Journal of Philosophy*, Vol. LXXII, No. 19, pp. 655–69. **[Ch. 10]**

Schön, D. A. (1987) *Educating the Reflective Practitioner*, Oxford, Jossey-Bass. **[Ch. 9]**

Scottish Executive (2000) *The Same as You? A Review of Services for People with Learning Disabilities*, Edinburgh, The Stationery Office. **[Ch. 2]**

Scottish Executive (2001a) *The Future of Care Homes in Scotland. A Consultation Paper*, Edinburgh, The Scottish Executive. **[Ch. 1]**

Scottish Executive (2001b) *National Care Standards* www.scotland.gov.uk/government [accessed June 2002] **[Ch. 11]**

Scottish Office (1999) *Aiming for Excellence: Modernising Social Work Services in Scotland*, Cm. 4288, Edinburgh, The Stationery Office. **[Chs 2, 3, 7]**

Scottish Office (2000a) *The Way Forward for Care – A Policy Position Paper*, Edinburgh, The Stationery Office. **[Ch. 7]**

Scottish Office (2000b) *Protecting Children – Securing Their Safety*, Edinburgh, The Stationery Office. **[Ch. 7]**

Seebohm, F. (1968) *Local Authority and Allied Personal Social Services*, Cmnd 3703, London, HMSO. [**Ch. 1**]

Senge, P. (1993) *The Fifth Discipline: The Art and Practice of the Learning Organisation*, London, Century Business. [**Ch. 11**]

Service User Engagement Project (2000) *Newsletter Winter 2000*, London, King's College London Community Care Development Centre. [**Ch. 2**]

Shakespeare, T. (2000) 'The social relations of care', in Lewis, G., Gewirtz, S. and Clarke, J. (eds) *Rethinking Social Policy*, London, Sage. (Reader for D860 *Rethinking Social Policy*) [**Chs 8, 10**]

Sheldon, B. and Chilvers, R. (2000) *Evidence-Based Social Care: A Study of Prospects and Problems*, Lyme Regis, Russell House Publishing. [**Chs 9, 11**]

Simons, K. (1998) *A Place at the Table: Involving People with Learning Difficulties in Purchasing and Commissioning Services*, Kidderminster, BILD Publications. [**Ch. 1**]

Sinclair, I., Gibbs, I. and Hicks, L. (2000) *The Management and Effectiveness of the Home Care Service*, York, University of York Social Work Research and Development Unit. [**Ch. 2**]

Social Care Institute for Excellence (SCIE) (2002) *Better Knowledge or Better Practice*. http://www.scie.org.uk/aboutscie/about.htm [accessed June 2002] [**Ch. 9**]

Social Services Committee (1990) *Community Care: Choice for Service Users*, Sixth Report, Session 1989/90, HC444, London, HMSO. [**Ch. 3**]

Social Services Inspectorate (1990) *Caring for Quality: Guidance on Standards for Residential Homes for Elderly People*, London, HMSO. [**Ch. 7**]

Social Services Inspectorate (1991a) *Purchase of Service: Practice Guidance and Practice Materials for SSDs and Other Agencies*, London, HMSO. [**Ch. 7**]

Social Services Inspectorate (1991b) *Inspecting for Quality: Guidance on Practice for Inspection Units in Social Services Departments and Other Agencies: Principles, Issues and Recommendations*, London, HMSO. [**Ch. 7**]

Social Services Inspectorate (1993) *Inspecting for Quality: Introducing the Inspection Division*, London, HMSO. [**Ch. 7**]

Social Services Inspectorate (2000) *Modern Social Services – A Commitment to People*, 9th Annual Report of the Chief Inspector of Social Services, London, Department of Health. [**Ch. 1**]

Social Services Inspectorate (2001) *Detained: SSI Inspection of Compulsory Mental Health Admissions*, CI(2001)I, London, Department of Health. [**Ch. 2**]

Social Services Inspectorate/Department of Health (2001) *Quality on the Way: A Report of an Inspection of Service Quality Improvements in Social Care*, London, Department of Health. [**Ch. 7**]

Sommer, R. T. (1969) *Personal Space: The Behavioural Basis of Design*, Englewood Cliffs, NJ, Prentice-Hall. [**Ch. 6**]

Southon, G. and Braithwaite, J. (1998) 'The end of professionalism?', *Social Science and Medicine*, Vol. 46, pp. 23–8. [**Ch. 3**]

Statham, D. (1996) *The Future of Social and Personal Care: The Role of Social Services Organisations in the Public, Private and Voluntary Sectors*, London, National Institute for Social Work. [**Ch. 1**]

Stevens, A. (2000) 'Women superintendents: the contribution of Margaret McDowall and other women managers of mental deficiency in institutions in England', *British Journal of Learning Disabilities*, Vol. 28, No. 2, pp. 71–7. **[Ch. 12]**

Stevenson, O. and Parsloe, P. (1978) *Social Service Teams: The Practitioner's View*, London, Department of Health and Social Services. **[Ch. 9]**

Stewart, J. and Walsh, K. (1992) 'Change in the management of public services', *Public Administration*, Vol. 70, pp. 499–518. **[Ch. 3]**

Swiss, J. E. (1992) 'Adapting Total Quality Management (TQM) to Government', *Public Management Review*, Vol. 52, No. 4, pp. 356–61. **[Ch. 7]**

Taylor, F. W. (1911) *Principles of Scientific Management*, New York, Harper. **[Ch. 5]**

Taylor, G. (1999) 'Empowerment, identity and participatory research: using social action research to challenge isolation for deaf and hard of hearing people from minority ethnic communities', *Disability and Society*, Vol. 14, No. 3, pp. 369–84. **[Ch. 2]**

Thornton, P. (2000) *Older People Speaking Out: Developing Opportunities for Influence*, York, Joseph Rowntree Foundation. **[Ch. 2]**

Timms, J. E. (1995) *Children's Representation: A Practitioner's Guide*, London, Sweet and Maxwell. **[Ch. 4]**

TOPSS (Training Organisation for the Personal Social Services) (1999) *Modernising the Social Care Workforce: The First National Training Strategy for England*, A consultation document.
www.topss.org.uk [accessed March 2002] **[Ch. 3]**

Trompenaars, F. (1993) *Riding the Waves of Culture: Understanding Cultural Diversity in Business*, London, Economist Books. **[Chs 1, 9]**

Tunstill, J. and Aldgate, J. (2000) *Services for Children in Need – From Policy to Practice*, London, The Stationery Office. **[Ch. 1]**

Turner, M. (2000) *Our Voice in Our Futures: Services and Support*, London, National Institute for Social Work/Shaping Our Lives. **[Ch. 2]**

Urry, A. (1990) 'The struggle towards a feminist practice in family therapy: premises', in Perelberg, R. J. and Miller, A. C. (eds) *Gender and Power in Families*, pp. 104–34, London, Routledge. **[Ch. 9]**

Utting, W. (1998) *People Like Us*, London, The Stationery Office. **[Ch. 1]**

Utting, D., Rose, W. and Pugh, G. (2001) *Better Results for Children and Families*, London, National Council for Voluntary Child Care Organisations. **[Ch. 11]**

Veitch, R. and Arkkelin, D. (1995) *Environmental Psychology: An Interdisciplinary Perspective*, London, Prentice Hall. **[Ch. 6]**

Vincent, A. and Plant, R. (1984) *Philosophy, Politics and Citizenship*, Oxford, Blackwell. **[Ch. 10]**

von Bertalanffy, L. (1971) *General Systems Theory: Foundations, Development, Application*, London, Allen Lane. **[Ch. 9]**

Ward, H. (1990) *The Charitable Relationship: Parents, Children and the Waifs and Strays Society*, Unpublished thesis, University of Bristol. **[Ch. 12]**

Ward, H., Skuse, T. and Pinnock, M. (1998) *Looking After Children: Using Data as Management Information: Interim Report to Research Advisory Group*, Unpublished report, Centre for Child and Family Research, Loughborough University. **[Ch. 11]**

Warr, P. (1987) *Work, Unemployment and Mental Health*, Oxford, Clarendon Press. **[Ch. 9]**

Warr, B. and Kelly, D. (1992) 'What is meant by quality in social care?', in Kelly, D. and Warr, B. (eds) *Quality Counts: Achieving Quality in Social Care Services*, London, Whiting and Birch/SCA Copublication. **[Ch. 7]**

Webb, S. and Webb, B. (1929) *English Poor Law History*, London, Longman. **[Ch. 1]**

Weber, M. (1947) *The Theory of Social and Economic Organization*, London, Free Press. **[Ch. 5]**

Weiner, M. E. (1994) *Human Services Management: Analysis and Applications* (2nd edn), Storrs, University of Connecticut. **[Ch. 1]**

Westwood, G. (2002) 'Promoting race equality in social care: The Race Relations (Amendment) Act 2000', Unpublished paper, Milton Keynes, School of Health and Social Welfare, The Open University. **[Ch. 1]**

Whipp, R., Kirkpatrick, I., Kitchener, M. and Owen, D. (1998) 'The external management of children's homes by local authorities', in *Caring for Children Away from Home: Messages from Research*, Chichester, Department of Health/ John Wiley & Sons. **[Ch. 6]**

Whitaker, D., Archer, L. and Hicks, L. (1998) *Working in Children's Homes. Challenges and Complexities*, Chichester, Wiley. **[Ch. 5]**

Willcocks, D., Peace, S. and Kellaher, L. (1987) *Private Lives in Public Places*, London, Tavistock Publications. **[Ch. 6]**

Wilmot, S. (1997) *The Ethics of Community Care*, London, Cassell. **[Ch. 10]**

Wilson, G. (1998) 'Neighbourhoods and exclusion', in Barry, M. and Hallet, C. (eds) *Social Exclusion and Social Work*, Lyme Regis, Russell House Publishing. **[Ch. 11]**

Wistow, G. (1991) 'Quality and research: the policy and legislative context', *Research Policy and Planning*, Vol. 9, No. 1, pp. 9–12. **[Ch. 7]**

Wollheim, R. (1971) *Freud*, London, Fontana/Collins. **[Ch. 9]**

Index